Killer
Diseases

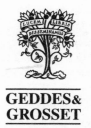

**GEDDES&
GROSSET**

This edition published 2000 by Geddes & Grosset,
an imprint of Children's Leisure Products Limited

© 2000 Children's Leisure Products Limited,
David Dale House, New Lanark, ML11 9DJ, Scotland

First published in this edition 2000

Cover photograph of Salmonella bacterium by USDA,
courtesy of Science Photo Library

ISBN 1 85534 968 X

Printed and bound in Europe

Contents

Introduction

Microorganisms, organisms that cannot be seen with the naked eye, are found throughout the environment. They include bacteria, viruses, protozoans and some algae and fungi. They are found in and on humans, in food, the soil, water and the air. Microorganisms have adapted to a wide range of environments and can be found in hot springs and in almost Arctic conditions. Some need oxygen to survive while others thrive where it is absent; yet more can live with or without oxygen. Some have very particular nutrient requirements.

Many microorganisms perform vital functions that contribute to the cycle of life. In particular, some bacteria and fungi are important in breaking down dead, organic material into simpler chemical substances that then enter the cycle again. Without this process of putrefaction the world would soon run out of nutrients to sustain life. Other bacteria are essential in the process of nitrification and nitrogen-fixation, both essential in providing amino acids – the building blocks of life and vital for both plants and animals. Yeasts and certain bacteria are important in fermentation processes and cheese-making.

Microorganisms are essential to life, but a very small proportion of them are pathogenic, that is, they are capable of causing disease. The effects of these particular microorganisms can be devastating, and epidemics of ill-health and death may result.

This book examines some of the microorganisms that are a cause of concern to the public today. Some of these have been around for some time, such as *Staphylococcus aureus* and *Escherichia coli*, but have surfaced as problems because of resistance to antibiotics, in the case of *Staphylococcus aureus*, and mutations into more virulent forms, as in the case of *Esherichia coli*. In addition, there are a number of previously unrecognized microorganisms, for example those that cause legionnaires' disease, Aids and the haemorrhagic fevers. These organisms may have existed for some time, but it is only changes in the way that we live, for example by the introduction of air-conditioning systems, that have provided the right environment for them to become pathogenic. Some of these changes have been brought about by rapid and easy access to most parts of the world, the continuing problems of poverty and warfare, and interference with the environment on local, regional and now global scales with the effects of global warming. It is not only viruses that change; bacteria and parasites are mutating. So when a new strain of influenza strikes, there is little or no resistance. In eastern Europe diphtheria is again active, yellow fever is once again troubling Africa, and even in the USA there are problems with a resurgence of tuberculosis.

Around 50,000 people die each day from disease. Malaria, plague, smallpox and other diseases were thought to be beaten; it was hoped that polio, typhoid, meningitis, diphtheria and others would soon join the list. However, this hope has been turned on its head and in addition there are new scourges, such as Aids, which the World Health Organization estimate may affect up to 30 million adults by the year 2000.

In a world that had until recently been congratulating itself on the near eradication of certain diseases, there is considerable cause for concern. Diseases from the past are reappearing and new ones are being discovered at an alarming rate. Resistance to antibiotics is increasing and viruses seem to be constantly changing and adapting, becoming more virulent. There has to be constant vigilance and a tackling of the massive problems facing the world if killer bugs are not to become the nightmare of the new millennium.

1

MRSA

Methicillin-resistant *Staphylococcus aureus* (MRSA) and the growth of antibiotic resistance

Staphylococci are among the hardiest non-spore-forming bacteria and can survive a range of environmental conditions. They are relatively heat-resistant and can tolerate high salt media and remain viable for several months in a dried condition. *Staphylococcus aureus* (*S. aureus*) has remained a major human pathogen despite the availability of a range of powerful antibiotics, improved public health conditions and hospital-infection control measures. *S. aureus* colonizes and infects both hospitalized patients with decreased host defences and healthy, immunologically competent people in the community. Most people carry *S. aureus* in their noses, mouth and on their skin where it does no harm. The human carriers in most cases are perfectly healthy.

On the surface of the body *S. aureus* can cause boils, abscesses, conjunctivitis, and Lyell's syndrome, otherwise known a 'SSSS' or the staphylococcal scalded skin syndrome, in which the skin peels off in sheets. Generally, the skin and mucous membranes are effective mechanical barriers against invasion by *S. aureus*. However, if this barrier is breached by surgery or a wound, *S. aureus* can gain access to the underlying tissue, creating a characteristic abscess lesion. This consists of dead tissue, fibrin (the clotting agent in blood) and a large number of live and dead white blood cells. The toxin released by the infection may affect the skin and other organs of the body and various types of skin rashes may develop. The liberated toxin may also cause toxic shock, including the toxic shock syndrome that has killed a number of women who used super-absorbent tampons during menstruation. At any time, the multiplying bacteria may overcome the body's natural defence mechanisms and gain access to the lymphatic system and bloodstream. The ensuing septicaemia is a dreaded complication, and it can lead to a variety of secondary infections, such as endocarditis, pneumonia, meningitis or osteomyelitis (infection of the bone marrow), and eventually to the patient's death.

The success of *S. aureus* as a cause of human infection is in part the result of its remarkable capacity to adapt to the presence of antibiotics in the environment by developing resistance to them. Today, approximately 90 per cent of hospital strains of the bacterium and 50 per cent of community strains are resistant to penicillin. The history of the resistance of *S. aureus* towards penicillin and other drugs demonstrates well the interaction between pathogenic organisms and antibiotics.

The development of antibiotics

In 1928 the British scientist Alexander Fleming discovered that the penicillium mould could kill *Staphylococcus* bacteria grown in Petri dishes in the laboratory. The lethal antibacterial chemical secreted by the mould was named 'penicillin'. This was the beginning of the antibiotic age.

Penicillin was introduced into general clinical practice in the mid-1940s, and the term 'miracle drug' soon passed into the vocabulary. Many other antibiotics with increasing potency were soon discovered and introduced into medical practice. In a very short time bacterial infections such as sore throats, skin boils and infected wounds, which were once considered very serious conditions and in some cases even fatal, instantly became trivial. Tuberculosis, which was once extremely dangerous and claimed many lives, was now considered an easily managed minor infection. By 1965 more than 25,000 different antibiotic products had been developed.

At this time the medical profession was very optimistic about the use of antibiotics and considered that it was only a matter of time before all the infectious diseases in the world would be eradicated. The mass experimental polio vaccination campaign introduced in the mid-1950s seemed to confirm this expectation. This campaign was so successful that cases of the disease in Western Europe and North America fell dramatically, from 76,000 cases in 1955 to fewer than 1,000 in 1967.

The same optimism surrounded the control of all infectious diseases in the developed and the developing world. A US Secretary of State, addressing the 1948 gathering of the Fourth International Congress on Tropical Medicine and Malaria, declared that the conquest of all infectious diseases was imminent. Through a combination of enhanced crop yields to provide adequate food and scientific breakthroughs in microbe control, it was predicted that all the earth's microscopic scourges would be eliminated.

In 1955, the World Health Organization decided to eliminate all malaria on the planet. At that time few doubted such an ambitious and lofty goal was possible – every infectious disease seemed conquerable.

However, even in these early days of optimism there were reports of bacteria that were resistant to chemicals. Cases of patients who could not be healed with antibiotics soon began to appear. Scientists were also finding colonies of *Staphylococcus* and *Streptococcus* that thrived in solutions rich in penicillin and a range of other antibiotics. It was soon found that the bacteria's ability to resist antibiotics was due to special characteristics found in their DNA (the genetic material found in each cell that determines the characteristics of the next generation). It was concluded that some bacteria were genetically resistant to penicillin or other drugs and had probably always possessed this ability, certainly long before the discovery of antibiotics.

In whatever environment bacteria are present, they are in constant competition with millions of others. In this competitive, rapidly changing environment bacteria evolved the ability to produce chemicals to fight off their competitors. To counter this, and in order for a particular bacterial population to survive, at least some of the individual members of the population must possess genetically coded resistance factors to resist chemical attack. It is these same genetic factors that enable the bacterial population to withstand attack by antibiotics.

The use of antibiotics on a population of bacteria may kill off 99 per cent of the organisms. However, the 1 per cent of resistant bacteria that remain then have free access to the available nutrients and can go on to multiply without competition. The bacterial population that remains is then resistant to that particular antibiotic.

So, a doctor may give a patient an antibiotic that would immediately kill off the majority of the infecting bacteria. The patient's own immune system would be left to to deal with the remaining resistant organisms. In very dangerous infections, a cocktail of two or three antibiotics would be administered together, on the basis that a particular strain of a bacterium might be resistant to one or even two antibiotics but was unlikely to be resistant to several widely divergent ones.

Resistance of S. aureus

S. aureus is the microbiological cause of most staphylococcal infections. The ubiquitous nature of this organism in the environment meant that prior to the use of antibiotics, surgery and many other procedures that are now commonplace carried a high risk of infection. The early golden age of antibiotics created wonderful opportunities for surgeons. Open-body surgery and other massive procedures became feasible for the first time because patients could be protected against what otherwise would be far too high a risk of dangerous or even deadly infections. Antibiotics could be used before, during and after operations to protect patients. At first, penicillin worked against S. aureus and many other bacteria that had made major surgery such a hazard in the pre-antibiotic era.

However, the extensive use of antibiotics in hospitals created the conditions in which bacteria could become superbugs. S. aureus became resistant not only to penicillin but also to other antibiotics such as streptomycin, tetracycline and erythromycin. By the end of the 1950s, Staphylococcus had become resistant to all the known antibiotics that were available at that time. In a period of fifteen years medicine returned again to the pre-antibiotic era where patients were dying of infections because there were no antibiotics to treat them. Once again Staphylococcus became a potentially lethal infection.

Most strains of Staphylococcus became resistant to penicillin by absorbing a small molecule of DNA (a plasmid) and incorporating this into their own DNA. This small piece of DNA, named the beta-lactamase plasmid, rendered penicillin harmless to the bacteria. Once the beta-lactamase plasmid was fully incorporated into the bacterium's genetic material, it was passed from one generation of the organism to the next.

Work began on looking for a new antibiotic that would be effective against this penicillin-resistant *S. aureus*. In the late 1950s, scientists working for the Beecham pharmaceutical company developed a new generation of semi-synthetic penicillins, which it was hoped would combat the progress of penicillin resistance. These new drugs included methicillin, the isoxazolyl penicillins (oxacillin, cloxacillin, etc) and nafacillin. These became best-selling drugs, specifically because they worked against the drug-resistant *S. aureus*. Predictably, the enthusiastic use of methicillin, the best known of the beta-lactamase-resistant penicillins, bred new strains of *S. aureus*. These were known as methicillin-resistant *Staphylococcus aureus*, or MRSA. Isolation of these methicillin-resistant strains was reported as early as 1961. Initially this did not cause undue concern because these resistant strains could be killed by other antibiotics that were available, so *Staphylococcus* infections were under control

Inevitably, *S. aureus* began to fight back. Soon MRSA strains were causing serious outbreaks of infection in hospitals. By 1976, a strain resistant to both gentamycin and methicillin was reported in Britain as well as increasingly causing outbreaks in the USA, Australia and the Republic of Ireland. In the early 1980s, strains of *Staphylococcus* emerged that were resistant to methicillin and the closely related antibiotics such as naficillin. This caused serious clinical concern.

Hospitals in London were devastated by a new strain of MRSA, sometimes called EMRSA (epidemic methicillin-resistant *Staphylococcus aureus*), defined as MRSA and isolated from two or more patients in at least two hospitals. This new strain, EMRSA-1, killed scores of patients. It is thought that it had spread from Australia because it had similarities to some of those strains responsible for major epidemics there in the late 1970s and early 1980s. This new superbug had evolved resistance to practically all antibiotics. Only vancomycin and sometimes chroramphenicol could work against it. Outbreaks of EMRSA occurred in hospitals in the Middle East, the United States, South Africa, continental Europe and the UK, where it was found in a London hospital and many other major hospitals.

A survey carried out by the Staphylococcus Reference Laboratory in 1987–88 over a six-month period showed that this strain was affecting 50 different hospitals but there were also 11 other epidemic strains, each affecting up to eight hospitals. In one outbreak in May 1982, in San Francisco, USA, a newborn baby on the neonatal ward died after infection with a strain of *S. aureus* that was resistant to the penicillins, cephalosporins and naficillin. This mutant strain had drifted about the hospital and the local community for three years, infected a nurse on the neonatal ward and then found its way to three babies. The only way the hospital could prevent further cases was to treat aggressively the ward staff and babies with antibiotics to which the bacteria remained susceptible, close the ward off to new patients, refit all items on which dormant *Staphylococcus* might lie, for example rubber fittings on equipment, curtains, sheets, etc, and scrub the entire ward with disinfectants.

Who is affected by MRSA?

Patients with underlying medical problems are most at risk from MRSA infection. Outbreaks of infection occur particularly on wards that house patients with immune systems that are least able to resist infection, for example people who have suffered major burns, premature babies, individuals with terminal cancers, those who have undergone major surgery, and intensive care patients. Serious infections can also occur in patients who have indwelling intravenous catheters or prosthetic heart valves. MRSA makes common operations like hip replacement surgery a hazardous procedure. *S. aureus* is a facultative aerobe, that is, it can live without air – and when it gets into surgical wounds that are then closed it can cause internal infections that ruin the effects of the operation.

Transmission of MRSA

MRSA is most probably introduced into a hospital by an infected or colonized patient or health worker. Many individuals can carry the bacterium without showing any symptoms of ill-health.

The organism may be present in the nose and mouth or on the skin. *S. aureus* that is present on the skin may enter the body via a tracheostomy site (a hole made in the trachea through which a breathing tube is inserted) or a wound. The transfer of the bacterium from one patient to another probably occurs via the colonized hands of health workers or via the inanimate environment, for example, surgical equipment, linen, clothing, etc.

Colonization of humans with *S. aureus* begins shortly after birth. Newborn babies are probably infected by humans around them, including their own mothers. *S. aureus* has been found around the umbilical stump, in the skin and sometimes the gastrointestinal tract. Up to 25 per cent of the adult population may be carriers, but unlike babies, the principal reservoir of *S. aureus* in adults is the nose. Some adults (20 per cent) may be long-term carriers of the organism, others (50 per cent) may only carry it intermittently. The number of individuals carrying the organism at any one time may vary according to the season and the level of infection in the environment, and it is not unusual for people to be colonized by several strains of the bacteria.

In certain groups of individuals the rate of colonization may be higher than in the general population. Thus 50 per cent of doctors, 70 per cent of nurses and up to 90 per cent of hospital ward attendants have been found to be carriers of *S. aureus*. Diabetics receiving insulin injections, patients on regular dialysis, those with a variety of skin conditions and users of illegal intravenous drugs all have a higher carriage rate than the general population. It is estimated that about 20 per cent of the population never carry the organism.

The carrier state is important in infection with *S. aureus*, because in addition to being a source of infection, when these individuals undergo surgery or suffer from particular skin conditions, they will experience more infection than non-carriers. On investigation it is found that these infections are caused by the same strain of the organism that colonized the patient on admission to hospital.

When patients are moved from one hospital to another they may carry the organism with them.

Treatment

At present the only treatment for MRSA infection is vancomycin. This drug is expensive and requires frequent measurement of serum drug concentrations to prevent toxic side effects. It can damage hearing and affect kidney function. The drug is unpleasant to administer as it has to be given through a drip for an hour at a time and can irritate patients' veins.

These undesirable qualities of the drug are probably reasons why it has remained effective against *S. aureus* years after the drug was first marketed. A cheaper, more easily administered drug would have been used more widely and *S.aureus* would probably have developed resistance to it.

Occurrence

The second UK national prevalence survey conducted in 1993–94 revealed that MRSA comprised 5 per cent of all infections, including 14 of the 228 surgical wound infections. Data from the Public Health Laboratory Sevice (PHLS) indicate increases in MRSA infections. The incidence of MRSA infection remained static (about 1.8 per cent) between 1989 and 1991 but increased to 8.1 per cent by 1994 and in the first half of 1995 was 13.5 per cent.

Control measures

Patients who are known to be infected or colonized with MRSA, or who have been transferred from a hospital known to have MRSA present, should be admitted directly to an isolation room. Swabs should be taken from relevant sites, such as the nose, mouth, throat, wounds or abnormal skin. These patients should be clearly identified on their case notes as either carriers or as infected with MRSA. Patients from abroad should be screened, especially if they come from countries with major problems with MRSA.

All staff and visitors entering isolation areas should receive instruction on effective hand-washing, etc. Gowns, and in some cases masks, should also be worn. Gloves should always be worn when handling contaminated dressings or linen. Patients should be discharged as soon as their clinical condition allows so as to reduce the risk of further infection.

In nurseries for the newborn, several strategies have helped prevent infections in the infants, including individual care by a limited number of people, umbilical cord care, arm and hand-washing by the staff with chlorhexidine and the wearing of clean gowns.

In critical areas such as surgery or intensive care wards, all staff and patients should be screened for MRSA so that appropriate measures can then be taken, which may include assigning staff to non-clinical duties or prescribing antibacterial compounds to which *S. aureus* is still sensitive. In less critical areas the screening programme should be modified as appropriate. The highest priority for isolation should be given to patients with clinical infections or who are highly likely to be dispersers of the organism, such as those with skin conditions that result in them regularly losing skin cells, for example. Lyell's syndrome, mentioned earlier.

Thorough, repeated hand-washing has been shown to reduce the number of bacteria on the hands and so can help lower the infection rate. The use of antiseptic detergents or alcohol (70 per cent) is recommended, together with appropriate training. All patients should use an antiseptic detergent for washing and bathing. When a ward has been closed to new admissions it should be emptied and cleaned, with special emphasis on dust-collecting areas.

Testing for carriers of MRSA, used as a method of controlling the infection, at present has not stemmed its relentless progress. Studies have shown that the incidence of MRSA infection has increased in recent years, causing 5 per cent of all hospital infections. Screening for MRSA and eradicating the carriage of the organism have been shown to be cost-effective, even in a large prolonged outbreak in Madrid, and have resulted in a seven-fold reduction in the number of infected patients. The costs of extended lengths of stay and the resources needed to treat infections far outweigh those costs of screening and control.

On the other hand, it is claimed that MRSA causes no more illness than MSSA (methicillin-sensitive *Staphylococcus aureus*) and that screening is costly, not only in terms of pharmacy costs but also in ward closures and the demoralization and stigmatization of staff who are found to be carriers. Even when carriers are identified, the organism may not be completely removed. Also, there are ethical arguments about giving carriers showing no symptoms of disease potentially toxic antibiotics.

There is general agreement that the cost of ignoring MRSA is higher than that of controlling it, particularly if potential legal action is taken into account. It is important for hospitals to demonstrate that well-documented and effective control measures are implemented. The main capital cost in attempting to control MRSA is the establishment of an isolation ward.

2

Creutzfeldt-Jakob Disease

Creutzfeldt-Jakob disease (CJD) and its related diseases, including bovine spongiform encephalopathy (BSE)

In recent years, a handful of illnesses have come to the attention of the public and have been the focus of fear and anxiety. Often these diseases are not new, and usually they are very uncommon, but the fear arises because they are perceived as untreatable killers. Creutzfeldt-Jakob disease, or CJD, can certainly be fitted into this category but with the added dimension that, at the time of writing (1997), no one really knows whether Britain is facing a major epidemic of this fatal illness.

Here, the historical background of medical and scientific research into CJD, and its related human and animal variants, is covered in some depth. This is relevant to current thinking and fears about the possibility of a link between a recently emerged 'new variant CJD' and the new disease of cattle called bovine spongiform encephalopathy (BSE) or, more sensationally, 'mad cow disease'. The nature of classic CJD and related illnesses is described, along with the development of BSE and its probable causes. New variant CJD is described and its probable relationship with BSE is explored, as are the potential risk factors and implications of a possible epidemic. The various public health measures that are currently in place are described and an attempt is made to evaluate all the available evidence.

The spongiform encephalopathies

Until comparatively recently, Creutzfeldt-Jakob disease was familiar mainly to members of the medical profession and those engaged in scientific research. It was known to be one of a linked group of neuro-degenerative disorders, (causing destructive changes in the brain), variously called slow-virus diseases, spongiform encephalopathies and transmissible dementias. These occur rarely in people but one form is quite common in sheep. Similar diseases have been induced experimentally in other animals.

The sheep form of spongiform encephalopathy, which also affects goats, called scrapie, was the earliest to be recognized and has been recorded for at least 200 years. The term 'Creutzfeldt-Jakob disease' was first used in 1922 and thereafter, to describe certain cases of degenerative brain disease in human beings. (It is now believed that some of these may not, in fact, have been cases of the illness that is now recognized as CJD.) By 1936, scientists researching scrapie had demonstrated that this disease could be transmitted between sheep by injecting a normal animal with infected material. The resulting illness took a long time to develop and it was thought that it must be caused by some kind of as yet unidentified virus. The term 'slow-virus infection', introduced in 1954, appropriately referred to the supposed organism and the prolonged development of the disease.

Additionally, in the 1950s and 1960s, there was considerable interest and research into an epidemic of a disease known as kuru, which occurred only among the Fore indigenous peoples of the highlands of Papua New Guinea. These people practised ritual cannibalism, which included eating the organs and brains of relatives who had died as part of ceremonial funeral rites. In many cases, women and children were affected, and it was they who had mainly taken part in the rituals. Those affected exhibited progressive mental and behavioural disturbances, muscle spasms with loss of coordination (ataxia) and dementia, which progressed inexorably to total unresponsiveness and death, usually within three to twelve months. The similarities between kuru and scrapie were recognized by 1959, both in the neuropathological changes that occurred in the brain and in the nature of the disease itself. In 1966, kuru was transmitted to a chimpanzee by injecting selected material directly into the animal's brain. By the end of the 1960s, similar experiments had demonstrated that both kuru and CJD could be transmitted to other animals, and the term 'transmissible dementias' was introduced. Also, it was concluded that the most likely explanation for the transmission of kuru was cannibalism, establishing that this spongiform encephalopathy was being passed by a dietary route, albeit between the same species of animal (human beings).

There was renewed concern that there might be a link between scrapie and human CJD, but no evidence for this has yet been found (although an alternative view has been expressed). CJD appears to be no more or less common in countries where scrapie is prevalent, even although in the past people must have eaten infected meat. However, scrapie-infected sheep have not been permitted to enter the human food chain in Britain for many years. More recently, intensive research on scrapie, involving injecting infected material into the brain of laboratory mice, has provided evidence that there are several strains of this disease. These have differing incubation periods and cause varying patterns of neuropathological damage. It has been demonstrated that some sheep have a genetic predisposition for scrapie, and it is thought that the infectious agent may be present in the placental fluid and swallowed by lambs while in the womb. It is further believed that scrapie may spread between sheep, and one route that has been suggested is feeding on grass contaminated with placental fluid containing the infection. If these assumptions are correct, there would appear to be parallels with both kuru and the familial forms of CJD (*see* below). A test introduced four years ago enables sheep that are more likely to be either resistant or susceptible to scrapie to be identified. It is hoped that, by careful breeding, the incidence of the disease will be reduced. The absence of evidence for a definite link between scrapie and human CJD was arguably the most significant factor in encouraging an over-complacent attitude to the development and emergence of BSE in the 1980s.

It has not been shown that normal occupational exposure to infected animals or people (for example, by farmers, veterinarians, abattoir workers, medical and health-care personnel, research scientists) poses any particular risk. Those handling or directly exposed to known or potentially infected material, whether human or animal in origin, must obviously take strict precautions to avoid accidental contamination.

Examination of infected brain tissue from both people and animals, including cattle with BSE, has revealed a characteristic pattern of damage, although the three typical features are not invariably present in all cases. These features, which can be seen when brain tissue is examined in the laboratory after death, are:

1. spongiform vacuolar proliferation – the appearance of holes (vacuoles) or spaces, which makes the tissue look spongy;
2. proliferation of astrocytes – an increase in certain large, star-shaped cells;
3. loss of neurones (normal nerve cells) and the formation of amyloid (starchy) plaques of waxy proteins, called glycoproteins.

Another human variant of CJD, called Gerstmann-Sträussler-Scheinker syndrome, was experimentally transmitted to laboratory animals in 1981. Since the 1960s, the Fore people have abandoned their cannibalistic rituals and the incidence of kuru has declined, although it has not disappeared entirely.

By the early 1990s, the human spongiform encephalopathies were recognized as representing a spectrum of illnesses. These sometimes arise rarely and sporadically for no apparent reason, although many researchers now believe that there are identifiable factors located at a particular gene site in those affected (*see* classic CJD, page 16). Also, it has long been recognized that some forms of CJD must be genetically linked as they tend to occur in a family context. Gerstmann-Sträussler-Scheinker syndrome is one such form. Additionally, it is known that in some cases classic CJD has been acquired as a result of certain medical procedures (*see* below). Kuru is believed to be an acquired form, transmitted through cannibalism, which is capable of developing rapidly (since children were affected) or more slowly (since the disease has not yet died out).

The infective agents

The nature of the agents responsible for the spongiform encephalopathies has long been the subject of intense research. As early as the mid-1960s, some scientists were questioning whether the causative agents could be viruses. It was discovered that the infective agents are extremely resistant to the methods that normally inactivate molecules, called nucleic acids, which are present in viruses (and the cells of all other life forms). Inactivation methods include the use of proteases (enzymes), ultraviolet radiation, heat, extremes of acidity and alkalinity (pH), and certain chemicals. It is now proposed that the causative agents of the spongiform encephalopathies are aberrant forms of naturally occurring brain proteins, which somehow become modified and which may lack nucleic acids. These aberrant proteins were called prion-proteins (PRP), or prions, in 1982, defined as 'small proteinaceous infectious particles that resist inactivation by procedures which modify nucleic acids' (S. B. Prusiner). Research into the inherited, familial forms of CJD has identified the gene that is involved in these diseases and that its normal product is a protease-sensitive protein, designated PSPs. The abnormal prion derived from it has been designated PRPsc ('sc' indicating scrapie). A number of pathogenic (that is, disease-causing) mutations have now been identified in the PRP gene, relating to various familial forms of CJD. Susceptibility for familial CJD can be passed on genetically and yet it is also transmissible to other animals by injections of the infective prion into the brain.

It is suggested that one way in which aberrant prions may operate is by setting off a chain reaction and gradually causing more and more normal protein to alter and build up in the brain. This abnormal material disrupts and damages the brain so it can no longer operate, shown by the symptoms of the disease. All the prion diseases studied, including BSE, share the characteristic of having infectious agents that are resistant to inactivation techniques that normally work on nucleic acids. Their mode of operation is not fully understood but there are similarities between them and they remain the subject of intense research.

Classic CJD

Classic Creutzfeldt-Jakob disease is an uncommon, fatal disease of the brain affecting middle-aged or elderly people, that is, those in the age range 40–65 years. The most common age of occurrence is the late 50s. It usually develops slowly so that by the time symptoms appear considerable irreversible changes have already taken place in the brain. There is rapidly worsening dementia, muscle seizures (myoclonus), Parkinson-like symptoms and inexorable mental and physical decline. Death usually follows after about three months to one year, although it may take longer, often as a direct result of a complication such as pneumonia.

CJD occurs throughout the world and sometimes arises spontaneously for no apparent cause. It has been known for many years, however, that some people have been infected through previous neurosurgical and medical procedures. These include transplants of cornea and dura mater (the outer, tough inelastic membrane surrounding the brain and spinal cord) and the use of contaminated brain electrodes. Similarly, it has been discovered that a number of adults who were treated for dwarfism during their childhood with growth hormone derived from pituitary glands extracted from corpses developed CJD. It is now thought certain that some of the pituitary glands used harboured the infective agent, which would have been able to withstand the purification methods that were in use at the time. Research in recent years, however, has provided strong evidence that, in many cases, both people who developed sporadic CJD and those who were infected by medical procedures showed a particular characteristic connected with the human prion (PRP) gene. This is believed to be similar to those that occur in familial CJD. Hence, those affected may have had an increased disposition for the development of CJD. A further piece of supporting evidence is that, of the many people treated with human pituitary gland extract, only 50 developed CJD and these usually showed the genetic factor. The practice of using hormones derived from human pituitary glands was discontinued some years ago. *It must be emphasized* that any children diagnosed today as having pituitary-related growth or development deficiencies are treated with synthetically manufactured hormones and are not at risk.

Bovine spongiform encephalopathy

The new disease of bovine spongiform encephalopathy (BSE) first appeared in British cattle in 1986 and rapidly reached epidemic proportions, peaking at the end of 1991 to early 1993, since when it has gradually declined. Over 160,000 cattle have developed the disease, which causes staggering, behavioural changes, loss of weight and fall in milk yields (but no 'madness') and from which there is no recovery, the only option being slaughter.

It is now widely believed that BSE arose from the earlier practice of rendering down the carcases of sheep, some of which would have been scrapie-infected, into meat and bone meal (MBM), which was made into pellets that were fed to cattle. More specifically, it is thought that the taking out of a particular stage in the rendering process, the removal of a solvent extraction technique, enabled the scrapie agent to retain its infectivity in MBM. The BSE epidemic arose only after the solvent-extraction process was withdrawn (in the early 1980s) even although MBM had been used as cattle feed for several years. Furthermore, in Scotland and the north of England, where the solvent extraction technique was often retained and where more cattle were fed traditionally and not given MBM, the incidence of BSE was much lower than in the south. (In some cases, instances of BSE in Scotland could be traced to cattle that had been moved from the south.) Cattle offal, including brain and spinal cord, was also recycled and made into MBM. It is thought that bovine material harbouring the infective agent was processed into MBM between 1984 and 1988 and that this intensified the BSE epidemic.

BSE has been recorded infrequently in other countries, but in many cases the cattle had been fed on MBM manufactured in the UK or they had been exported from Britain. Spongiform encephalopathy with strong similarities to BSE has also occurred in exotic zoo animals (nyala, gemsbok, Arabian oryx and eland) that were fed on MBM.

The feeding of MBM to ruminant animals such as cattle and sheep was banned in 1988, although not rigorously enforced. It is now known that the practice continued and feed was used up rather than being totally withdrawn. Controls were tightened in 1989–90, when specified bovine offals (SBO), which include brain, spinal cord, thymus gland, spleen, intestine and tonsil, were banned from all animal feeds. The use of MBM has now been discontinued. It is thought that, with BSE, vertical transmission of the infection from cow to calf or from a bull to its offspring is negligible, while this almost certainly occurs in sheep with scrapie.

When the BSE epidemic arose there was undoubted concern that human beings might have been exposed to the infection and that it could have passed into the human food chain. It was thought that even if this had occurred, there was little risk to human health as it was assumed that, like scrapie, the disease would not pass to people. It is now recognized that BSE-infected material did indeed enter the food chain prior to 1989–90.

Recent investigations have revealed that not only were the guidelines at first not strictly enforced but also that the practices in some abattoirs left a great deal to be desired. Intensive experimental research has discovered only one strain of BSE, unlike scrapie in which there are, apparently, several strains. The BSE agent is known to occur in infected cattle offal, especially brain and spinal cord. Experiments demonstrated that disease could be produced in laboratory mice that were fed on this material. Also, cases of spongiform encephalopathy in cats, which were first noted in the 1980s, have been attributed to BSE-infected material in tinned food. The same strain as in BSE has been demonstrated. (At the time of writing, April 1997, scientists are examining the brain of a dog that is believed to have died of BSE. If confirmed, this will be the first recorded case of the illness in dogs.) Feeding laboratory mice with muscle meat, milk, blood and other tissues derived from BSE-infected cattle has not produced disease. Also, disease has not been induced by injecting this material directly into the brain of experimental animals.

There is now general agreement that BSE entered the human food chain via infected offal (brain and spinal cord), which may have been used in such products as hamburgers and beefburgers. It is thought that muscle meat, milk, etc, in which the BSE agent has not been found was probably not involved.

New variant CJD (nvCJD)

From 1986 to early 1996, the general view, and the one voiced by the United Kingdom government, was that BSE posed no risk to human health (although there were notable exceptions). From 1994 onwards, however, news began to emerge that a new type of CJD was occurring that was affecting teenagers and younger adults, under 45 years old. In March 1996, the then Health Minister, Stephen Dorrel, announced that the ten people so far identified as victims of 'new variant CJD' had possibly contracted it through eating BSE-infected beef. Swift action followed from the European Union, which imposed a complete ban on the export of British beef and a consequent severe consumer crisis and slump in sales.

What are the differences between nvCJD and the classic disease?
Although based on very few cases (11 now diagnosed), two sets of

factors suggest that nvCJD is different. First, it is extremely rare (although not unknown) for younger people to be afflicted with classic CJD. Secondly, nvCJD seems to present a different pattern of symptoms, which is probably reflected in its neuropathology. Also, since some people in their teens and twenties have been affected, nvCJD appears to be able to develop much more rapidly than classic CJD (perhaps showing similarities with kuru).

What are the symptoms of nvCJD?
The illness seems more likely to begin with behavioural changes, mood swings, anxiety and depression followed by loss of balance and coordination, inability to concentrate and memory loss. The person deteriorates rapidly and becomes progressively more physically and mentally incapable, with death usually occurring within a few months.

Is it certain that nvCJD has arisen from eating BSE-infected beef?
An absolute link between nvCJD and BSE has not been established entirely but a great deal of evidence points to that conclusion. Building on the knowledge that has been gained from many years of research, as well as the most recent studies, the evidence can be summarized as follows:

BSE can be transmitted both by intracerebral inoculation and by a dietary route to animals other than cattle, and the same strain of disease seems to be present in all cases. Recent experiments involving the injection of monkeys with BSE have produced a disease that appears to be very similar to nvCJD. Transgenic mice, which have been genetically altered so that they express the human PRP gene, have now been injected with infected brain material from victims of nvCJD and with BSE tissue. If these experiments, the results of which are expected within three years, demonstrate the same pattern and strain of disease as BSE then the evidence will be compelling. All the victims of nvCJD so far identified, ate beef.

If the link is established, who is now at risk?
Scientists have put forward the view that, because material derived from cattle has been so widely used in food manufacturing, every person in the UK, with the possible exception of strict vegans, has eaten some BSE-infected food. The most gloomy scenario (voiced

in 1996) is that half a million or more people could succumb to nvCJD and that the cases so far represent the start of an epidemic. More recently, the figure has been revised downwards but could still be as high as 80,000 people or as low as a few dozen.

On an individual level, it is probably always going to be impossible to say who may be at risk. A number of factors are likely to prove significant, and one of these may be the amount of infected material that an individual has eaten. It is known that a 'species barrier' exists in the transmission of all the spongiform encephalopathies, including BSE, but also that it can be overcome. Also, there may well be a genetic susceptibility in individual people to the development of nvCJD, as has been shown to be the case with some of the classic forms of the illness. It is not possible for any individual person to discover whether he or she may be susceptible, only that this may be a factor. There have been only 11 confirmed cases of nvCJD so far, and while these are enormous tragedies for the families involved, the disease is at present very rare. Each individual in Britain is at greater risk of premature death from many causes other than CJD. Of course, if an epidemic of the disease occurs, these assurances will change.

Is it now safe to eat beef?
Experts agree that eating British beef now poses little or no risk to human health. This conclusion is based on a number of different factors, the most important ones being the strict controls that are now being rigorously enforced on beef and cattle. These are:

1. A total ban on any specified bovine offal (which is the only part in which the infectious BSE agent has ever been found) from entering either human or animal food.
2. No cattle aged over 30 months are allowed to be slaughtered for human or animal consumption. It is only older cattle that could possibly have been exposed to BSE-infected MBM as calves, as this has been banned from cattle feed for some time. Hence, the current policy of slaughtering and destroying all older cattle should deal with any animals that might, conceivably, be incubating BSE. (This policy is controversial and many farmers are bitterly opposed to it, maintaining that it is 'overkill' and that perfectly healthy cattle are being destroyed.)

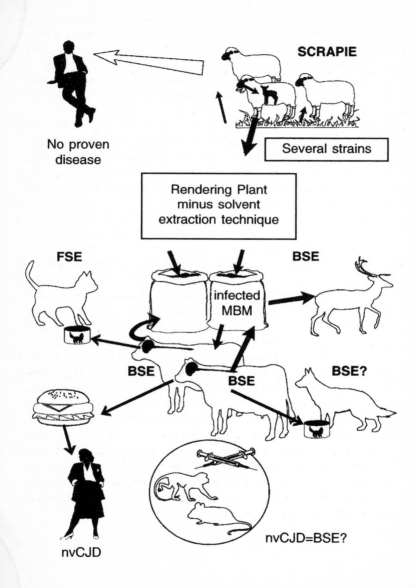

The possible route of infection of BSE

3. The incidence of BSE in cattle has declined markedly since the MBM feed ban was imposed, so it is assumed that there are now far fewer potentially infected animals. Controls on any farm where there has been a case of BSE in the past are stringent.
4. All butchers now sell only beef from cattle certified to be free of BSE. There are many farms and beef herds that have never had a case of BSE.

In addition, milk is subject to strict controls, even although the best evidence is that it is non-infective. Any milk from dairy cattle suspected of harbouring BSE has to be destroyed. At present, the European Union remains unconvinced, and exports of British beef and its derivatives are still banned.

When will it be known if Britain is facing an epidemic of nvCJD and what are the implications of this?
At present, it is too early to know whether an epidemic of nvCJD is likely to occur, and the cases so far may or may not represent the beginning of such an event. There are many unknown factors, such as how much infective BSE material has to be eaten to produce disease in a person and how many people might be susceptible or more resistant to nvCJD. Also, the incubation period of nvCJD is significant. It appears to be short, since younger people have been affected, but if it can be longer, any epidemic may not have materialized yet. Most scientists believe that matters will become clearer within the next few years and, if the number of cases does not begin to rise significantly, the risk of a full-scale epidemic may recede. However, if it does occur on the scale that has been envisaged, the consequences could be severe. There is no treatment other than supportive care for victims of CJD, and an overstretched health service could be faced with caring for many more young, terminally ill people with all the consequent emotional and psychological stresses that this would engender.

3

Escherichia coli

The *Escherichia coli* (*E. coli*) bacterium is a normal inhabitant of
the intestines of people and many domestic animals. Normally this
bacterium serves a useful function in the body by suppressing the
growth of harmful bacteria species and by synthesizing appreciable
amounts of vitamins. However, there is a minority of strains of
E. coli that are capable of causing illness in human beings.

The *E. coli* organisms can be classified into four broad groups
and within each of these groups there are many serotypes
(subgroups). The first group, enteropathic *E. coli* (EPEC), cause
outbreaks of diarrhoea in infants and are a particular problem when
they occur in hospital neonatal or paediatric wards. The enteroin-
vasive *E. coli* (EIEC) cause a dysentery-like syndrome in older
children and adults. Enterotoxigenic *E. coli* (ETEC) produce toxins
and watery diarrhoea rather like that which occurs in cholera. They
are a common cause of diarrhoeal illness amongst infants in tropical countries and in adult travellers to such areas. They are one
of the causes of travellers' diarrhoea and are acquired by contact
with contaminated food and water.

The fourth group, the verocytotoxin-producing *E. coli* (VTEC),
produce toxins that can cause severe illness in humans. The toxins
are closely related or identical to the shiga toxin produced by
Shigella dysenteriae, the bacterium that causes dysentery. The most
important of the VTEC *E. coli* associated with human disease is
E. coli 0157:H7, or enterohaemorrhagic *E. coli*, which produces a
particularly potent toxin when it enters the human gut and can
cause severe damage to the lining of the intestine. If the toxin is
absorbed into the bloodstream, it can cause damage to the lining
of other organs of the body, most notably the kidneys. In some
cases this can lead to permanent kidney damage and/or death.

Haemorrhagic colitis is the name of the acute disease caused by *E. coli* 0157.

It is the verocytotoxin of *E. coli*, and in particular *E. coli* 0157:H7, which has been responsible for the recent well-publicized outbreaks of *E. coli* infection in Britain. These infections are also recognized to be an important problem in North America, Europe, South Africa, Japan, southern South America and Australia. The true frequency of haemorrhagic colitis is not known. It is likely that only the most serious cases are reported. Less severe cases, the majority of which go unreported, are likely to be more numerous.

It is thought that *E. coli* 0157:H7 is second only to salmonella as a cause of bacterial diarrhoea, and in some parts of the USA and Canada infection with *E. coli* 0157:H7 may be more common than salmonella infection. It is also a potentially more dangerous form of food-borne infection than salmonella because of the severity of the disease it can cause.

The majority of cases of *E. coli* 0157 infection are sporadic, although outbreaks, some very large, do occur. Infections usually peak in the summer when temperatures rise and the rate of bacterial growth increases.

All age groups are believed to be susceptible to haemorrhagic colitis. Children under four, however, show the highest rate of infection, followed by the 5–14-year-old age group and then those over 65. Most of the larger outbreaks have occurred in institutional settings such as homes for the elderly.

Source of infection

The main reservoir of *E. coli* 0157 is in the stomach and intestines of cattle, but it has also been found in sheep, pigs and, more recently, in a goose. There is no evidence yet that it is carried by other domestic fowl. Recent evidence indicates, however, that seagulls contribute to the spread of *E. coli* by feeding on slurry, rubbish tips and sewage and spreading the bacteria in their droppings. Gulls often roost on farmland and their droppings can get into animal feed and troughs of water. The *E. coli* bacterium can then enter the food chain. It is not known how widespread *E. coli* 0157 is in cattle in Britain nor the potential for infection.

How are people infected?

Humans are most commonly infected by the consumption of contaminated food. The usual source of infection is via uncooked or undercooked meat or meat products, particularly minced beef, often in the form of hamburgers. Other meat products that have also been implicated in various outbreaks include sausages, meat pies and dry cured salami. The other main source of infection is milk, both unpasteurized and that contaminated after pasteurization. Milk products such as cheese and yoghurt made with contaminated milk are also potential sources of infection. A large outbreak in Scotland in 1994 was associated with the consumption of contaminated milk. More than a hundred people were affected and one child died.

Other outbreaks of *E. coli* 0157 infection have been attributed to apple juice, raw vegetables and water. One outbreak has been traced to apple cider made from apples contaminated by cow manure. In 1996, there was a large outbreak of *E. coli* 0157 infection in Japan that affected thousands of schoolchildren. Radish sprouts served in school meals were identified as the possible source of infection. Eleven people died in this outbreak.

Cross-contamination, that is, uninfected meat coming into contact with contaminated material and so becoming infected, is important in the transfer of *E. coli* bacteria. Cold cooked meats kept in close proximity to raw meat has long been recognized as a cause of cross-contamination and source of food poisoning. Slaughterhouses are now also recognized as cross-contamination sites. Carcasses can become contaminated by contact with intestinal contents at slaughter. Dirty animals being taken for slaughter can also contribute to the risk of cross-contamination.

Infection may also occur via direct contact with infected animals. Sporadic cases and outbreaks have been linked with handling of animals, particularly cattle, and therefore there are risks associated with visitors, especially children, to farm centres. Person-to-person spread by the faecal-oral route also occurs and is particularly associated with institutional settings such as hospitals, nursing homes and other institutions where the inhabitants are in close contact with each other. Pre-school children are at particular risk, and outbreaks of *E. coli* 0157 infection have been reported in nurseries.

There have also been limited outbreaks of infection associated with contaminated water. In one outbreak people were infected after swimming in a crowded lake, and in another infection was caused by drinking contaminated unchlorinated municipal water.

Although the minimal dose needed to cause infection is not known, it is suggested that because of the organism's ability to be passed from person to person in nursing homes, etc, the dose required to cause infection is very low and may be as little as a hundred or even ten organisms.

Symptoms of infection with *E. coli* 0157

The incubation period of *E. coli* 0157 is uncertain, but it is usually between 12 to 60 hours before symptoms of infection begin to become evident. In some cases, however, it may be up to 14 days before the symptoms manifest themselves.

Haemorrhagic colitis, the condition caused by *E. coli* infection, is marked by an acute onset of severe abdominal cramps and diarrhoea, which is initially watery but may become very bloody within 24 hours. Vomiting may occur and there may be a slight fever. The lack of fever in most patients can help differentiate this illness from dysentery and shigellosis (a specific form of dysentery).

The symptoms last on average eight days in cases with no complications. In 2–7 per cent of cases of haemorrhagic colitis, infection is complicated by the development of haemolytic uraemic syndrome (HUS). Children under five and, to a lesser extent, elderly people are at particular risk. The syndrome is characterized by haemolytic anaemia (breakdown of the red blood cells and consequent loss of oxygen-carrying capacity of the blood), thrombocytopenia (reduction in platelet count – important in blood clotting) and acute kidney failure. The disease may lead to permanent loss of kidney function, resulting in the victim leading a life on kidney dialysis if a transplant is not available or is not suitable.

In the elderly, HUS, plus two other symptoms, fever and neurologic symptoms, give rise to a condition known as thrombotic thrombocytopenic purpura (TTP). Both HUS and TTP typically develop in the second week of illness and may be heralded by rising temperature and white blood cell counts. *E. coli* 0157 infection complicated by TTP can have a mortality rate in the elderly as high as 50 per cent.

Treatment

There is no specific treatment for *E. coli* infection. Each phase of the disease is treated symptom by symptom. Typically, the mainstay of treatment is supportive care with fluids and electrolyte replacement when diarrhoea is watery or there are signs of dehydration.

Patients who develop complications such as HUS and TTP are likely to require intensive care, including dialysis, plasmapheresis (complete body plasma exchange) and other specific clinical care.

Although the organism is sensitive to most commonly used antibiotics, the use of these has not been shown to improve symptoms, reduce spread of the organism or prevent complications. The *E. coli* verotoxin works by binding to cells in the kidney and destroying them. Research is being carried out to find a chemical agent that absorbs the free verotoxin within the gut and so prevents it reaching the kidneys and the onset of HUS.

An important step in this search for a chemical agent has been taken by scientists at St Andrew's University in Scotland. They have recently revealed that they have uncovered the molecular structure of verotoxin. Armed with this knowledge, the scientists' next step will be to design a drug that will mimic the structure of cells within the kidney so that the toxin will bind to these and attract the verotoxin away from the kidney. If this proves to be effective it may prevent the onset of HUS and consequent kidney damage.

Outbreaks of *E. coli* O157:H7

The relatively harmless *E. coli* has been around for some time. In the early 1980s the strain of *E. coli* O157:H7 began to emerge as a source of infection and illness. *E. coli* had undergone a mutation that enabled it to produce a powerful and dangerous poison when ingested into the human body. Research by the US Food and Drug Administration (FDA) suggests that strains of *E. coli* O157:H7 mutate with abnormally high frequency.

The first outbreaks caused by this strain were identified in North America, three of them in 1982. Two involved hamburgers from a national fast-food chain. The third outbreak occurred in a home for the elderly in Ottawa in Ontario, Canada. Sandwiches eaten by the residents were implicated as the source of infection. Nineteen people died. Since then several large outbreaks have been recorded, largely involving nursing homes and day-care centres.

In 1986 an outbreak of haemorrhagic colitis caused by *E. coli* O157:H7 occurred in Walla Walla in Western Australia. Thirty-seven people, aged 11 months to 78 years, developed diarrhoea, and 17 were hospitalized. One four-year-old patient developed HUS and three patients, all in their seventies, developed TTP. Two people with TTP died. Minced beef was implicated as the food vehicle.

In Britain there were only a handful of cases of *E. coli* O157:H7 in the 1980s. Since the late 1980s the number of confirmed cases has been increasing. By 1995, 1,039 cases were confirmed in the UK. The incidence of *E. coli* 0157 infection is variable throughout the United Kingdom (*see* Table 1). The highest rate of infection is in Scotland, but the gap between the number of cases in Scotland and those in England and Wales is narrowing. It has been suggested that a particularly virulent sub-clone of *E. coli* 0157:H7 may be responsible for the outbreaks in Scotland.

One of the world's worst outbreaks of *E. coli*, and the largest in the United Kingdom, was centred on the town of Wishaw in central Scotland in 1996–97. More than 400 people were affected. Twenty-seven victims developed HUS or TTP and nineteen people died. The source of infection appeared to be a butcher's shop in the town of Wishaw. The shop, in addition to its local butcher retail trade, also had substantial wholesale and retail outlets involving the production and distribution of raw and cooked meats and bakery products. Microbiological evidence showed that the outbreak consisted of several separate but related incidents: a lunch attended by about a hundred people in a local parish church; a birthday party held in a public house; and retail sales in a wide geographic area around Wishaw. All cases were caused by the same strain of *E. coli* 0157. The age range of those who died was 69 to 93 years. Eight of these people attended the parish church lunch and six were residents of a nursing home.

This outbreak was shortly followed by a second unrelated one in Tayside, Scotland. Six people in a nursing home were identified as showing symptoms of disease and were confirmed as being infected with *E. coli* 0157. Three deaths have been associated with this outbreak.

Table 1: Number of reports of *E.Coli* infection and rates of infection per 100,000 population 1989–96

Year	England and Wales Number of cases	Rate	Scotland Number of cases	Rate
1989	119	0.23	87	1.70
1990	250	0.49	173	3.39
1991	362	0.71	202	3.98
1992	473	0.97	115	2.25
1993	390	0.76	119	2.32
1994	411	0.80	242	4.73
1995	792	1.52	247	4.8
1996	660*	1.26*	488*	9.5*

* provisional figures

Prevention

The eradication or even control of *E. coli* 0157 in cattle and other potential animal carriers is difficult, so control measures must be employed at every level of the food chain in an effort to prevent infection.

Storage and preparation of food

Raw meat and products like sausages and hamburgers carry no risk from *E. coli* if the product is thoroughly cooked until the juices run clear. This is because the bacteria are killed in the cooking process. To avoid risk from *E. coli* contamination, the following advice should be followed in the storage and preparation of food:

• Kitchens should be kept clean and all surfaces, utensils, chopping boards and cloths washed thoroughly after use.
• Raw and cooked foods should be kept apart.
• The same utensils and chopping boards should not be used for preparing raw and cooked meat.
• Controlling temperature helps control bacteria. The coldest part of a refrigerator should be not more than 8°C.

- Raw foods should be kept separately at the bottom of the refrigerator in covered containers so that they cannot contaminate other foods.
- All frozen meat should be thoroughly defrosted before cooking.
- Poultry, sausages, chopped or minced meats and burgers should be cooked thoroughly so that the juices run clear.
- It should be ensured that food is piping hot when served.
- Leftovers should not be left out in the kitchen.
- Hands should always be kept clean to avoid the spread of the bacteria.

Personal hygiene

Individuals can become infected with the *E. coli* bacteria without showing symptoms of the disease. However, they then become potential carriers and can pass on the bacteria to others with whom they come into contact. An obvious example would be other members of the family. The highest standards of personal hygiene should therefore be observed to prevent passing the infection from person to person. It is advised that:

- Every family member should maintain good personal hygiene by washing hands immediately after using the toilet, before eating or touching food and after handling raw meat.
- Fingernails should be kept clean as they can harbour food-poisoning germs.
- Parents should supervise young children who are unable to wash their hands thoroughly.
- Adults should take extra care when handling nappies, potties, soiled clothing or bedding and always remember to wash their hands immediately afterwards.
- Avoid touching the face and nose while preparing food.

   If these measures are followed, cases of secondary infection can be reduced or avoided altogether.

Public health measures

The early involvement of local health authorities to identify the source of infection is essential. Specific measures can be taken by the appropriate authorities to apply particular preventative measures. In some countries there is a legal obligation to notify authorities of such infections.

As a result of the outbreak of *E. coli* infection in central Scotland already mentioned, a group was set up by the Government to report on the circumstances of the outbreak, the implications for food safety and the lessons to be learnt. The group was led by Professor Hugh Pennington. The report stressed the importance of the Hazard Analysis and Critical Control Point (HACCP) system, which ensures that the potential hazards in a system are identified and that staff are trained to deal with the hazard. In this way every risk is identified at each step of the food chain. This system was first introduced by a European directive in 1995 but has never been properly implemented and monitored.

Thirty-two recommendations were made in the report, many of which rely on the implementation of the HACCP system. There is also great emphasis on training in food hygiene, starting with children in school, and particularly for all those involved in food preparation, especially those preparing meals intended for the young or the elderly.

The recommendations covered all stages of meat production:

Farms and livestock
It was recommended that education programmes be carried out to ensure that farm workers were aware of the existence and nature of *E. coli*, that they knew how it was spread and the consequent need for scrupulous personal hygiene. Also that they were aware of the need for care in the use of untreated slurry or manure and of the absolute requirement for the presentation of cattle in a clean condition for slaughter.

Slaughterhouses
Slaughterhouses were identified as the second most critical point in the meat production process. Again there was a need for education and awareness among staff of the hazards of *E. coli*. In addition, it was recommended that abattoirs should be graded according to standards of hygiene and that those that consistently fail to meet the requirements should lose their licence. Emphasis was also placed on the elimination of the risks of cross-contamination, particularly between skinned carcasses coming into contact with those that were

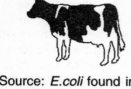

Source: *E.coli* found in gut of farm animals, especially cattle

Found in meat, particularly mince, and unpasturized milk and cheese

Secondary infections may be caused by person-to-person contact

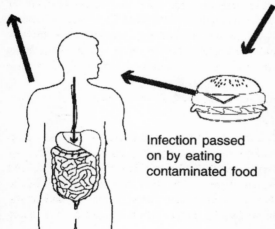

Infection passed on by eating contaminated food

Bacteria contaminate the surface of meat and are killed when cooked at high heat. When meat is minced, the bacteria are distributed throughout – so the meat should be cooked until the juices run clear and the meat loses its pink colour

Toxins produced by the bacteria in the intestines enter the bloodstream, destroy red blood cells and potentially cause fatal kidney failure

How Escherichia coli 0157 is spread

yet to have the hide removed. There was strong evidence that contaminated meat was entering butchers' shops from abattoirs.

Butchers' shops, kitchens and meat processors
It was recommended that selective licensing arrangements for premises not covered by the Meat Products (Hygiene) Regulations 1994 should be introduced. This would include butchers and producers who handle raw and cooked meats, whether retail, preparation or wholesale and also canneries not covered under other legislation. It was recognized that when HACCP has been fully implemented in all premises, licensing may become unnecessary.

It was also recommended that raw and cooked meats be kept separate at all times, including the use of separate refrigerators, production equipment and work areas, and that, where possible, separate staff should be employed to handle cooked and raw meat. If this was not possible, staff should be trained to wash their hands after serving raw meat and before serving cooked meat to prevent cross-contamination. All staff should also undertake at least a basic food hygiene course.

4

Necrotizing Fasciitis

Necrotizing fasciitis is a term given to a progressive infection that causes the destruction of soft tissue just below the skin. It may also include the destruction of deeper subcutaneous tissues and muscle. The process is usually rapid and can lead to a toxic shock syndrome and death. Rapid early diagnosis and aggressive treatment are required to avoid a fatal outcome. Several cases in Great Britain received much publicity in the media in 1994. The condition was popularized as an infection caused by 'flesh-eating bacteria'.

Necrotizing fasciitis can be divided into two types. Type 1 comprises infections caused by a mixture of bacteria, including *Esherichia coli*, *Pseudomonas aeruginosa*, *Klebsiella pneumonia* and other streptococci but not *Streptococcus pyogenes* (*S. pyogenes*). Type 2 includes infections in which only *S. pyogenes* is involved, or those in which both *S. pyogenes* and *Staphylcoccus aureus* (*S. aureus*) are the causal organisms.

In the USA, necrotizing fasciitis usually refers to any infection spreading along layers of soft tissue. In Britain and Europe, the term focuses on the more rapidly developing type 2 infections. This chapter will concentrate mainly on type 2 infections, which are the ones that have received most media attention.

Streptococcal necrotizing fasciitis, also known as streptococcal or hospital gangrene, was first extensively reported during the American Civil War. A Confederate Army surgeon, Joseph Jones, is generally credited with having provided the first modern description of necrotizing fasciitis. At that time the only treatment available was surgery, and the death rate from the infection was high. Death usually occurred some time after the onset of infection.

It has been reported that the number of Streptococcus (Type A) invasive infections has been increasing worldwide. There is no explanation for this phenomenon as yet, but there are some indications to suggest that this group of organisms may be acquiring greater virulence.

Source of infection

S. pyogenes is carried in the throat by many individuals without producing any symptoms of illness. It is estimated that up to 10 per cent of children up to the age of 15 years, 2.5 per cent of those aged 15–45 and about 0.5 per cent of those aged 45 and over carry the organism.

How are people infected?

When *S. pyogenes* enters the body through the lining of the upper respiratory tract or through a break in the skin, a local lesion may occur or the infection may spread along the tissues or lymphatic system. Although in some cases the disease seems to develop spontaneously, further investigation usually reveals some minor break in the skin through which the organism has obtained entry to the underlying tissue.

It is thought that nasal carriers of the organism and those with septic lesions are important in its spread. Particles of dried secretion or infected skin scales may be disseminated the length of a hospital ward. Streptococci dispersed in the air or transferred to inanimate objects may remain viable for several weeks, but it is likely that the most recently shed organisms are more infectious.

In a cluster of cases of necrotizing fasciitis in Gloucester in 1994, the source of infection in two of the cases was thought to be a nasopharyngeal carrier of the organism among the theatre staff.

Who is at risk?

Necrotizing fasciitis occurs principally in individuals who have undergone surgery or who have sustained a minor injury. It is also more likely in those who have an underlying condition that reduces their resistance to disease, such as diabetes mellitus or cancer, and also in patients with peripheral vascular disease, in which there is poor circulation to the body's extremities. Patients with a history of intravenous drug problems are particularly vulnerable. However, this infection can also occur in young, previously healthy individuals.

Symptoms

Although necrotizing fasciitis can occur in any region of the body, the abdominal wall, the perineum and the legs and arms are the most common sites of infection.

In two-thirds of cases, the organism has entered the body via the skin and the site of infection is apparent, but in the remainder it may not be apparent.

Symptoms begin with swelling and inflammation or redness of the skin, which may be accompanied by itching or pain. Fever then develops. A purple or bronze discoloration of the skin appears, followed by blisters containing bloody fluid. Initially, the outer layers of the skin remain intact, and it is this lack of skin findings in the early stages of the disease that makes diagnosis difficult. About one week after onset, necrosis of the skin occurs. Investigations of the deeper layers of the skin and subcutaneous fat show areas of necrosis. In some cases there is also evidence of a spread of infection away from the primary site and deep muscle may be affected, showing signs of necrosis even although there is no evidence of a penetrating injury.

Survival is usually between five and 12 days from the onset of symptoms. Some patients have survived longer, in one case up to 44 days, but death often occurs. In some rare cases, septicaemia and systemic toxic effects may develop rapidly and lead to multi-organ failure and death within a very short time – 24 to 96 hours. Patients with shorter survival times have usually been those who have undergone major surgery or who were diabetic, but rapid progression to death has also been reported occasionally in otherwise healthy people.

Treatment

The key to successful treatment of this disease is early diagnosis and removal of infected tissue. A diagnosis of necrotizing fasciitis should be considered with any soft tissue infection that is accompanied by marked swelling and signs of toxicity. Most reports show that the patient's chances of survival are greatly improved with an early diagnosis.

Early and complete removal of all infected tissue is vital in increasing the chances of survival by stopping the infection from developing into a septicaemia and spreading throughout the body. In some cases, removal of infected tissue may be so extensive as to lead to amputation of a limb. In one report, excision (cutting out) of 35 per cent of the total body area was required. Survivors of such aggressive surgical treatments often need extensive skin grafting for reconstruction.

As well as surgery, administration of broad spectrum antibiotics is initiated as soon as the diagnosis is suspected.

Death rates as high as 76 per cent have been reported. Delays in diagnosis and/or treatment contribute to this mortality, with the cause of death being overwhelming toxic shock syndrome and/or multiple organ system failure.

Recent outbreaks

The first cluster of cases of necrotizing fasciitis in the UK recorded this century occurred in Gloucestershire in 1994. Between January and June that year, there were six cases (five confirmed, one probable) of *S. pyogenes* necrotizing fasciitis. Two people died. The patients ranged in age from 46 to 48 years. Two of the patients probably acquired their infections during the course of routine surgery performed in the same operating theatre. It is likely they acquired the infection from a symptomless carrier of *S. pyogenes* among the theatre staff. The remaining cases were community-acquired infections.

5

HIV and Aids

Aids is Acquired Immune Deficiency Syndrome, which was first recognized in Los Angeles, USA, in 1981. The causal agent was identified in 1983 and designated the Human Immunodeficiency Virus, or HIV. Recently, in Britain at least, it has dropped out of the limelight to a certain extent because of the advent of the BSE/CJD crisis. This may be partly due to the fact that although the numbers of people affected have been distressingly high, the early doomsday predictions of deaths on an apocalyptic scale have not been fulfilled.

However, there is no room for complacency – the virus is the cause of enormous human suffering and premature death on a huge scale throughout the world. It affects people of both sexes, all ages and in every walk of life, and there were over 100,000 deaths from HIV infections and Aids in 1990 alone. At the present time, there is no cure and the expected outcome for those who develop Aids is premature death.

Human Immunodeficiency Virus

HIV is a ribonucleic acid (RNA) retrovirus that is able to introduce its genetic material into the DNA of body cells. The virus is found in blood and body fluids such as semen and vaginal secretions. It is transmitted mainly by sexual intercourse but can be passed on in any circumstances where secretions containing HIV are transferred to the body of a non-infected person. HIV affects white blood cells, known as T-lymphocytes, which are vital to the effective operation of the immune system. Natural immunity declines, leaving the person increasingly vulnerable to the development of certain opportunistic infections and tumours. Hence the parts of the body initially involved in HIV and Aids are the immune system, including T-lymphocytes, lymph nodes and glands, bone marrow, the spleen and also the liver.

Symptoms and signs

Early symptoms include the enlargement of the lymph glands and spleen, fever, fatigue, ready bruising and bleeding, thrush-type fungal infections, diarrhoea, weight loss, dermatitis and respiratory illnesses. Later, as a person develops full-blown Aids, further serious infections and cancers usually occur. These include herpes and salmonella infections, pneumonia, meningitis, Kaposi's sarcoma and non-Hodgkin's lymphoma. A number of illnesses, known as Aids indicator conditions, are particularly associated with Aids. Alternatively, some people infected with HIV develop a series of severe symptoms and manifestations but not the infections and cancers associated with Aids. This is called the Aids-related complex, or ARC.

Diagnosis and treatment

A blood test is used to detect the presence of HIV and, at the time of diagnosis, a person may be an asymptomatic carrier of the virus. It is generally accepted that a person with HIV will eventually develop infections and illnesses related to the virus, although there may be a period of several years when he or she remains well. During this period, the person may be treated with anti-retroviral therapy to delay the onset and lessen the impact of HIV infections.

Drugs that are used include zidovudine, or ZDU, which was formerly called azidothymidine, or AZT. This potent drug has proved to be effective in increasing the survival time of some patients with Aids or ARC. It can also delay the onset of illnesses and apparently works by slowing down the replication rate of the virus. However, results can be variable and in some patients resistance develops, reducing the effectiveness of ZDU. A similar drug, dideoxyinosine, or DDI, may be given, which acts in a similar way. Both ZDU and DDI have been in use since 1991 and have produced encouraging results, although both have a range of toxic side effects. A huge research effort by the drug companies continues to be directed towards the development of new drugs. An example is dideoxycytidine (DDC), which it is hoped will produce fewer side effects.

Other treatment is directed towards the particular infections and cancers that may arise. For many of these, chemotherapy and other treatments have greatly improved the short-term outlook and the quality of life of Aids victims. It is hoped that it will eventually prove possible to hold HIV in check and reduce the decline in natural immunity that it causes, with the ultimate aim of restoring the immune system to normal. In addition, intense research effort is being devoted to developing an effective vaccine against the virus.

Who is most at risk?

As has already been stated, HIV is no respecter of persons and anyone can be infected if certain circumstances prevail. Fortunately, outside these circumstances, HIV is not easily passed on. It is generally accepted that ordinary family or social contact with a person who has HIV or Aids poses no risk of transmitting the virus. Infants and children who are infected almost always became so during birth. An infected mother has a high risk of passing on the virus to her baby during the final stages of labour and delivery. HIV has also been detected in breast milk, but transmission of the virus by breast-feeding is not thought to be a significant route of infection.

Anyone who has unprotected sexual intercourse with an HIV-infected partner is at risk, but the use of condoms, reduces this considerably. Intravenous drug users are at risk through the sharing of contaminated needles and equipment. A great effort has been made to address this problem by issuing registered addicts with sterile, disposable needles. Unfortunately, the drug habit often causes people to take risks and to continue to share contaminated needles and so gives HIV a chance to claim more victims.

Medical, nursing, dental and other health care staff are at greater risk, particularly from accidental 'needlestick' injuries when dealing with infected blood or body secretions. Strict procedures are in place in all hospitals, clinics and surgeries to protect staff, and these must be closely followed at all times. Infection in the opposite direction, from a doctor, nurse or dentist with HIV to a patient, has occurred but is exceedingly rare.

Infected donated blood was once a means of transmission of HIV. In all developed countries, such blood is now screened for the presence of the virus. In addition, donors are asked detailed and searching questions about their lifestyle (in the form of a printed questionnaire) before they give blood. Any doubts about possible exposure to HIV are revealed by this process and the person is discreetly asked not to be a donor. He or she will also be given confidential counselling and told how to go about obtaining an HIV test. The combination of questioning donors and screening blood works well in Britain and hence the risk of infection via transfusion is extremely small. On exceedingly rare occasions, an infected donation has 'slipped through the net'. This is believed to have occurred because of the existence of a 'window' of about three weeks between a person being infected with HIV and his or her body producing detectable antibodies to the virus that then appear in the blood. It is possible for blood donated during the short window period to give false-negatives when tested for HIV but, as stated above, this is extremely rare. Anyone who has received a blood transfusion, which is itself only given for good medical reasons, should not feel anxious in any way.

On an individual level, sexually active people can take sensible precautions to minimize personal risk. A person may wish to avoid numerous casual sexual relationships and should always practise safe sex, which means using barrier methods of contraception. These minimize the risk of infection but cannot remove it altogether. A person who fears that he or she might have been infected, or who simply wants reassurance on this point, should have an HIV blood test. This is freely available and completely confidential and there is no need even to consult your general practitioner if you do not wish to do so. All waiting rooms at surgeries, clinics and hospitals have leaflets and posters to advise people of where they can obtain an HIV test. Many people fear the social, as well as health, consequences of a positive result, and obviously these can and have been considerable in some cases. The climate of public sympathy towards victims of HIV and Aids is moving towards removing the stigma and prejudice that have undoubtedly been attached to sufferers in the past.

It is in many Third World countries, which lack health and educational resources and where people are frequently malnourished, that Aids is at its most devastating. In the worst instances, Aids has removed many of the young adults on whom the economy of a country largely depends. Their children are left orphaned and many will develop the disease in their turn. It is up to all the inhabitants of the 'global village' to do what they can to end the scourge of HIV and Aids.

6

Meningitis

Meningitis is one of the most feared of illnesses in the British Isles and throughout the world, particularly for those who are parents or who are involved with children and young people. The reason for this fear is that it can be a severe and violent infection, striking suddenly and without warning, which can cause a child who was seemingly perfectly well to die within 24 hours. It is these chilling facts, usually widely reported in the media, that make meningitis so terrifying. It is perhaps worth stating at this stage that the illness just described is rare and is only one form of the disease, called acute bacterial meningitis. It is most commonly caused by three species of bacteria, which are responsible for about 80 per cent of all cases of the illness in the British Isles. These are meningococcus (*Neisseria meningitidis*), haemophilus influenzae type B and pneumococcus (*Streptococcus pneumoniae*). This report concentrates on the meningococcal disease as its main example, as it is one of the most common forms of meningitis in young people and children. However, a broader description may also prove to be helpful.

General information

Meningitis means inflammation of the meninges or membranes of the brain (cerebral meningitis) or spinal cord (spinal meningitis). The inflammation may affect either or both regions. If it affects the dura mater or pachymeninx membrane, which is the outer, fibrous, tough and inelastic layer surrounding the brain and spinal cord, it is known as pachymeningitis. This is a fairly uncommon form and often arises as a secondary inflammation resulting from the presence of disease elsewhere, for example tuberculous and syphilitic meningitis, both bacterial in origin.

Meningitis can also affect the inner two membranes, the arachnoid mater and pia mater, sometimes collectively called the pia-arachnoid or leptomeninges. This form, called leptomeningitis, is relatively more common and may be either a primary or a secondary infection.

Meningitis can also be classified as acute, sub-acute and chronic. Acute meningitis is the severe form described above, with a rapid appearance and development of symptoms. Sub-acute meningitis lasts more than two weeks, and chronic meningitis for more than one month. The symptoms can be very severe but develop over weeks not days. These forms usually arise as a result of the presence of an existing disease or condition, including various forms of cancer, such as leukaemia and lymphoma (involving lymph nodes), Aids, tuberculosis, syphilis, Hodgkin's disease, Lyme disease and fungal infections (especially in Aids patients).

Meningitis may also be classified according to its causal organism, usually bacteria (bacterial) or viruses (viral) but also fungi and, rarely, others, for example, amoebae. Some bacteria have already been mentioned, and there are a number that can cause meningitis, especially if particular factors are present. Haemophilus influenzae type B, or Hib, is the most common cause of meningitis in newborn babies under four weeks old. It does not usually arise in adults unless particular circumstances apply, for example, if the person has suppressed immunity or has sustained a head injury. Pneumococcus is a common cause of meningitis in adults and poses a particular risk for those with a head injury, ongoing or chronic middle ear infection or sinusitis, pneumococcal pneumonia, sickle-cell anaemia, or those with a depressed immune system and in alcoholics. It often arises as a secondary infection.

Other bacteria that can be involved, especially after some forms of surgery or in those with a suppressed immune system, are Gram-negative organisms such as *Escherichia coli*. *Staphylococcus* bacteria can also cause meningitis, particularly in neurosurgical patients or those with a penetrating head wound. Meningitis may arise with the acute infectious disease leptospirosis (Weil's disease), caused by *Leptospira* bacteria. Similarly, it may arise in listeriosis caused by the Gram-positive bacterium *Listeria monocytogenes*, particularly in those with renal failure or who have been treated with steroid drugs.

All patients with bacterial meningitis are treated in hospital with intensive courses of appropriate antibiotics and supportive nursing care. A person with suspected or confirmed bacterial meningitis is normally looked after in an isolation room.

Most cases of viral meningitis are relatively mild, and these are treated with bed rest, painkilling drugs and the drinking of plenty of fluids until recovery takes place. However, some viruses can cause severe illness, and these include poliovirus, echovirus, arbovirus and Coxsackie virus. In cases of serious illness, the person needs to be treated intensively in hospital with the antiviral drug acyclovir and supportive nursing care.

Aseptic meningitis describes all forms of the illness in which bacteria are not the cause. The usual cause is viral infection, but other agents may be involved, including fungi, reactions to antibiotic and other drugs, vaccines or diagnostic dyes, and poisons such as lead. Also included in this category are the cancers mentioned previously. Fungal infections have become more common with the advent of Aids and are particularly likely to arise in patients who have received treatment with immunosuppressive drugs. Fungal meningitis can occur in those suffering from Aids or HIV-related illness, Hodgkin's disease, lymphoblastic leukaemia and other forms of cancer affecting the central nervous system. The most common causal fungus is *Cryptococcus*, but *Candida* (a yeast-like organism responsible for thrush), *Actinomyces* and others may be involved. Fungal meningitis can be very severe, requiring treatment in hospital with appropriate intensive drug therapy and supportive care. Amphotericin B, flucytosine, fluconazole and penicillin are drugs that may be given depending upon the organism involved.

In all forms of meningitis there is a rise in intracranial pressure accompanying changes in the constituents and appearance of the liquid bathing the brain and spinal cord (cerebrospinal fluid). Hence a lumbar puncture to obtain a sample of the fluid is normally carried out in all suspected cases, and the causal organism, especially if it is bacterial, can usually be identified by this or other techniques.

Meningococcal meningitis

Meningococcal meningitis is one of the most severe and common forms of the illness and may occur in epidemics. These were formerly common in many areas, affecting large numbers of people, but in countries with an effective health care system are now usually contained. This has been made possible by the use of antibiotics, which revolutionized treatment and greatly improved the chances of survival for individuals affected. Those most at risk of death, in meningococcal and many other forms of meningitis, are infants and young children and the elderly. Incidence is greater in winter and spring (February to April) although cases can occur at any time.

The bacteria

Meningococci, or *Neisseria meningitidus*, are common bacteria that routinely inhabit the back of the throat and nose of many people within the population of the British Isles. It is extremely rare for any of these people to contract meningitis. They are carriers of the organism and since they remain healthy, the presence of the bacteria is not suspected. It is thought that most people may be carriers at some stage in their lives, with about 5 to 10 per cent of the population being affected at any one time.

Meningococci can be divided into various groups. In Britain, nearly two-thirds of all cases of meningococcal infection are caused by group B bacteria and the remainder by group C. The latter is more likely to be the cause of infection in younger people.

People at highest risk

The people at most risk of contracting a meningococcal infection are children under the age of four and especially babies around six months old. It is thought that this may be because their immune system is vulnerable as it is immature. The second most affected group are teenagers and young adults in the age range of 15 to 20. Infection of an epidemic nature is especially likely where young people live in close proximity to each other, as in a boarding school, a hall of residence or military establishment.

Route of infection

The most common means by which the bacteria are spread is in nasal discharges (coughs and sneezes) from a person who is a carrier or who is incubating the infection. Fortunately, the bacteria are not at all hardy and can survive for only a very short time in the air or environment. They cannot be picked up from objects, clothing or furnishings but must be breathed in from the air. In fact, evidence shows that they are likely to be passed on only if there is close contact between people, and even then the risk of infection is low. It is more likely that bacteria picked up in this way will be destroyed by a person's immune system or he or she will become a carrier. In a very few people, the body's natural defences are overcome, resulting in the development of a meningococcal infection. It is not known why some people are more susceptible than others, but it is believed to be related to individual differences in immunity. Gathering together in an enclosed space with poor ventilation may be factors that favour the spread of the bacteria.

The risk for each individual remains very small. For every 100,000 people in the United Kingdom, about four develop a meningococcal infection. Overall, there are about 2,000 cases of bacterial meningitis each year, of which 150 to 200 prove to be fatal. The incidence is higher in some years than in others, and the chances of recovery improve with prompt diagnosis and treatment. Improving public awareness of the signs and symptoms of meningitis is vitally important in the fight against this disease.

Forms of meningococcal disease

Meningococci cause two forms of illness, which can arise separately or together, and these are meningitis and meningococcal septicaemia (blood poisoning). There is probably greater public awareness of meningitis than of septicaemia. Both are serious, with a rapid development of symptoms, but septicaemia and septicaemia with meningitis are the most severe. With prompt diagnosis and appropriate intensive treatment, 90 per cent of patients recover from meningitis, depending on their age and other factors, such as state of immunity. With meningococcal septicaemia, 50 to 80 per cent of people recover, depending, once again, on age, severity of symptoms and immunity. Both types of illness produce a range of symptoms, which may vary slightly in the time of their appearance but are usually present. The symptoms of meningitis are characteristic of all acute forms of the illness. Generally, the incubation period (that is, the time that elapses between the start of infection and the appearance of symptoms) is short, about two to five days. However, it may be up to ten days before symptoms first appear. The bacteria enter the bloodstream from the back of the nose and throat and, overcoming the defences of the immune system, proliferate rapidly, releasing toxins causing the onset of symptoms.

Unfortunately, the early signs can easily be mistaken for those of influenza or other common illnesses, and meningitis is often preceded by a sore throat, respiratory symptoms and slight malaise. This is sometimes the cause of a delay in seeking early medical treatment, especially if an ordinary viral type of infection is known to be 'doing the rounds' in a community. However, a person with meningitis rapidly becomes severely ill. Symptoms include vomiting, severe headache, stiff neck, fever, intolerance of bright lights (called photophobia), rash (not always present) and changes in consciousness. The latter range from confusion and irritability to drowsiness, unconsciousness and coma.

The symptoms are caused by inflammation of the meninges as a result of a rapid proliferation of the bacteria with release of their toxins, increasing intracranial pressure because of changes in the quantity and components of the cerebrospinal fluid and a build-up of pus-like material from damaged cells and tissues. This causes obstruction of the channels through which the cerebrospinal fluid normally passes and damages nerve pathways, for example, those of the cranial nerves. If the latter occurs, there may be the development of facial nerve palsy and disturbance of vision because of damage to the (oculomotor) nerves operating the eyes. Rarely, deafness can also arise.

Depending on the nature and extent of the irritation of motor nerve roots within the central nervous system, other signs affecting nerves and muscles may be present. A doctor may test for the presence of these, which are called Kernig's sign and Brudzinski's sign. Kernig's sign is the inability of someone with meningitis to straighten the legs at the knees when the thighs are flexed against the abdomen or at right angles to the body and the person is in a supine position. Brudzinski's sign is an involuntary bending of the knees, hips and arms when the patient's neck is passively and suddenly flexed while he or she is in a supine position. Both these signs are characteristic of meningitis but are not necessarily present. In infants and young children under two years old, symptoms include fretfulness, shrill high-pitched crying, refusing of feeds, fever, vomiting and a tight or bulging fontanelle. The child's skin may be pale or develop a blotchy rash, although this is not always present. The child may become lethargic, and convulsions are quite common. The development of hydrocephalus, that is, an enlarged head as a result of fluid collection, may eventually occur. Small children can become severely and dangerously ill within a few hours and adults within 24 hours.

Symptoms and signs of meningococcal septicaemia

In the bloodstream, the bacteria multiply at a very high rate, releasing toxic substances that cause damage, inflammation and disintegration of the walls of blood vessels, allowing blood to escape. This causes the characteristic symptom of a red, blotchy rash that can develop anywhere on the body. This may be paler at first but soon becomes red, and, if pressed hard with a glass tumbler, the rash remains the same colour and does not blanch. This is also the case with the rash that occurs with meningitis. Additional symptoms are pains in joints, muscles, chest and abdomen, changes in level of consciousness and possibly coma. There may be shallow, rapid breathing, cold feet and hands, vomiting and possibly diarrhoea. The damage to blood vessels can rapidly lead to a fall in blood pressure and the development of shock.

Action to take

If a person has any of the signs or symptoms of meningitis or septicaemia, seek medical help immediately. Do not wait to see what happens or worry about being wrong. Remember that with this illness time saves life and the sooner a person receives medical treatment the greater the chances of recovery. If the patient's condition is causing worry, which is always the case with meningitis, then it is far better to call your doctor so that you can have the reassurance that the person will receive the appropriate treatment. In cases of suspected or even possible meningitis, a general practitioner will normally arrange for the patient to be admitted to hospital for observation, tests and treatment. The doctor may also give the patient an injection of an antibiotic, usually a form of penicillin.

Hospital treatment

On admittance to hospital, the patient is usually placed in an isolation room and a sample of cerebrospinal fluid is obtained as soon as possible by means of a lumbar puncture. The sample is examined immediately in the laboratory, and a technique known as the Gram stain can usually distinguish between the bacteria that commonly cause meningitis, that is, meningococcus, pneumococcus and haemophilus influenzae. The sample is cultured and the organisms grown so that they can be positively identified. The patient may be given an intravenous injection of antibiotic immediately, before the results of the laboratory tests are available, and one will be used that is effective against the common meningitis bacteria, usually cephalosporin, penicillin G or ampicillin. Further antibiotic treatment depends on the type of organism involved. Penicillin G is usually given to combat meningococcal meningitis and septicaemia. In addition, the patient will receive intensive supportive therapy and nursing care, which may include fluid and electrolyte replacement and measures to control fever and pain. With this combination of treatment, the majority of patients start to improve, with the first few hours being critical. Further samples of cerebrospinal fluid are obtained and examined regularly. Antibiotic treatment is usually continued for some time and for at least one week after symptoms have declined and the cerebrospinal fluid appears normal, with no trace of bacteria. This is to ensure that all the organisms have been eradicated and that there is no danger of the infection flaring up again.

Most people make a complete recovery, although it may take some time to regain full strength. Occasionally, there can be long-term brain damage, mental retardation, occurrence of fits and problems connected with the cranial nerves.

Public health measures

Meningitis and meningococcal septicaemia are notifiable diseases
and when a case is confirmed the appropriate authorities are
informed. Usually, if only one person has been infected, then preventative antibiotics are given to his or her immediate family and those
living under the same roof and other close contacts such as a
boyfriend or girlfriend. If there have been two or more cases (known
as a cluster) within a few weeks of each other and in a connected
group, antibiotics are offered to contacts who may be at risk. If
young children are involved, as in a nursery or primary class, the
recommendation is to treat all pupils and teachers. In a secondary
school, university, college or military establishment, those in direct
contact, for example, those in the same year or class, are usually
given antibiotics. Other people may also be offered them if they are
possibly at risk, and this is determined by the doctor working for
the public health authority.

When a case of meningitis occurs in a community, particularly
if a child or young person is involved, or there has been a fatality,
there is naturally a great deal of anxiety. There is a tendency for
people to demand antibiotic treatment and to be resentful if this is
not offered. Usually, this is based on misconceptions about the role
of antibiotic prophylaxis and the nature of meningitis itself.

Firstly, and most importantly, as has already been noted, meningitis is not easy to catch and the risks are small, even for those who
have been in direct contact with a person who has developed the
disease. Hence there is no benefit for indirect contacts, such as a
'friend of a friend' of a meningitis victim, receiving antibiotics.

Secondly, bacteria are notoriously adept at mutating to produce
antibiotic-resistant strains. At the present time, while there are some
strains of meningitis bacteria that are resistant to certain antibiotics,
the problem is not too great. There is a fear, however, that overuse
of preventative antibiotics would favour the development of resistance, hence lessening the effectiveness of treatment and decreasing
the chances of survival for meningitis victims. Finally, the antibiotics
that are given are powerful drugs, which kill not only the meningitis bacteria but other organisms that may be beneficial. Also, there
is a risk of allergic reactions and side effects so these antibiotics are
given only if they are really needed. The health and best interests

of the people concerned are always the governing factors, and decisions rest with the public health doctors involved. Anyone who continues to feel anxious should talk things over with his or her general practitioner.

Vaccination

A vaccine is available to combat meningitis caused by haemophilus influenzae type B, and this is normally given to babies. A vaccine also exists for group C meningococcal infections, but it is not effective in young children aged under 18 months. Unfortunately, this is the age group most at risk from the infection. Hence, for reasons outlined above, the vaccine is not used widely but only when an outbreak has occurred attributable to this strain of bacteria. The immunity given lasts for about three to five years. A great deal of research is being devoted to developing new vaccines for both group C and group B infections and it is hoped that these will eventually become available.

7

Hepatitis

Hepatitis is inflammation of the liver, and it can range from a mild to a very severe, fatal illness. It can arise from a number of different causes, both infectious and non-infectious, and can produce a range of symptoms that may arise suddenly or develop insidiously, depending on the form of the illness.

The most common causes are viral, as a result of infection by a number of different viruses, excess alcohol consumption, various drugs, toxic substances and poisons. The most frequent cause in the British Isles is alcohol abuse, and in some susceptible individuals, especially women, a modest daily intake over a prolonged number of years is enough to cause damage. Viral hepatitis is also common in many countries, posing a significant risk to human health.

Acute hepatitis produces an attack of symptoms, which include abdominal pain, nausea, loss of appetite and weight, fever, skin rashes, itching, jaundice, passing of pale-coloured stools and diarrhoea. Chronic active or aggressive hepatitis has a similar range of symptoms, which develop more slowly. This condition may persist for years, eventually leading to cirrhosis, liver failure and early death. Cirrhosis causes the formation of fibrous tissue as a result of damage and death of cells, and the liver becomes yellow-coloured and nodular in appearance. It can arise in connection with both alcohol-related and some forms of viral hepatitis and may also be an auto-immune disorder related to complex factors in a person's immune system.

Fulminant hepatitis is the most severe form and usually the cause is viral (hepatitis B virus), drug-related, for example, paracetamol overdose or alcohol abuse. The condition can progress rapidly, with massive death of liver tissue (acute yellow atrophy), bleeding, loss of consciousness and kidney failure. A liver transplant may then offer the only chance of survival, but the outlook is poor for adults and somewhat better for children. Patients who survive normally make a complete recovery.

Many viruses can cause hepatitis, including Epstein-Barr (responsible for glandular fever or infectious mononucleosis), cytomegalovirus, HIV and yellow fever virus. A number of parasitic infestations can cause inflammation of the liver although not true hepatitis. These include malaria, schistosomiasis, toxoplasmosis (in newborn babies) and amoebiasis. Liver inflammation can similarly result from bacterial infection, for example, in tuberculosis, liver abscess, leptospirosis (Weil's disease) and in connection with a number of other diseases and disorders.

However, the so-called hepatic viruses, designated A, B, C, D and E, are the main cause of viral hepatitis, causing significant ill-health and premature death on a worldwide basis and transmittable from one person to another. These will be considered individually.

Hepatitis A, epidemic hepatitis, infectious hepatitis

Hepatitis A virus (HAV) is shed in the faeces of an infected person. The infection spreads easily when water or food becomes contaminated, which commonly occurs in conditions of poor hygiene and sanitation. It is also possible, although less common, for it to be passed by oral or anal sex. The virus is shed prolifically during the incubation period, that is, the time between infection and appearance of any symptoms, when the person is perfectly well. This is therefore the period when the person is most infective and by the time symptoms appear, virus numbers are decreasing and infectiveness starts to decline. Also, many people do not exhibit symptoms at all or these are so mild that they are disregarded. Of course, they still shed the virus and are a potential source of infection to others. It can be seen that these factors facilitate the easy spread of the virus, as by the time hepatitis A infection is suspected, infective material has inevitably been passed to the environment.

People most at risk

Children and adolescents are most likely to be infected. Many adults have been exposed previously and have developed immunity to further infection.

Symptoms (acute hepatitis)

The incubation period varies between two and six weeks and usually begins with loss of appetite, feverishness, nausea, sickness and malaise. A person who smokes may develop an aversion to cigarettes. Also, there may be headaches, abdominal pain, pale-coloured stools and diarrhoea. After about one week, the urine becomes darker and jaundice appears, and some people may develop itchiness or skin rashes. The jaundice often intensifies for a further week, although the patient begins to feel better and other symptoms subside. It may take two weeks to a month for the jaundice to disappear and for recovery to be complete. Most people suffer no further ill-effects and develop antibodies to the virus, which provide long-term immunity. These are called IgG Ab, or anti-HA. They develop a few weeks after infection and usually provide lifelong protection against future attacks. Studies on blood have shown that in some countries three-quarters of adults tested possess these antibodies, indicating previous exposure to HAV.

Diagnosis and treatment

Hepatitis is diagnosed by examining samples of blood in a laboratory. In the case of hepatitis A, a type of antibody, known as IgMAb, is produced early in the infection in response to the presence of viral antigen (Ag), but this disappears within a few weeks. Hence its presence in the blood is indicative of an acute HAV infection. Usually no specific treatment is needed other than plenty of rest, fluids and a nourishing diet as appetite allows. Alcohol should be avoided. Strict standards of hygiene should be maintained, especially with regard to the washing of hands, and it is probably advisable for an infected person not to prepare food intended for others. If the patient is an infant, care should be taken in handling nappies. HAV infection does not lead to more severe forms of hepatitis or cirrhosis and the virus does not remain in the body. It is rare for there to be any long-lasting effects. Occasionally, there may be a chronic benign disorder called chronic persistent hepatitis, but this rarely produces symptoms and is not life-threatening. (Compare chronic active hepatitis, which is described on page 53.)

Preventative measures

People intending to travel to countries where hepatitis A is very common can take certain precautions. A blood test can determine individual immunity to HAV by testing for the presence of IgG Ab. If necessary, a person can be given an injection of human immunoglobulin containing antibodies to HAV, which gives up to 12 weeks' protection. Also, vaccination is now available, although the two injections of vaccine necessary to complete the course must be separated by a twelve-month interval. Vaccination affords protection for ten years or even longer.

It is sensible to be careful about food and water when visiting a country where hepatitis A is prevalent. Uncooked shellfish should be avoided and also salad vegetables and unpeeled fruit, which may have been in contact with contaminated water. Ice cubes should not be added to drinks, and boiled or bottled water should be used for drinking and cleaning teeth. Hands should always be thoroughly washed before food is prepared or handled.

Hepatitis E (HEV)

Hepatitis E infection is similar in most respects to HAV and can occur in epidemics, being transmitted via contaminated food or drink. The symptoms, recovery and prognosis are apparently the same, although less is known about this virus which was identified only quite recently. HEV is prevalent in Third World countries, although rare in the British Isles, and can pose a threat to the health of travellers. There is evidence to suggest that HEV may be responsible for some deaths in pregnant women in the countries where it is common.

Hepatitis B (HBV) serum hepatitis B

The hepatitis B virus is responsible for a broad range of illness, varying from an attack of acute symptoms to chronic (type B) aggressive disease leading to cirrhosis and early death (especially in Africa and Asia). HBV is also associated with liver cancer (hepatocellular cancer), which is common in populations where the virus is prevalent. At the other extreme, some people are infected with HBV and subsequently eliminate the virus from their bodies without showing signs of illness, or the symptoms are so mild that they are disregarded. (Blood tests can reveal the presence of anti-HB antibodies, which indicates past HBV infection.) HBV is highly infectious and is carried in blood and body fluids, such as vaginal and rectal secretions, semen, saliva and urine. It can persist in the body for many years, and a proportion of people who recover from HBV illness become chronic carriers of the virus and provide a reservoir of infection.

The virus is transmitted by the infected blood or body fluid of someone with HBV coming into contact with that of a non-infected person. This can occur as a result of unprotected sexual intercourse, both heterosexual and homosexual, and anal and oral sex. In western countries, all blood and blood products are screened for the presence of HBV so transfusion poses no risk. The main route of infection involving blood is the sharing of contaminated needles by injecting drug addicts. Tattooing, ear piercing and minor dental and surgical procedures are also further areas of potential risk. Health care workers are at risk of 'needlestick injuries', that is, being accidentally pierced by needles, scalpels, etc, during the course of their work. In the British Isles, people involved with drugs or prostitution or who have unprotected sex or who are in a closed institution, such as a prison, are at greatest risk of HBV infection. Also, particularly in countries where HBV is prevalent, the virus may be passed from an infected mother to her child during pregnancy or childbirth. Finally, there is a possibility that bloodsucking insects may transmit the virus, although the significance of this is not clear.

People most at risk

People of any age can be infected, with those most at risk belonging to the groups described above.

Symptoms

The incubation period for HBV is longer than for HAV and is usually between six weeks to six months. Symptoms, when they occur, are typical of acute hepatitis but are generally more severe than with HAV infection. They include anorexia, headache, fever, malaise, pains and chills, nausea, sickness, skin rashes, painful, swollen wrists and ankles before the appearance of jaundice and the passing of dark urine and pale-coloured stools. Most people gradually make a complete recovery, although this may take several weeks, and they may be abnormally tired for some months. A small proportion of people go on to develop chronic active hepatitis, which is described on page 53.

Diagnosis and treatment

Hepatitis is diagnosed by examining samples of blood in a laboratory. In the case of hepatitis B, a number of antigen-antibody systems may be looked for, although one antigen is commonly used to make a diagnosis. This is called hepatitis B surface antigen (or Hbs Ag) and is also known as Australia Ag. It is associated with the surface coat of the virus and usually appears in the blood between one and six weeks before the onset of symptoms during the incubation period. It indicates the presence either of acute HBV infection or a person who is a carrier.

As the illness progresses, Hbs Ag normally declines as the body mounts an immune response and manufactures anti-HB antibodies. However, in a few people (about 10 per cent), HBV surface Ag persists in the blood and no anti-HBs are produced. These patients either become carriers of the virus without displaying further symptoms or they may go on to develop chronic hepatitis. Anyone who is diagnosed as having a hepatitis B infection will require further blood tests after recovery to determine their status with regard to the virus. While HBV surface Ag remains in the blood, a person is infective and must take precautions to avoid passing on the virus (*see* Preventative measures, overleaf). When there is no HBV surface Ag but anti-HB is present in the blood, the person is no longer infective and is immune, probably for life, against future infection.

Depending on the severity of symptoms, treatment is usually much the same as for HAV infection. The person should have plenty of rest and fluids and should eat a normal balanced diet, as appetite allows. Alcoholic drinks should be avoided, and most people make a gradual recovery. However, those who develop more severe chronic hepatitis require hospital treatment with various drugs, which may include antiviral interferon. The mortality rate is between 1 and 5 per cent but can be as high as 10 to 15 per cent, for example, in elderly patients or those who are debilitated.

Preventative measures

For individuals, precautions that can be taken to limit the risk of HBV infection involve personal and behavioural modifications and vaccination. In addition, health care workers should adhere strictly to the high standards of safety and hygiene in place in all modern hospitals, health centres and dental surgeries. Measures include practising 'safe sex' by using barrier methods of contraception, for example, condoms. Drug users should never reuse or share needles or syringes and disposable items should be used. Ideally, used items should be handed in to a hospital clinic dealing with addiction so that they can be disposed of safely. Children should be educated about the dangers of handling syringes and needles and taught never to touch them. Anyone who collects these for safe disposal must wear protective gloves and clothing. People seeking acupuncture, ear piercing or tattooing should ensure that the premises they attend are properly run and meet current safety standards. Disposable needles should be used or instruments sterilized in an autoclave. People should not share toothbrushes, razors or other items connected with personal hygiene.

People who may have been accidentally exposed to HBV can be protected by injections of immunoglobulin (IG) or hepatitis B immunoglobulin (HBIG) and may also require vaccination. HBV vaccine is given to those who are considered to be at potential risk of infection, and three injections are given over an interval of six months. Six weeks after the course is completed, a blood sample is taken so that immunity can be tested. A few people (about 5 per cent) do not respond to vaccination by manufacturing antibodies and so remain at risk, but the reasons for this are not known. Also, vaccination is less effective in patients with compromised immunity, receiving kidney dialysis or with cirrhosis of the liver. Booster injections are needed every three to five years for those who receive vaccination.

In the British Isles, vaccination is not routinely offered to all the population but is available for those who may be at risk. Vaccination and/or immunoglobulin (HBIG) is normally given to:

1. Newborn babies of mothers who are HBV surface Ag positive. HBIG is effective in preventing the development of chronic hepatitis in 70 per cent of infants.
2. People who suffer accidental 'needlestick' injury involving known infected blood.
3. Sexual partners of a person with confirmed HBV infection.
4. Victims of rape or sexual assault.
5. Injecting drug addicts and their sexual contacts.
6. Prostitutes, homosexual and heterosexual people with many sexual contacts.
7. Doctors, nurses, dentists and all health workers who may be at risk.
8. Residents and staff in closed institutions.
9. People planning to travel to a country where HBV infections are prevalent.

Any person who fears that he or she may have been exposed or may be at risk should contact his or her general practitioner. Blood tests and vaccination can provide reassurance in many cases and the outlook is better for those who seek early medical advice and treatment.

Hepatitis C (HCV), non-A, non-B hepatitis, serum hepatitis C

Hepatitis C is believed to be less common than HAV or HBV infections, but it is responsible for 80 per cent of cases of hepatitis that arise after blood transfusion. Less is known about HCV, but it has now been identified as a likely cause of hepatitis in patients who have formerly received multiple transfusions of blood. HCV is transmitted in the same way as HBV, and it is hoped that recently developed tests for the screening of all donated blood will reduce the incidence of infection worldwide. HCV is also known to be responsible for a substantial number of cases of acute hepatitis. It usually produces a mild attack of symptoms, or even none at all, but around half of those infected go on to develop chronic hepatitis. In some of these (20 per cent), the illness is the serious form of chronic active hepatitis and HCV is also implicated in cirrhosis and hepatocellular carcinoma (liver cancer). A number of people become carriers of HCV without showing any symptoms of illness. It is believed that a proportion of these may eventually develop some form of liver disease.

In the British Isles, HCV is now most commonly transmitted between injecting drug users through the sharing of contaminated needles and syringes. It can also be passed sexually from one person to another, in the same way as HBV, although there is some evidence that it is less likely to be transmitted in this way. HCV can also pass from an infected mother to her baby during childbirth.

People most at risk

People of any age group can be infected with HCV, but drug users and those who have previously had many blood transfusions may be at greater risk.

Symptoms

The incubation period is usually about two months but varies between two weeks and four months before generally minor symptoms appear. Often these are in the form of fairly mild, 'flu-like symptoms in which jaundice is not a feature (particularly in posttransfusion cases). This is called aricteric hepatitis, and it is thought that it may be far more common than is generally realized but is usually not diagnosed. Acute HCV hepatitis may also produce the more typical symptoms described previously. About half the people infected recover from the initial illness, although this may take some time. Antibodies to HCV usually appear in the blood after several months, but as time passes these slowly decline. During the recovery phase the infection can assume a 'roller-coaster' nature of fluctuating levels of activity, resulting in relapses and the return of symptoms, known as recrudescent hepatitis. A number of these patients may then go on to develop chronic hepatitis. The long-term prospects for those identified as having HCV infection or who are carriers is difficult to predict.

Diagnosis and treatment

Diagnosis is made by examining blood serum for the presence of the virus. HCV antigen can also be detected in infected liver cells. Treatment for the initial mild illness is the same as for HAV and HBV. Those who develop chronic active hepatitis require treatment in hospital with a variety of different drugs, including interferon.

Preventative measures

There is no vaccine currently available against HCV, and, since antibody levels decline, exposure may not provide immunity to further infection. Hence, preventative measures, as described for HBV infections, are of vital importance to limit individual risk.

Hepatitis D (HDV, delta agent)

HDV is unusual in that it is a defective RNA virus which can proliferate only in the presence of hepatitis B virus. In general, its effect seems to exacerbate an HBV infection and this can occur in a number of different ways. One of the most serious is to cause severe acute symptoms of hepatitis in those infected with HBV. It is believed that HDV in conjunction with HBV may be responsible for half the cases of serious fulminant B hepatitis. HDV may cause chronic B hepatitis to follow a more aggressive route than would otherwise have been the case. In a person who is a carrier of HBV, HDV may be responsible for a flare-up of the symptoms of hepatitis or a super-infection.

The prevalence of HDV varies widely from one country to another, with injecting drug users being at high risk of infection. The same preventative measures that are employed against HBV are also effective against HDV. The fact that HDV has the potential to render HBV infections more severe or even fatal means that vigilance must always be maintained.

8

Legionnaires' Disease

Legionnaires' disease derived its name from the 182 cases of pneumonia that occurred amongst nearly 4,000 delegates attending an American Legion convention in Philadelphia, USA, in 1976. The episode attracted widespread publicity, particularly since 147 of these cases required hospital treatment and the episode resulted in 29 deaths. An intense investigation of this outbreak was carried out and led to the discovery of a bacterium now called *Legionella pneumophila* (*L. pneumophila*). This bacterium, which was previously unrecognized, was isolated from the water in the air-conditioning system in the hotel in which the convention was taking place. Since then over 30 species of *Legionella* have been identified and at least 19 have been implicated as agents of pneumonia in human beings.

Retrospective studies have identified cases of the disease as early as the 1940s. The first case occurred in 1947 and the first documented outbreak in 1957. The first epidemic of the disease occurred in 1965 at a psychiatric hospital in Washington DC. In this episode 81 people contracted a respiratory illness and 15 died. Legionnaires' disease has now been identified in Australia, Africa, South America and Europe. In the USA, the US Center for Disease Control and Prevention (CDC) estimated that each year between 2,000 and 6,000 people had been dying of legionnaires' disease. This had probably been happening for decades, certainly since the advent of air-conditioning technology and probably long before that as a result of indoor plumbing. Prior to the dramatic Philadelphia outbreak, these cases had probably been classified as 'pneumonia of unknown aetiology', that is, pneumonia of unknown cause.

The most common agent of human disease is *Legionella pneumophila*, followed by *L. micdadei* and then *L. bozemanii* and *L. dumoffii*. These organisms are similar in form, share biochemical characteristics and cause similar diseases. The majority of *Legionella* infections present in two different forms: Pontiac fever, which is a self-limiting, influenza-like illness without pneumonia; and legionnaires' disease, which in the initial stages is similar to Pontiac fever but patients characteristically go on to develop pneumonia. This is the most serious and frequently recognized form of the disease. There is a third and very rare form that results in a localized infection of soft tissue.

Legionnaires' disease accounts for 1 to 8 per cent of all pneumonias and about 4 per cent of lethal pneumonias acquired in hospital. These rates may increase substantially in areas or hospitals where the disease is endemic. Most cases are sporadic and are more likely to occur in the late summer and early autumn. However, numerous outbreaks similar to the original one in Philadelphia tend to occur in buildings, especially hospitals and hotels, or within certain geographical areas.

Source of infection

The natural habitat of *Legionella pneumophila* and other species is water, and it has been found in lakes, ponds and rivers. It has also been found in mud and polluted and silty water. *L. pneumophila* can survive in a wide range of environmental conditions, for example, in temperatures ranging from 0 to 63°C and in water with pH values of 5.4 to 8.2. The organism is inhibited by sodium chloride and is not found in sea water.

Legionella has also been found in cooling towers, water-driven condensers, steam turbines, shower heads, whirlpool spas, decorative fountains and in a wide variety of humidifiers and other devices that create water aerosols. The major sources of the bacterium in outbreaks of the disease have been attributed to organisms in aerosols from evaporative condensers of air-conditioning systems or tap water used through contaminated shower heads. However, the evidence is not entirely clear. One community outbreak of legionnaires' disease in the USA was linked to an ultrasonic mist machine in a grocery shop.

In the Philadelphia outbreak, it was noticed that most of the legionnaires' disease sufferers had spent time in the five cocktail suites run by the candidates for leadership of the veterans' group. Further analysis revealed that the bacteria thrived in the hotel's cooling tower, and it was from that water supply that the hotel derived its air-conditioning. The *Legionella* organisms were hidden in the biofilm 'scums' along the edges of the cooling tower and were actively pumped into the hotel's hospitality suites during the hot month of July.

Legionella has also been found in allegedly clean water sources. One study of tap water showed that the organism could survive for over a year in water pipes, emerging in a wholly infectious form once the tap had been turned on with full force. Even distilled water samples have been found occasionally to contain small numbers of *Legionella* organisms. Consumption of water by many of the individuals who developed legionnaires' disease in the Philadelphia outbreak in 1976 was significantly associated with the acquisition of the disease – an association that has often been overlooked.

Natural aquatic bodies usually contain only small numbers of *Legionella*. Treatment of water sources with chlorine is not effective in killing the *Legionella* organism as it has developed a tolerance to this. Resistance to such water-treatment processes means it can pass into the water distribution system. However, at this stage the organism exists only in small numbers. The subsequent growth and proliferation of the organism occurs in those man-made habitats, such as cooling towers and water distribution systems, which can provide the right conditions for it to grow. Essentially these include favourable water temperatures, physical protection and nutrients.

The ubiquitous distribution of *L. pneumophila* in man-made aquatic reservoirs is paradoxical considering the difficulties in growing the organism under laboratory conditions. It has been well established that the presence of symbiotic microorganisms, including amoebae and water bacteria, are necessary for optimal growth of *Legionella*. *L. pneumophila* can infect and multiply within amoebae and other unicellular microorganisms. When these host microorganisms rupture, large numbers of motile *Legionella* are freed. This ability of *L. pneumophila* to infect and exist within other unicellular organisms may explain its capacity to survive in otherwise inhospitable environments.

It has been found that the colonization of the water distribution system by *L. pneumophila* is dependent on a combination of several factors. These include water temperature, sediment accumulation and the presence of microorganisms that can provide essential nutrients. Water temperature appears to be a particularly critical factor. The organism is most readily found at the bottom of hot water tanks.

Transmission

It is likely that there are several modes of transmission of *L. pneumophila*. There is evidence that transmission may be by inhalation of droplets from air-conditioning plants, shower heads, etc. Taps and shower heads produce very localized aerosols. Water droplets (drift) contained in the airstream released from a cooling tower may be carried a considerable distance, exposing a greater number of people to risk Large extensive outbreaks affecting people not only in a building but also in the vicinity are typical of a cooling tower source. For example, passers-by in the Philadelphia outbreak were found to be infected. Other modes of transmission have not been established conclusively, but it appears unlikely that person-to-person transmission of the organism is important in spreading the disease. Infection via consumption of water containing the organism has not been ruled out. There is also some epidemiological evidence that suggests that airborne dust from excavation sites may also be a possible route of transmission.

Symptoms

Pneumonia is the predominant clinical manifestation in legionnaires' disease and in serious cases can lead to multi-system failure.

The incubation period is between two and ten days and most often between five and six days. For Pontiac disease, the incubation period ranges from five to six days and more usually 24 to 48 hours. The attack rate for those exposed is quite high and is estimated to be greater than 90 per cent.

Legionnaires' disease may occur at any age but most patients have been middle-aged males. The disease is extremely rare in the under twenties. Cases are more frequent in males than females in a ratio of 2.5:1. Cigarette smoking, chronic lung disease, diabetes, advanced age and immunosuppression have consistently been implicated as risk factors for legionnaires' disease. Excess alcohol intake and renal failure have also been noted as additional ones in some studies. People who have undergone surgery are more likely to acquire the infection than others, with transplant patients being at highest risk. Hospital-acquired infection in paediatric cases has also been reported in newborn babies, immunosuppressed patients and in children with underlying lung disease. In the hospitals in which these cases occurred, investigations showed a link with the hospital water supply. *Legionella* is now being recognized in patients with acquired immunodeficiency syndrome (Aids).

The initial stage of both legionnaires' disease and Pontiac fever resembles influenza and is characterized by anorexia, general malaise, muscle pain and headache. In Pontiac fever there is a nonproductive cough, and dizziness, and nausea sometimes occurs. Chest X-rays remain clear and patients usually recover spontaneously within two to five days without treatment. Pontiac fever is not associated with pneumonia or death. The clinical symptoms may represent reaction to the inhaled antigen rather than bacterial invasion.

In legionnaires' disease, following the initial 'flu-like symptoms, the patient becomes progressively more ill, with rapidly rising fever associated with chills. Temperatures may reach 39–40.5°C (102–105°F). A cough usually develops, which initially is dry but subsequently produces mucoid sputum. The sputum may be streaked with blood in 20–40 per cent of cases. A common associated symptom, in 25–50 per cent of cases, is abdominal pain and diarrhoea which is watery rather than bloody. In a few cases an altered mental state may also be apparent, with associated confusion, lethargy or delirium. Shaking chills are common in patients in advanced stages of the pneumonia. Chest pain can be a prominent feature for some patients. Chest X-rays show that virtually all patients have radiographic abnormalities by the third day of onset of the disease. Initially, only the lower part of one lung is usually involved. As the disease progresses, both upper and lower areas of both lungs may be affected. Ultimately, respiratory failure results. Occasionally patients develop lung abscesses and multiple rounded densities within the lung tissue, suggesting septic emboli. The case fatality rate from legionnaires' disease may be as high as 39 per cent in hospitalized cases and is generally higher in those with compromised immunity.

Diagnosis

The *Legionella* bacterium has peculiar dietary needs. The standard laboratory culture media does not support growth of the organism. It requires supplements of the amino acid cysteine, vitamins and minerals, particularly iron. *Legionella* prefers dark, nutrient-rich almost anoxic (deficient in oxygen) environments. As already described, *Legionella* also enjoys living inside the cytoplasms of larger one-celled organisms. These conditions hampered all the early investigations. It was impossible to see through microscopes with standard techniques. However, when treated with silver, the organism clearly revealed itself.

There are four diagnostic studies employed to detect the *Legionella* species:

- culture of the organism;
- a direct fluorescent antibody (DFA) stain of exudate;
- serology using the indirect fluorescent antibody (IFA) assay;
- urinary antigen assays.

All are reasonably specific but none is particularly sensitive, so if only small numbers of the organism are present they may be missed. There are numerous species within the genera, most of which have been implicated in causing a similar type of lung infection.

Culture of the organism is the definitive method for diagnosis of *Legionella* infection, since the bacteria are not part of the normal body microflora. The organism may be recovered from expectorated sputum, respiratory secretions, lung biopsies, pleural fluid or blood. Cultures from sputum samples are less successful than other samples. The preferred medium for culture is charcoal yeast extract.

Demonstration of the bacterium by direct fluorescent antibody staining of sputum, lung biopsy or post-mortem lung examination provides a more immediate result but this technique requires considerable expertise and depends on large numbers of the organism being present.

Serology, using the indirect fluorescent antibody (IFA) assay, was at one time the most commonly used diagnostic test. This has now been largely superseded by the use of cultures and more specific tests. The urinary antigen test is a relatively new diagnostic test for *Legionella*. Its results are available more rapidly than those of other tests. It has the additional advantage of using urine samples rather than sputum, the former being easier to obtain from sick patients.

Treatment

Erythromycin is the preferred drug used to treat legionnaires' disease. Patients with mild illness receive the drug orally every six hours. Seriously ill patients are treated with erythromycin intravenously. A clinical response, including a feeling of wellbeing, occurs within three to five days. Treatment is usually continued for at least three weeks to prevent relapses, although intravenous therapy can be changed to oral therapy when the fever and other acute symptoms have resolved.

With appropriate antibiotic therapy, mortality is low in patients who are immunocompetent. Without treatment, the mortality rate ranges from 15 to 25 per cent in community-acquired cases and is much higher among immunosuppressed or hospitalized patients with the disease. Most patients treated with erythromycin respond, but convalescence may be slow and X-ray abnormalities usually persist for up to a month.

Incidence

The incidence of legionnaires' disease is dependent on the degree of contamination by the organism in the aquatic reservoir, susceptibility of the persons exposed and the intensity of the exposure. The discovery of the infection is dependent on availability of special laboratory tests and to these being applied as soon as possible.

The first recorded case of legionnaires' disease in England occurred in Nottingham in 1977. In the months of August and September that year, a small but unusual cluster of patients with severe lobar pneumonia came to light. The illness was relatively mild at first, with fever and a nonproductive cough. Despite initial chemotherapy at home, the cough worsened and became productive, and signs of pneumonia with amnesia or mental confusion developed. In hospital, infection in the lung spread and patients did not respond to antibiotics that were ordinarily effective in pneumonia. Intensive care was needed, with assisted ventilation for long periods. Initially, no pathogen, bacterial or viral, was identified. In all, 15 were involved in the outbreak, with ages ranging from 17 to 63 years.

This cluster of severe pneumonia was unusual in Britain because it arose in summer and, additionally, so many patients needed assistance with ventilation. With assistance from the Center for Disease Control (CDC) in Atlanta, USA, these were confirmed as the first cases of legionnaires' disease in England. None of the patients had travelled abroad, there was no secondary infection in hospital or at home, nor were there any other unusual circumstances. There was no contact between patients. Six people died in the outbreak. The disease was severe, and the survivors required prolonged convalescence.

Other notable outbreaks of the disease in Great Britain include one in the Stafford District General Hospital in 1985, in which there were 101 cases and 28 deaths, and also an outbreak in 1988 in the British Broadcasting Corporation (BBC) building in London, which resulted in 79 cases and two deaths.

In Great Britain, the greater proportion of cases of legionnaires' disease is associated with travel abroad. The number of hospital-acquired infections has been declining in recent years.

Since 1979, there have been 2,800 cases of legionnaires' disease reported in residents of England and Wales to the Public Health Laboratory Service (PHLS). Of these, 46 per cent were associated with travel, 8 per cent were acquired within hospitals, and the remainder were assumed to be community-acquired. Table 8:1 overleaf shows the number of cases of legionnaires' disease reported in England and Wales between 1985 and 1995.

In 1995, 160 cases of legionnaires' disease were reported, 13 per cent of which were fatal. Ninety (56 per cent) of these were associated with travel, four were acquired in hospital, and 66 were community-acquired. One hundred and twenty-three of these cases were sporadic occurences. There were three community outbreaks, and one that occurred on an industrial site.

	Table 2: Cases of Legionnaires' Disease in England and Wales 1985–95	
	Total confirmed cases	*Associated with travel abroad*
1985	210	56
1986	189	89
1987	209	109
1988	278	82
1989	240	91
1990	188	91
1991	112	52
1992	146	64
1993	129	60
1994	158	77
1995	159	86

Prevention

Legionellosis is acquired from environmental water sources by the inhalation of water droplets. At first all the cases were attributed to exposure of the drift escaping from cooling towers of recirculating cooling systems. Now it is known that domestic and industrial piped water can be the source. As *Legionellae* are ubiquitous in natural waters, there are three aspects to consider in reducing the risk of legionellosis:

- measures to minimize colonization, growth and release of *Legionellae* into the atmosphere;
- physical or chemical treatment of water to kill the bacteria;
- the protection of maintenance personnel who work on contaminated water systems.

Stringent cleaning and hygiene regimes for cooling towers and large-scale air-conditioning systems have been implemented all over the world in the wake of the Philadelphia outbreak.

In Britain, statutory requirements for dealing with the risk of legionnaires' disease were set out in an Approved Code of Practice, *The Prevention or Control of Legionellosis (including Legionnaires'*

Disease) in 1991. This code applies wherever water is stored or used in a way that may create 'a reasonable foreseeable risk of legionellosis'. Examples include:

- recirculating water systems incorporating a cooling tower or evaporative condenser;
- hot-water systems with a volume greater that 300 litres;
- hot and cold water systems of any size, serving a particularly susceptible population;
- water systems that create a spray and are likely to exceed a water temperature of 20°C;
- whirlpool baths.

It is recommended that, in any building or environment, systems that could be colonized by *Legionellae* must be identified and their potential risks assessed. A scheme for prevention and control can then be prepared. It is essential to avoid holding water at temperatures between 20 and 40°C, which is the range in which *Legionella* multiplication occurs. Other general precautions include:

- prevention of water stagnation;
- avoidance of plumbing and engineering materials that can provide nutrients for bacterial growth;
- preventing the concentration of sediments in the water by cleaning and good maintenance;
- the use of chemical or other water treatment, where appropriate and safe, to prevent bacterial growth;
- reduction or prevention of aerosol dispersion.

The implementation of the control scheme and maintenance programme must be monitored and records kept of all procedures, treatments and test results.

In November 1992, the Health and Safety Executive in Great Britain introduced regulations requiring wet cooling towers to be registered with local authorities with the intention of improving the standard of maintenance of cooling towers and facilitating the investigation of outbreaks.

The use of biocides and hyperchlorination is not recommended in the disinfection of cooling towers as they have been ineffective in eradicating *L. pneumophila* from cooling towers and they have been only marginally effective in reducing the number of organisms. Likewise, the treatment of water distribution systems with high levels of chlorine is no longer recommended. This treatment has proved not to be effective because chlorine decomposes at the higher temperatures found in hot-water systems and *Legionella* is relatively chlorine-tolerant. The other major disadvantages of hyperchlorination include the expense of this treatment, the corrosion of the plumbing system and the production of carcinogenic byproducts.

The second report of the committee of inquiry into the outbreak of legionnaires' disease in Stafford in April 1985 recommended dry cooling equipment for air-conditioning plants. There are a number of disadvantages to this type of cooling equipment, however, including its inability to cool sufficiently in hot weather. Recent improvements in wet cooling system designs have made them easier to clean. In addition, drift eliminators have been improved to reduce the number of droplets released into the atmosphere. The number of bacteria released has consequently fallen.

Routine environmental culturing for *Legionella* should be performed in hospitals in which organ and bone marrow transplants are performed, given the high risk of disease in these patients. The disease is not contagious from person to person so isolation of patients is not necessary.

9

Botulism

Botulism is an uncommon illness caused by the bacteria *Clostridium botulinum* (*C. botulinum*). Although botulism is not very common, it is important as the bacteria produce a very potent toxin that affects the nervous system, leading to difficulties in swallowing, talking, breathing, double vision and paralysis, in addition to vomiting and diarrhoea. Recovery from the illness takes several months, but it is often fatal if not treated immediately and properly.

Types of Botulism

C. botulinum is an anaerobic bacillus which can produce spores that are heat resistant and can survive in foods that are minimally or incorrectly processed.

There are seven types of botulism (A, B, C, D, E, F and G). The different types are recognized by the toxins produced by each strain. Strains A, B, E and, rarely, F cause botulism in humans. Type A and B toxins are highly poisonous proteins that are resistant to digestion by enzymes of the intestine. Strains C and D are responsible for most cases of botulism in animals. The animals most commonly affected are wild fowl, poultry, cattle, horses and some species of fish. Strain G botulism has been isolated from soil in Argentina, but there have been no outbreaks identified involving this type.

There are four distinct forms of botulism: food-borne botulism, infant botulism, wound botulism, and a fourth type whose classification has not been determined.

Food-borne botulism is the name of the disease caused by the consumption of foods containing the neurotoxin produced by *C. botulinum*.

Infant botulism typically affects infants under 12 months and was first identified in the USA in 1976. This form of botulism occurs when spores of *C. botulinum* colonize the infant's gut. The spores then start to produce the toxin within the infant's intestinal tract. To date, honey has been the only confirmed source of the bacterial spore linked to infant botulism. Other potential environmental sources of the botulinum spore are cistern water, dust and other foods. The number of confirmed infant botulism cases has increased significantly as a result of greater awareness by health workers of this form of botulism. Cases have now been identified in the United Kingdom as well as in Australia, Asia and South America.

Wound botulism is the rarest form and occurs when *C. botulinum*, by itself or with other microorganisms, infects a wound and produces toxins. These toxins then travel via the bloodstream to other parts of the body. Foods are not involved in this type of botulism.

The fourth and undetermined category of botulism involves adult cases in which a specific food or wound source cannot be identified. In some cases this form of botulism appears similar to that of infant botulism and may result from the intestinal colonization of adults with the subsequent production of the toxin within the gut. In many of these cases, the patients had previously undergone surgical alterations of the gastrointestinal tract and/or had a course of antibiotic therapy. It may be that these procedures altered the normal gut flora, allowing *C. botulinum* to colonize the intestinal tract.

C. botulinum spores are highly heat-resistant. They may survive several hours at 100°C, but exposure to moist heat at 120°C for 30 minutes will kill the spores. Toxins, on the other hand, are readily destroyed by heat, and cooking food at 80°C will destroy the toxin. Toxin production, especially Type E, can occur at temperatures as low as 3°C and does not require strict anaerobic conditions.

Source of infection

In adverse conditions *C. botulinum* can form spores that protect them from high temperatures, drying and disinfection. Spores are the resting phase of the bacteria; they do not reproduce in this phase and can exist in the environment for many years. When favourable conditions return, the spore releases the bacterium and it can start to grow and multiply.

C. botulinum and its spores are widely distributed in nature. They are ubiquitous in soil worldwide, occurring in both cultivated and forest soils, and bottom sediments of streams, lakes and coastal waters. They are also found in the intestinal tracts of fish and mammals, and in the gills and viscera of crabs and other shellfish. The spores of *C. botulinum* are frequently recovered from agricultural products, including honey.

The types of food involved in botulism vary according to food preservation and eating habits in different regions. Any food that is not very acidic (pH above 4.6) can support the growth of this bacteria and the subsequent production of the toxin. If the food process allows spore survival and this food is then not heated before consumption, botulism can result.

The usual vehicles of infection are vegetables of low acidity, mostly home-canned and home-preserved food. This is particularly so in the USA, where home canning is more common. Other vehicles of infection include highly preserved or semi-preserved fish, vacuum-packed, dried or smoked sausages, smoked meat, home-made raw ham, patés, salted fish and a wide variety of other insufficiently heated or pickled food, such as olives and peppers. Newer varieties of certain garden foods, such as tomatoes, formerly thought too acidic to support the growth of *C. botulinum*, may no longer be considered safe for home canning. In many outbreaks the food vehicle is not known.

The botulin toxin is extremely potent, and only a very small amount is required to cause illness. The minimum lethal dose is estimated to be just a few nanograms (that is, a few thousand millionths of a gram).

Symptoms

Food-borne botulism

The onset of symptoms is abrupt in this form of botulism. Symptoms usually begin to develop 18 to 36 hours after the consumption of the food containing the toxin. However, cases have indicated incubation periods ranging from four hours to eight days. Generally, the shorter the incubation period the more severe the disease and the higher the fatality rate. The most common initial symptoms and signs include a dry mouth, double vision, general weakness and diminished or total loss of pupillary light reflex. Nausea, vomiting, abdominal cramps and diarrhoea then follow. Speaking and swallowing become progressively more difficult. Muscles of the extremities and trunk and those involved in respiration become progressively weaker. There are no sensory disturbances, and the victim remains alert until shortly before death. Fever is usually absent unless a complicating infection occurs. Constipation is frequent after neurologic impairment appears. Major complications that can appear include respiratory failure, as a result of paralysis of the diaphragm, and pulmonary infections.

Wound botulism

Wound botulism shows the same symptoms of impairment of the nervous system as in food-borne botulism but there are no symptoms of the intestinal tract, such as diarrhoea and vomiting, nor is there any evidence implicating food as a cause. Patients exhibiting wound botulism often have a history of a traumatic injury or deep puncture wound in the preceding two weeks before the onset of symptoms.

Infant botulism

Infant botulism is seen most often in infants of two to three months. Clinical symptoms typically begin with constipation, which occurs in two-thirds of cases. This is followed by neuromuscular paralysis, which begins with the cranial nerves and proceeds to the peripheral and respiratory musculature. This is followed by poor feeding, listlessness, weakness, pooled oral secretions, and wail or altered cry. There is a striking loss of head control. In some cases there are severe respiratory difficulties and arrest.

Infant botulism can show a wide spectrum of clinical severity, ranging from mild illness with a gradual onset to sudden infant death. It is estimated that this form of botulism may cause 5 per cent of cases of sudden infant death syndrome in the USA.

Affected infants have characteristically been normal before the onset of illness and have usually been breast-fed. However, they have generally been exposed to foods other than milk and spores are common in the environment.

Diagnosis

Food-borne botulism

The pattern of neuromuscular disturbances (described above), together with the recent consumption of a likely food source, provides an important clue in the diagnosis of this form of botulism. The simultaneous occurrence of two or more cases after eating the same food simplifies the diagnosis. Confirmation of the diagnosis can be demonstrated by isolating botulinal toxin in the blood serum or faeces of the patient or by discovering the organism itself. Identification of the organisms in the suspected food source is helpful, but as spores are ubiquitous in nature, the identification of the toxin is more significant in confirming the source of infection. Pets may develop botulism from eating the same contaminated food.

Wound botulism

Finding the toxin in blood serum or isolating the *C. botulinum* organism on anaerobic culture of the infection site confirms the diagnosis.

Infant botulism

Finding *C. botulinum* toxin or organisms in the faeces establishes the diagnosis.

Treatment

Treatment of botulism involves the administration of an antitoxin and intensive care, including support with breathing. If correct care is given promptly and effectively then fatalities can be reduced.

To eliminate any toxin remaining in the gastrointestinal tract, the induction of vomiting, gastric lavage and enemas are recommended. It is recommended that botulinal antitoxin is given as soon as possible in cases of food-borne botulism. Antitoxins can be prepared for active immunization of people at particular risk, for example, those working with C botulism or its toxins.

Paralysis associated with food-borne botulism progresses symmetrically down the body, usually starting with the eyes and face then moving to the throat, chest and extremities. When the diaphragm and chest muscles become involved, respiration is inhibited. This difficulty with breathing and possible complications present the greatest threat to life from botulism, and ultimately death from asphyxia can result. The progressive nature of the paralysis prevents patients from showing visible signs of respiratory distress while their vital capacity decreases. Respiratory impairment requires management in an intensive care unit where vital signs can be monitored and help with breathing, such as tracheostomy, intubation or mechanical ventilation, is available. Intravenous nutrition may also be required. Improvements in such care have reduced mortality to less than 10 per cent of cases. However, the illness may persist for up to six months and recovery may be slow.

Use of antitoxins

A trivalent antitoxin for use against botulism A, B, E and another polyvalent antitoxin for specific outbreaks caused by C, D or F are also available. Antitoxin will not release toxin that is already bound, so pre-existing neurological damage will not be reversed. At best it will slow or halt further progress of the disease. Antitoxin should be given as soon as possible after botulism has been diagnosed. It is unlikely to be of benefit if given more than 72 hours after the onset of symptoms. Since these preparations are derived from horse serum antitoxins, there is a risk of serum sickness or anaphylaxis. Thus the risks of administering the antitoxin must be weighed up against the benefits. The use of antitoxin in infant botulism has not been adequately studied and at present is not generally recommended.

Antibiotics do not improve the course of the disease and some may worsen it. They should be used only to treat secondary infections that may occur.

Prevention

Proper home and commercial canning and adequate heating of home-canned food before serving are essential. Canned foods showing any evidence of spoilage should be discarded. Infants under 12 months old should not be fed honey. Anyone known or thought to have been exposed to contaminated food must be carefully observed.

Outbreaks of *C. botulinum*

Outbreaks occur when food products are prepared or preserved by methods that do not destroy spores and permit toxin formation. Cases rarely result from contaminated commercially processed products. However, with these products there is potential for a correspondingly greater impact where ingredients from several suppliers are blended and foods are widely distributed. Outbreaks have occurred from contamination from cans that were damaged after processing. In the USA, two separate outbreaks of botulism involving commercially canned salmon have occurred in the last ten years.

Restaurant foods such as sautéed onions, chopped bottled garlic, potato salad made from baked potatoes and baked potatoes themselves have been responsible for a number of outbreaks. Also, smoked fish, both hot- and cold-smoked (for example, Kapchunka), have caused outbreaks of type E botulism.

An outbreak of botulism involving Kapchunka, an un-eviscerated, dry-salted, air-dried whole whitefish, occurred in the USA in 1987. Several cases resulting from the same source were also confirmed in Israel. Eight cases of type E botulism were reported, two in New York City and six in Israel. All eight patients had consumed Kapchunka. The product was made in New York City and some of it was transported by individuals to Israel. All eight patients with botulism developed symptoms within 36 hours of consuming the fish. One woman died, two patients required breathing assistance, three were treated therapeutically with antitoxin and three recovered spontaneously. The Kapchunka involved in this outbreak contained high levels of type E botulinal toxin despite salt levels that exceeded those sufficient to inhibit *C. botulinum* type E outgrowth. One possible explanation was that the fish contained low salt levels when air-dried at room temperature, became toxic and then were re-brined. As a result of this outbreak, regulations were brought in to prohibit the processing, distribution and sale of Kapchunka and Kapchunka-type products in the United States.

Most recently, a bottled chopped garlic-in-oil mix was responsible for three cases of botulism in Kingston, New York. Two men and a woman were hospitalized with botulism after consuming a mix that had been used in a spread for garlic bread. The bottled chopped garlic relied on refrigeration for safety and did not contain any additional antibotulinal additives or barriers. The Food and Drug Administration (FDA) ordered companies to stop making the product and to withdraw from the market any garlic-in-oil mix that did not include microbial inhibitors or acidifying agents and did not require refrigeration for safety.

Botulism is rare in the United Kingdom, there having been nine outbreaks between 1922 and 1989 involving a total of 46 persons. Some outbreaks have involved only single contaminated items, such as in the Loch Maree episode in 1922 when eight people died after eating duck paste, the 1978 outbreak in Birmingham involving four people who ate tinned salmon, and one case in 1989 following a meal on a commercial airliner.

The largest recorded outbreak of food-borne botulism in the United Kingdom occurred in 1989. There were 27 cases of botulism and one death. The outbreak was associated with contaminated hazelnut purée added to commercially produced yoghurt. Most of the potentially contaminated cartons could not be accounted for, suggesting variability in attack rate or the failure to diagnose mild symptoms.

10

Listeriosis

Listeria, or more correctly listeriosis, is the name given to the general group of disorders caused by the bacterium *Listeria monocytogenes* (*L. monocytogenes*). The bacteria are found widely in the environment throughout the world and can cause disease in humans and in many domestic and wild animals.

The manifestation of the disease varies according to its development, the site of infection and the age of the patient. Two other strains of the family Listeriaceae, *L. ivanovii* and *L. seligeri*, may also cause infection in humans, but these are rare. Cases of illness attributed to *L. monocytogenes* are relatively rare, but these organisms have attracted a lot of attention, partly because the illness can be serious or even fatal but also because they are one of the few pathogenic bacteria that can grow at refrigeration temperatures.

Source of infection

L. monocytogenes is distributed widely in the environment throughout the world. It has been found in at least 37 species of mammals, both domestic and feral, as well as in 17 species of birds. There is also some evidence that the organism is found in some fish and shellfish.

The organism has been isolated from the faeces of apparently healthy animals and people. Some studies suggest that 1 to 10 per cent of humans may be intestinal carriers of *L. monocytogenes*. In addition, the bacteria have been isolated from soil, silage and other environmental sources. Seasonal use of silage as animal fodder is frequently followed by an increase in the incidence of cases of listeriosis in animals. Considerable numbers of the organism have been found in sewerage sludge. Listeria have been found to survive longer than salmonella on land sprayed with sludge.

L. monocytogenes is quite resilient and can resist the deleterious effects of freezing, drying and heat remarkably well for a bacterium that does not form spores. It is known to have survived for two years in soil and 10 to 12 years in silage.

The main reservoir of the bacteria for human infections is not clear. There is circumstantial evidence that suggests that the contamination of food materials and food production areas probably derives from environmental sources. Animal disease is probably a less important pathway for infection to humans than that of food. However, the reported variable incubation period of one to 90 days makes it difficult to associate outbreaks of listeriosis with a specific food source or to link together sporadic cases of the disease.

How are people infected?

Listeriosis is primarily a food-borne disease in humans, but it may also be acquired by hospital patients and also by individuals directly exposed to infected material during the course of their work. Food-borne listeriosis *L. monocytogenes* has been associated with foods such as raw milk, supposedly pasteurized fluid milk, cheese (particularly soft ripened varieties such as Brie and Camembert), ice cream, raw vegetables, paté, salami, continental sausages, raw and cooked poultry, all types of raw meats, and raw and smoked fish. Pre-packed salads in dressings such as coleslaw and cooked chilled meals have frequently been found to be contaminated with listeria.

An outbreak in 1981 in Nova Scotia provided the first reported evidence for the transmission of listeriosis by food. Forty-one cases (7 adult and 34 in pregnant women) resulted from the eating of coleslaw produced by one manufacturer. When unopened packages of coleslaw were examined, they were found to contain the same strain of *L. monocytogenes* implicated in the outbreak. It was established that cabbages incorporated without heat treatment into coleslaw had been obtained from fields that had been treated with manure from a flock of sheep known to have had cases of listeriosis.

The increase in availability and popularity of cook-chill meals is a potential source of increase of cases of listeria food poisoning. This organism's ability to grow at temperatures as low as 3°C permits multiplication in refrigerated foods. As recent research has shown that approximately 20 per cent of such meals are infected with *L. monocytogenes*, it is essential that care is taken when reheating these foods. (Cook-chill is a type of food production system in which food is prepared, cooked, rapidly cooled and kept for a limited period under chilled storage prior to reheating.)

Infection may also occur by direct contact from a mother with the disease to her child, either before or during birth while the child passes through the birth canal. As a result, the Department of Health advises pregnant women and others with reduced immunity not to eat foods that are liable to be contaminated with high levels of the *Listeria spp*. These include:

- all types of paté;
- soft ripened cheeses such as Brie, Camembert and blue-veined cheeses;
- cook-chill meals and ready-to-eat poultry, unless thoroughly reheated until piping hot before they are eaten.

In occupationally acquired listeriosis, papular lesions (blisters) on the hands and arms may occur from direct contact with infectious material. Veterinary surgeons are at risk while attending listerial abortions in livestock, as are butchers and abattoir workers who slaughter infected animals.

Hospital-acquired listeriosis

Both person-to-person and food-borne spread of the infection have been suspected in outbreaks in hospitals amongst adult patients with reduced immunity. Poor hand hygiene, close contact between infected infants and their mothers, contaminated equipment, such as rectal thermometers and resuscitation equipment, or substances, including mineral oil used to bathe newborn infants, have all been implicated in reports of listeriosis developing among newborn babies.

Outbreaks of listeriosis have also occurred in nurseries, and these have been attributed to contaminated equipment or materials. However, outbreaks resulting from this cause of infection are rare.

Who is affected?

The vast majority of people who eat food contaminated with *L. monocytogenes* will be unaffected or, at worst, may have a mild fever for a short time. Listeria is mainly a danger to people whose immune system is impaired (about two-thirds of cases) or to the very young, the very old and pregnant women. It is an important cause of neonatal septicaemia and meningitis. Listeria infection in pregnant women may also cause the foetus to be aborted.

The 'at risk' groups are therefore:

- pregnant women;
- people whose illness or treatment affects their immune system, for example, those on corticosteroids or anti-cancer drugs, or transplant patients undergoing graft suppression therapy, or patients with Aids;
- cancer patients, particularly those with leukaemia;
- patients with diabetes, asthma, liver conditions and ulcerative colitis;
- the elderly;
- neonates;
- others – some reports suggest that normal, healthy people are at risk. A listeriosis outbreak in Switzerland involving cheese suggested that healthy uncompromised individuals could develop the disease, particularly if the foodstuff was heavily contaminated.

Clinical features

L. monocytogenes can cause a wide range of clinical conditions, ranging from a carrier of the infection with no outward signs of disease or a mild influenza-like illness to a fatal septicaemia. The normal host who acquires the infection may exhibit only an acute mild illness with fever; in some cases influenza-like symptoms will also be apparent. This mild form of the illness may be especially dangerous in pregnant women if it is not identified because of the grave risks for the foetus.

Clinical conditions associated with listeriosis include:

Meningitis

Meningitis (*see* page 43) is the most common form of listeriosis in adults but occurs rarely in pregnant women. The onset of the disease may either be sudden, with fever, intense headache, nausea, vomiting and signs of meningeal irritation, or it may be more gradual, particularly in someone who has reduced resistance to disease (immunocompromised) or in an elderly person. Delirium and coma may appear early; occasionally there is collapse and shock. Granular lesions in the liver and other organs, localized internal and external abscesses, blisters on the skin and other skin lesions may also occur.

Endocarditis

Endocarditis (inflammation of the endocardium, heart valves and muscle) is a rare manifestation of listeriosis.

Typhoidal listeriosis

This is also a rare form and results in bacteraemia (the presence of bacteria in the blood) and high fever with no localizing symptoms and signs.

Listerial dermatitis

This may follow direct contact with infected, aborted tissues.

Maternofoetal listeriosis

This can occur at any time during pregnancy. The mother may develop a fever, with headache and muscle and back pain. The infection may be carried from the mother to the foetus across the placenta. This may cause the amniotic fluid to become infected and in turn lead to either spontaneous septic abortion or premature labour with the delivery of an infected foetus or baby.

Neonatal listeriosis

In pregnant women, listeriosis may manifest itself as intrauterine or cervical infections. In the foetus and newborn, clinical presentation depends on the timing and route of infections. Usually the mother has influenza-like symptoms before the onset of labour but in some cases may show no symptoms of infection. Infection may be apparent within hours or days of birth, or it may be delayed for up to several weeks. Infants who show an early onset of the disease are frequently of low birth weight, have associated obstetric complications and show evidence of sepsis with circulatory or respiratory problems, or both. Early onset usually results from intrauterine infection, while later onset is probably caused by infection from the mother's genital tract during birth, but there have been reports of the infection spreading in nurseries and labour suites. Those infants with delayed onset are usually full-term, previously well and presenting with meningitis or sepsis. In 10 to 50 per cent of cases neonatal listeriosis proves fatal. The fatality rate is higher the earlier the onset of the disease.

The onset of all the above disorders is usually preceded by influenza-like symptoms, including persistent fever. It was recently reported that gastrointestinal symptoms, such as nausea, vomiting and diarrhoea, may precede more serious forms of listeriosis or may be the only symptoms shown. The gastrointestinal symptoms are usually associated with use of antacids or cimetidine (a drug that blocks the action of histamine).

The onset time to serious forms of listeriosis is unknown but may range from a few days to three weeks. The onset time to gastrointestinal symptoms is also unknown but is probably greater than 12 hours.

The minimal dose of *L. monocytogenes* necessary to cause disease has not been quantified but is believed to vary with the particular strain and the susceptibility of the victim. From cases contracted through raw or supposedly pasteurized milk, it is safe to assume that in susceptible persons, fewer than a thousand organisms may cause disease. *L. monocytogenes* may invade the lining of the gastrointestinal tract.

Once the bacterium enters the host's white blood cells, the infection can spread throughout the body (septicaemia). Its presence within white blood cells permits access to the brain and also probable migration across the placenta to the foetus in pregnant women. The success of *L. monocytogenes* in causing disease centres on its ability to survive and multiply in the host's phagocytic cells (defensive cells that usually engulf bacteria and cell debris and remove them from the body).

Most healthy people infected with *L. monocytogenes* show no symptoms. The 'complications' as described above are the usual clinical expressions of the disease. When listeric meningitis occurs, as many as 70 per cent of cases may be fatal, in cases of septicaemia 50 per cent, and in prenatal/neonatal infections the death rate is greater than 80 per cent. In infections during pregnancy, the mother usually survives.

Treatment

For meningitis in adults, successful treatment with intravenous penicillin or ampicillin has been reported. Trimethoprim-sulfamethodazole (TMP-SMX) or erythromycin have been shown to be effective in patients allergic to penicillin. For endocarditis and typhoidal listeriosis, penicillin given intravenously and continued until four weeks after the fever has begun to subside is recommended. In cases of neonatal listeriosis, initial treatment with ampicillin and an aminoglycoside is preferred. After a clinical response has been observed, ampicillin alone may be given. A 14-day course is usually satisfactory, but the optimum duration of medication is unknown. Other adjuncts should also be given to the newborn with bacterial sepsis. Ampicillin together with an aminoglycoside can be given to newborn babies as a precaution if the infective organism is found in the meconium.

Prevention

Pregnant women and other 'at risk' groups should avoid food products that may be contaminated by *L. monocytogenes* (as already listed). In July 1989, the Chief Medical Officer for England issued a warning to pregnant women and other vulnerable people not to eat meat paté.

It is important to observe the storage instructions, the 'eat by date' on the packet and the heating instructions for cook-chill meals and ready-to-eat poultry, including plain roast chicken. Listeria does not form a spore, so thorough heating will ensure that the food is safe to eat. If a microwave oven is used, the food must be cooked uniformly for the required length of time on the stated power setting and in the correct position. Instructions for standing times must also be observed because the food continues to cook by conduction during this period.

Pregnant women who have previously given birth to infected infants should have cervical and stool cultures performed during the latter stages of pregnancy to ascertain whether they are a carrier for *L. monocytogenes*. If the mother is recognized as a carrier, preventative treatment can be given before delivery or during birth to block transmission of the infection to the newborn. However, the usefulness of these measures has not been established. Vets and farmers should take proper precautions when handling aborted foetuses and sick or dead animals, especially sheep that have died of encephalitis.

Despite antibiotic therapy, the mortality of septicaemia and meningoencephalitis (inflammation of the brain and the meninges) caused by *L. monocytogenes* remains high (20–50 per cent). Survivors may experience long-term ill-health and take a long time to recover completely. It is important, therefore, that efforts should continue to be focused, firstly, on the prevention of this infection by the improvement in the microbiological safety of methods of food production and preparation, and, secondly, by education, so that vulnerable people can avoid high-risk foods.

It is interesting to note that the warning in July 1989 by the Chief Medical Officer to pregnant women and other vulnerable groups not to eat paté was followed by a decline in the number of cases of listeriosis reported (*see* Table 3).

Recent outbreaks

In 1985, one outbreak in California was caused by Mexican-style cheese and led to numerous stillbirths. As a result of this episode, the Food and Drug Administration (FDA) in the USA has been monitoring domestic and imported cheeses and has taken numerous actions to remove these products from the market when *L. monocytogenes* is found.

Table 3: Number of Reported Cases of Listeria in England and Wales 1988–1995	
Year	*Number of Reported Cases*
1988	281
1989	244
1990	116
1991	127
1992	106
1993	102
1994	112
1995	91

11

Salmonella

Salmonella bacteria

A salmonella organism was first identified in 1885 by D.E. Salmon, an American veterinary pathologist. Later, many other types of the bacteria came to be recognized, and they were all classified as species of the genus *Salmonella*. It is now considered that these bacteria all belong to one species, *Salmonella enterica*, and that the rest (over 2,500) are strictly serotypes of the same organism. Each serotype of the bacteria produces characteristic, slightly differing sets of antigens (the foreign substances that provoke the production of defensive antibodies in the body) involved in causing the symptoms of illness. It is convenient to refer to salmonella by their old, specific names, for example, *S. enteritidis*, *S. typhi* (typhoid) and *S. paratyphi* (paratyphoid), according to the type of illness that they cause. Also, many scientists now classify salmonella into three groups:

1. Those that almost invariably occur only in humans, including *S. typhi* and *S. paratyphi*.
2. Those that primarily occur in specific host animals but can infect humans. Examples include *S. cholerae-suis* in pigs (the type that was identified first in 1885) and *S. dublin* in cattle.
3. Those that do not have a preference for any particular host. Bacteria in this group are usually the ones involved in salmonella food poisoning (85 per cent of all known cases in the USA).

Salmonella food poisoning

Salmonellosis or salmonella food poisoning is common throughout the world and is one of the most significant problems for public health. Outbreaks of salmonellosis can also have grave economic consequences, potentially causing a collapse in consumer confidence if a particular product is involved and probable closure of food-serving or manufacturing premises or hospital wards while decontamination procedures are carried out, and also loss of production and earnings along with legal action on the part of victims. These may cause the failure of businesses in some cases, but of far greater significance is the suffering of affected individuals. While it is generally true that most people recover completely from an attack of salmonella food poisoning, this is by no means invariably the case. Death can occur, especially in the elderly, in newborn babies or where complications (focal infections) arise (*see* below) or in those with certain medical conditions. In any outbreak, where a number of people are known to be affected, a fatal outcome for one or two of the victims cannot be ruled out and, to a certain extent, this depends upon the virulence of the strain of bacteria involved.

In Western countries, the incidence of diagnosed cases has steadily risen in recent years, particularly since 1985, and this has been traced to the increasing prevalence of *S. enteritidis*. In Britain and Europe, these bacteria have become a particular problem in poultry and can pass from hens to eggs. The public acknowledgement of this by one particular government minister caused a political storm and a consumer crisis with regard to eggs, with the sort of far-reaching economic consequences described above.

It remains a fact that of the 2,250 known salmonella serotypes that can potentially cause food poisoning, *S. enteritidis* and *S. typhimurium* are responsible for over 75 per cent of diagnosed cases in Britain and elsewhere. It is believed that many cases are not identified, but for those diagnosed, salmonellosis occurs at a rate of 50 to 70 people in every 100,000 each year. In Britain outbreaks are more likely to occur in the late summer or early autumn.

Sources of infection

The primary sources of infection are the gastrointestinal tract and faeces of a wide variety of animals, including human beings. Of particular importance in Britain are poultry and cattle, but also pigs and, of lesser significance, domestic pets including terrapins and turtles, and wild birds and animals. In general, salmonella is less

likely to be passed to humans from live animals. It is far more likely
to occur when animal products have entered the human food chain.
Because of the ubiquitous nature of the organism, the potential for
contamination of raw meat and animal products with salmonella is
very great. The bacteria are destroyed by thorough cooking, and
usually it is only if large numbers are ingested that there is a risk
of food poisoning. Unfortunately, it is easy for salmonella to be inadvertently passed from a raw product to a cooked one, where it can
multiply to a disease-causing level on food before it is eaten. This
not only occurs quite easily in a home kitchen but also in commercial premises and food-manufacturing plants. In such premises, some
outbreaks of salmonellosis have been traced to contamination of a
product after it has been through the treatment process, and
equipment can easily harbour the organism.

In other cases, there may have been a failure to reach a sufficiently high temperature to destroy the bacteria during a
heat-treatment process. In general, the foods considered to be most
likely to be contaminated are poultry, eggs (both hen and duck) and
raw meat. However, salmonella can easily be transferred to many
other foods. Also, high-fat foods such as cheese, chocolate and salami
pose a particular risk as it has been shown that far fewer organisms
than normal (about 50) are sufficient to cause illness.

Once an infection has begun, it is possible for it to spread from
one person to another by faecal contamination of food. In western
countries with high standards of hygiene and sanitation, this is less
likely to occur. However, it can be a problem in hospital children's
wards, maternity units, old people's homes and institutions caring
for those who are mentally impaired. Unfortunately, some of these
people are also in vulnerable, higher risk groups with regard to
salmonella infection. Recurrent or persistent outbreaks can sometimes occur in an institutional setting by the human faecal-oral route.
One complicating factor is that some people can be infected with
salmonella without showing any signs of illness. These people nevertheless excrete the bacteria in faeces, as do those who become ill,
for about two to four months.

Symptoms

The incubation period is usually about 12 to 48 hours but may be shorter or longer depending on the number of bacteria ingested. Symptoms arise suddenly and vary in severity, but usually begin with nausea, malaise, abdominal cramps, watery diarrhoea and headache. Vomiting may occur but is usually not persistent. In those who are mildly affected, symptoms subside in two or three days and the person gradually recovers. It may take some time to regain an appetite and to feel back to normal.

Complications and focal infections

In some people, more severe symptoms arise that can result in life-threatening illness. The diarrhoea may contain blood or become green and foul-smelling, resembling cholera and indicative of inflammatory colitis. Pains, fever and shivering are common and, in severe cases, may resemble enteric fever (which is typical of typhoid and paratyphoid). These complications can rapidly lead to the development of dehydration and even uraemia, indicative of kidney failure. Death may occur, particularly in elderly or very young patients.

Following salmonella food poisoning and apparent recovery, a systemic focal infection can arise almost anywhere in the body. This may or may not be associated with bacteraemia (bacteria in the blood) and is more likely to occur in some vulnerable patients (see paragraph below). Infections include acute appendicitis and colitis, septic arthritis, osteomyelitis and meningitis. Abscesses may occur in the gastrointestinal tract, soft tissues, lungs, liver, gall bladder, spleen, uterus, heart valves and other membranes, especially with *S. typhimurium* and *S. cholerae-suis*. Occasionally, already existing solid tumours may develop abscesses, and these conditions may prove to be life-threatening.

Those most at risk

Apart from the elderly and the very young, certain medical conditions make individuals more vulnerable to salmonella infections and complications. These include those who have had partial gastrectomy (removal of the stomach) or splenectomy (spleen), those with sickle-cell anaemia and people who produce little or no hydrochloric acid in gastric juice, a condition known as achlorhydria. Also any other factor that lessens stomach acidity, such as taking antacids and some treatments for gastric ulcer. Patients with a suppressed immune system, as in leukaemia, lymphoma, Aids or HIV, are vulnerable, as are those with cirrhosis of the liver. Certain tropical illnesses such as malaria, bartonellosis (sandfly fever) and relapsing fever (transmitted by lice and ticks) increase susceptibility to salmonella infections. Persistent or focal salmonella infections are quite common in those with Aids or HIV and may indicate hitherto unsuspected illness.

Diagnosis

Salmonella food poisoning is a notifiable illness, although it is believed that many cases go unreported. Diagnosis is made by laboratory culture of samples of faeces to identify the bacteria and the serotype involved. In the case of an outbreak in which a particular food is suspected, this is normally submitted for laboratory testing. Outbreaks are generally identified in an institutional setting and usually further tests within the premises are necessary.

Treatment

Antibiotic treatment is not normally given to individual patients with mild disease as there is a considerable problem of resistance among the salmonella strains. Such treatment is not necessary as the patient recovers with rest, fluids and a light diet. Appropriate antibiotics are given to those with more severe symptoms or who are in a vulnerable group. They may also be given to people in an institution in order to control the spread of the infection. In the home, a high standard of personal hygiene must be maintained, and it is possible that the person may have to submit samples for testing. For those who are more severely ill or who develop complications, hospital treatment is required. Intravenous fluid and electrolyte replacement may be needed, and barrier nursing and isolation may be required. Careful laboratory monitoring of the antibiotics given and the analysis of samples is needed, possibly for several weeks. Antibiotics that may be used include ampicillin, amoxicillin and ciprofloxacin.

Public health measures

In the event of an outbreak in a public institution, various measures may be needed, including the exclusion from the workplace of any person who prepares food and who has symptoms of illness. It may be necessary to impose restrictions in infant schools, day-care centres, hospital wards, etc, until the infection is brought under control. It is not usually considered to be necessary to exclude well or asymptomatic people from school or work, but each case is considered individually. Antibiotic treatment may be recommended for people directly involved.

Preventative measures

In order to prevent salmonella food poisoning, action is needed in animal husbandry, abattoirs, food manufacturing and in the home. In animal husbandry, continued efforts should be made to exclude salmonella, for example, by heat treatment of feeds (which can harbour infection) and the testing of herds. In addition, the treatment of food animals with antibiotics, which encourages bacterial resistance and reduces the choice of effective drugs to treat human disease, should be limited. In abattoirs, high standards of hygiene are needed. Animals should be clean before slaughter and every effort must be made to avoid faecal contamination of raw meat. These measures are also highly relevant to the control of *E. coli*. The highest standards must be adhered to at all times in food-manufacturing plants. Irradiation of poultry carcasses before freezing or sale would be highly effective but is, at present, unpopular with the general public.

There is much that can be done by individuals to lessen the risk of salmonella infection. First, every person should endeavour to be well informed and to maintain high standards of hygiene in the home. Pets should be excluded from the kitchen and kept away from food. Food that is left out must always be covered. In the fridge, raw meat or poultry should be kept on the bottom shelf, well wrapped and completely separate from cooked foods. All food must be kept covered and eaten within its 'use by' date. The fridge must not be overloaded and should be cleaned regularly. Utensils and surfaces for the preparation of raw meat must be thoroughly washed and disinfected after use. Particular care should be taken with dish cloths, tea towels and chopping boards. It is safest to use separate chopping boards for raw and cooked foods. Hands must always be washed after handling raw meat or poultry. Hot, partly used foods should be covered and cooled as quickly as possible before being placed in the fridge when cold.

As indicated previously, poultry pose a particular risk with regard to salmonella, especially the incomplete thawing of frozen birds. It is necessary to thaw completely a frozen bird in a cool room, being especially careful if it is large (for example, the Christmas turkey), before cooking. Once thawed, the bird should be transferred to the fridge and cooked and eaten within 24 hours. Cooking must be thorough, right down to the bone, and the giblets should be removed before the bird is placed in the oven. Stuffing the bird hinders the cooking process. It is best to cook stuffing separately. All the above applies equally to the defrosting, preparation and cooking of meat.

Before the advent of pasteurization, milk was a common source of salmonella food poisoning, so no one should be tempted to drink

Table 4: Food Poisoning: Notifications 1982–1995	
Year	*England and Wales*
1982	14,253
1983	17,735
1984	20,702
1985	19,242
1986	23,948
1987	29,331
1988	39,713
1989	52,557
1990	52,145
1991	52,543
1992	63,347
1993	68,587
1994	81,833
1995	82,041*
* provisional	

this 'straight from the cow'. Other precautions include not repeatedly reheating meals. Reheating should always be thorough and eggs well cooked. It is best to avoid recipes containing raw egg. In general, one should be cautious about food and err on the side of safety. It is far better to throw out something suspect than to risk a bout of salmonella food poisoning.

Table 4 overleaf shows the incidence of food poisoning notifications for England and Wales for the 14 years up to 1995. It shows, unfortunately, an inexorable rise and a six-fold increase over the period.

12

Leptospirosis – Weil's Disease, Canicola Fever, Infectious Spirochaetal Jaundice

Spirochaetal jaundice

Leptospirosis is an all-embracing term for a number of acute infectious illnesses caused by spirochaete bacteria belonging to the genus *Leptospira*. *Leptospira* are characteristic, highly coiled spiral bacteria that naturally inhabit a wide variety of mammals, where they normally do not cause harm. If they are transmitted to humans, they cause a range of symptoms varying from a mild, 'flu-like illness to aseptic meningitis, high fever, liver and kidney damage and possibly death. It is believed that there are many undiagnosed cases of the milder forms of the illness each year. In the British Isles, two types of animal are implicated in passing the illness to people – rats (Weil's disease) and dogs (Canicola fever).

The bacteria are present in urine and are continually excreted over long periods of time by infected animals. They may gain access to a person directly via a cut or through the mucous membranes of the nose, eyes or mouth. Alternatively, infective urine may pass into standing water, and people can similarly acquire the organism from this, with some occupations (sewage and farm work) posing a greater risk. Veterinarians and abattoir workers may also be exposed to the infection, but leptospirosis is quite often acquired through recreational activities, particularly swimming in contaminated water.

Weil's disease is the most severe form of leptospirosis, and the bacteria are transmitted in rat urine. There are a number of cases of the infection each year in Britain, a few of which prove to be fatal.

The bacteria involved have been named *L. icterohaemorrhagiae* but are possibly, more correctly, serotypes of the organism *L. interrogans*. There are about 170 known serotypes (producing slightly varying antigens) which are responsible for the different degrees of illness.

Symptoms

The incubation period is normally between one to two weeks but has a broad range of two days to three weeks. Symptoms characteristically appear in two phases in all forms of leptospirosis, and the first of these is known as the leptospiremic phase. The illness arises suddenly, with headache, chills, fever, muscular aches and pain, and malaise. Round the third or fourth day, the eyes often become bloodshot and, in Weil's disease, the liver and kidneys become involved about three to six days into the illness. There is liver enlargement, jaundice, protein (proteinuria) blood (haematuria) and white blood cells (pyuria) in the urine along with capillary haemorrhages, especially in the skin and mucous membranes. The failure of the kidneys to filter waste products effectively frequently leads to azotaemia, in which there is a build-up of nitrogenous substances (urea) in the blood. Anaemia usually develops and also lapses in consciousness.

The second, or immune phase, of leptospirosis usually occurs about six to 12 days into the course of the illness. In most forms there has been a fluctuating fever, but in Weil's disease this is continuous. Meningitis may arise, and if symptoms have been overwhelming, death can occur. During the immune phase, antibodies to the organism begin to appear in the patient's blood. Normally there is no long-lasting liver damage following recovery.

Diagnosis and treatment

Diagnosis is made by examining samples of blood, urine or cerebrospinal fluid in order to detect the leptospires. The biphasic nature of the illness is characteristic of leptospirosis and helps to eliminate other possible causes of the symptoms. A person with Weil's disease requires treatment in hospital, with intensive courses of antibiotics along with supportive nursing care and intravenous replacement of

fluids and salts. Penicillin G or ampicillin may be given intravenously. Doxycycline or amoxicillin may be given by mouth in
less severe cases of illness. Doxycycline has been shown to be effective in preventing leptospirosis (among soldiers undergoing military
training in Panama).

Preventative measures

There were 72 cases of leptospirosis, of which 39 were Weil's
disease, in 1981 in the British Isles, resulting in seven deaths. It is
essential that those in the high-risk occupations noted previously
should be aware of the risk of Weil's disease and take necessary
precautions. These include wearing good protective clothing, rubber
boots and gloves when working in areas that might be contaminated
with rat urine. Cuts on the skin must additionally be well covered
with waterproof dressings. If any signs of influenza-like illness
develop, medical advice should be sought immediately as early
antibiotic treatment gives a better chance of a good recovery.
Members of the public should be aware of the possibility that pools
of standing water, particularly if they occur on farm land, might be
contaminated. Fortunately, Weil's disease is uncommon and sensible
precautions with regard to outdoor swimming and bathing help to
minimize the risk of infection.

13

Anthrax

Anthrax is an acute bacterial disease that usually affects the skin and in some rare cases affects the lungs or gastrointestinal tract. Anthrax is caused by the aerobic bacillus *Bacillus anthracis* (*B. anthracis*). It can form heat-resistant spores capable of surviving in the soil and animal products for decades. Anthrax is primarily a disease of herbivorous animals but all mammals may be susceptible to infection.

The word 'anthrax' derives from the Greek *anthrakos*, meaning 'coal' and refers to the characteristic sore, or 'eschar', with its coal-black centre. The earliest known description is found in the book of Genesis – the fifth plague, which appears to have been anthrax, was described as killing the Egyptians' cattle. Other descriptions involving both animals and humans have appeared in the early literature of the Hindus, Greeks and Romans.

In the seventeenth century, a pandemic referred to as 'the black bane' swept through Europe, causing many human and animal deaths. Later the disease in humans was described as 'the malignant pustule'.

Occurrence

Although anthrax is an important animal disease, it is now rare in humans, mainly occurring in countries without public health regulations that prevent industrial or agricultural exposure to infected animals. Anthrax is primarily a disease of herbivores; humans and carnivores are incidental hosts. It is an infrequent and sporadic human infection in most industrialized countries.

In the United Kingdom, anthrax is almost entirely an occupational disease, affecting workers handling infected animals and includes abattoir, agricultural and wildlife workers and veterinarians or those exposed to imported animal products. Goats, cattle, sheep and horses may all be infected with *B. anthracis*, as may products of these animals, such as carcasses, hides, hair (especially from goats), wool, bone and bone products such as bone meal.

Human anthrax is endemic in those agricultural regions of the world where anthrax in animals is common, including countries in South and Central America, southern and eastern Europe, Asia and Africa. In some parts of Africa and Asia, animals that have died of the disease are still skinned and eaten, the value of the carcass as meat far outweighing the perceived hazard of cutting it up and eating it. New areas of infection in livestock may develop through the introduction of animal feed containing contaminated bone meal. Environmental events such as floods may provoke epizootics (epidemics spread by animals).

Cases of anthrax are very rare in Britain, nine cases occurring in the ten years up to the beginning of the 1990s. One epidemic was recently reported in Switzerland. Within a period of less than three years, 25 workers in one textile factory contracted the disease. There were 24 cases of cutaneous anthrax and one case of inhalation anthrax. The infection was found to be imported in goat hair from Pakistan. The rarity of the illness in Europe contributed to a general lack of experience of the disease and therefore hindered the recognition of clinical symptoms. In addition, repeated attempts failed to identify the pathogenic agent conclusively.

Source of infection

Both domestic and wild animals, normally herbivores, shed the baccilli in terminal haemorrhages or spilt blood at death. The vegetative non-spore form of the bacillus is not a hardy organism. If an animal dies of anthrax and its body is left lying in summer heat at a temperature greater than about 25°C, anthrax bacilli may not be found in it after three to four days, having been overwhelmed by other microorganisms that break down the corpse. At lower temperatures, breakdown will take place more slowly, allowing the vegetative anthrax baccilli to persist for longer periods.

On exposure to the air, the bacilli can form spores, particularly at temperatures greater than 20°C and in high humidity. The spores of *B. anthracis* are very resistant to adverse environmental conditions, including extremes of heat, cold, desiccation and chemicals that would kill most other living things. These spores can remain viable in the soil long after the animal source of the infection has died. Dried or otherwise processed skins and hides of infected animals may harbour spores for years and are the way in which the disease may be spread worldwide.

How are people infected?

There are three forms of anthrax: the cutaneous (skin) form, the pulmonary or respiratory form and the gastrointestinal form.

Human infection with *B. anthracis* usually occurs either by direct contact of the skin with either contaminated material or, less commonly, with an animal dying of the disease. This contact may be with cattle, sheep, pigs, goats, horses or others. Infection by this route leads to the cutaneous form of the disease. *B. anthracis* is not an invasive organism and requires a break in the skin (a lesion) through which to establish infection. The head, forearms and hands are the most common sites of infection. It is also thought possible that infection may occur via insect bites. The insects feed on infected animals and then pass it on to their next victim. Contact with soil associated with infected animals is another possible source. Sometimes gardeners using unsterilized bone meal can become infected.

Pulmonary anthrax results from the inhalation of spores in industrial processes such as tanning of hides, or wool or bone processing, where aerosols of *B. anthracis* spores may be produced. This form of anthrax is also known as woolsorter's disease, reflecting its historic context. It is often fatal.

The gastrointestinal form of the disease usually follows consumption of undercooked and contaminated meat. There is no evidence that milk from infected animals transmits anthrax.

Anthrax spreads among grazing animals through contaminated soil and feed, and among omnivorous and carnivorous animals via contaminated meat, bone meal or other foodstuffs. Vultures have been reported to spread the organism from one area to another. Accidental infections may occur among laboratory workers.

In 1979, an outbreak of largely pulmonary anthrax occurred in Yekaterinburg (formerly Sverdlovsk) in Russia. On this occasion 66 individuals were documented as having died of anthrax and 11 infected persons are known to have survived. Many other cases are presumed to have occurred. Investigations disclosed that the cases occurred as the result of a plume emanating from a biological research institute and led to the conclusion that the outbreak had resulted from an accidental aerosol generated in work related to biological warfare.

Symptoms

The incubation period varies from 12 hours to five days but generally symptoms appear between three to five days after infection.

In the cutaneous form of anthrax, itching of the exposed skin surface occurs first. A skin lesion then develops, usually about two to four days after local infection. The lesion becomes papular, that is, pimple-like. The red-brown papule enlarges and there is considerable inflammation around the lesion, which becomes vesicular (blistered) over a period of several days. Sometimes secondary, smaller vesicles may also appear. After rupture of the vesicle, a deep-seated ulcer appears, with extensive swelling of the surrounding skin. Pain is unusual and, if present, is the result of swelling or secondary infection. The ulcer then becomes covered with a thick, dark, leathery scab – the characteristic eschar. At one time this was referred to as 'malignant pustule', although it was neither malignant nor pustular. Pus is only present if there is a secondary infection; alternatively, the presence of pus may indicate that the cause is not anthrax. Most anthrax sores are about 2 to 3 cm across, but some may be up to 6 to 7 cm in diameter or occasionally even larger.

The lymph nodes in the area surrounding the sore become enlarged and may be tender. Occasionally there is general malaise, joint pain, headache, fever, nausea and vomiting. Often the body temperature rises to 38.3° to 38.8°C and in some severe cases may reach 40°C. If the ulcer is left untreated, the infection can spread to the bloodstream, leading to septicaemia. This can be fatal in 5 to 20 per cent of cases. With effective treatment, however, the number of deaths can be reduced. In cases coming late to treatment and in the rare one that is overwhelming from the onset, there may be circulatory collapse and bleeding. In some cases the meninges – the membranes surrounding the brain – may also be involved.

Pulmonary anthrax follows rapid multiplication of spores in the mediastinal lymph nodes, that is, the lymph nodes in the area between the lungs. Severe haemorrhagic necrotizing lymphadenitis (inflammation of the lymph nodes with escape of blood) develops and spreads to the adjacent organs, which may include the heart, the aorta, the trachea and the thymus gland.

Pulmonary anthrax begins insidiously, with no symptoms or with mild nonspecific symptoms of slight fever and malaise which resemble influenza. Within a few days fever increases, severe respiratory distress develops, followed by cyanosis, shock and coma. As the temperature soars, the pulse becomes rapid and feeble. Lung X-rays may show diffuse patches of infection and the mediastinum is widened because of enlarged haemorrhagic lymph nodes. The chest is described as full of 'moist sounds'. There is nothing specific to point to a diagnosis of anthrax except, perhaps, the patient's occupation. Without early specific and generalized supportive treatment, a fatal outcome can ensue within two to three days.

Gastrointestinal anthrax is now very rare. This form is analogous to the cutaneous form, with the anthrax sore developing on the lining of the intestinal tract instead of on the skin. It occurs most often in the large intestine, in the ileum or caecum, but the duodenum and stomach are also sometimes affected in the same way. Gastrointestinal anthrax follows the ingestion of contaminated meat. Usually a break occurs in the pharyngeal or intestinal mucosa, allowing the invasion of the intestinal wall. Symptoms of mild to severe gastroenteritis may occur but not in all cases. As with pulmonary anthrax, the sudden onset of acute illness follows the benign incubation period of two to three days, with fever, shock, collapse and death occurring within a few hours.

Diagnosis

The occupational history is obviously an important factor in arriving at a diagnosis for anthrax. The organism may be observed with the aid of a microscope in sample material obtained from the undersurface of the eschar in the cutaneous form and from throat swabs and sputum in the pulmonary form.

Treatment

A human anthrax vaccine is available for those at high risk, for example, vets, laboratory technicians, employees of textile mills processing imported goat hair.

The cutaneous form can be treated with procaine penicillin given intramuscularly for seven days. This will prevent the systemic spread of the disease and induce the gradual resolution of the sore, which will become sterile within 24 to 48 hours. In severely toxic or late cases, the first doses may be given intravenously. Tetracycline, gentamicin and erythromycin are also effective in the treatment of cutaneous anthrax.

Although antibiotics have a rapid effect on *B. anthracis*, the eschar takes a long time, sometimes several weeks, to pass through its cycle of development and to heal. The scar should not be removed prematurely as this may lead to permanent scarring. There are no live anthrax bacilli in the lesion after a course of treatment with antibiotics and therefore there is no need to keep the patient in hospital until the scab separates. A patient is usually left with a pale scar after the lesion has resolved. Very occasionally surgical repair is required.

For pulmonary and gastrointestinal anthrax, early and continuous intravenous therapy with penicillin may be lifesaving. It has been used in combination with streptomycin given intramuscularly. In addition to antibiotics, the patient also needs intensive care. In the late stages of infection, even if treatment overcomes the bacteraemia, toxin-induced shock may still lead to death.

Prevention

In highly developed countries, anthrax is a very uncommon disease. Well-supervised disposal of carcasses from the occasional cases of anthrax that occur in cattle, sheep, etc, and of materials contaminated by these carcasses is essential in containing the disease. The disinfection of affected premises, together with immediate vaccination of other members of an affected herd, can also help to ensure the containment and control of the disease. In Britain, when a case of anthrax occurs in a herd, all the animals are kept under close observation and antibiotics are administered at the first sign of fever.

This is not possible in less developed countries where animals may roam over vast tracks of land and the veterinary services are severely limited.

The following preventative measures are recommended to control and contain the disease:

1. Vaccination of workers in conditions where they are exposed to the risk of infection. This is effective in preventing cutaneous and probably pulmonary anthrax. It is recommended for laboratory workers routinely working with *B. anthracis* and those handling potentially contaminated industrial raw materials. Annual booster injections are recommended if exposure continues.
2. Workers who handle potentially infected material should be trained in personal cleanliness and treatment of minor injuries and educated about the ways in which anthrax is transmitted.
3. In industries that handle raw animal materials, dust should be properly controlled and adequate ventilation should be maintained. There should be continuing medical supervision of employees with prompt investigation of all suspicious skin lesions. Protective clothing and adequate facilities for washing and changing clothes after work are essential. Eating facilities should be located away from places of work.
4. Thoroughly washing, disinfecting or sterilizing hair, wool and bone meal or other feed of animal origin is recommended prior to processing.
5. Hides of animals exposed to anthrax should not be sold nor their carcasses used as food or feed supplements (for example, as bone or blood meal).
6. Early diagnosis of affected animals or people and treatment with appropriate antibiotics is essential, as is the rapid identification of outbreaks.
7. Anthrax spores may survive in the soil for decades, so burial of the carcasses is not recommended. The preferable disposal technique is to incinerate the carcasses at the site of death, if possible, or have them removed to a rendering plant, taking care to ensure that there is no contamination en route. Should these methods not be possible, the carcasses, together with any contaminated material, should be deeply buried in quicklime at the site of

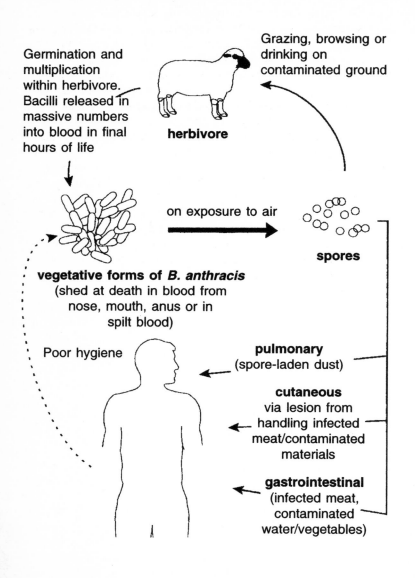

Grazing, browsing or drinking on contaminated ground

Germination and multiplication within herbivore. Bacilli released in massive numbers into blood in final hours of life

herbivore

on exposure to air

spores

vegetative forms of *B. anthracis*
(shed at death in blood from nose, mouth, anus or in spilt blood)

Poor hygiene

pulmonary
(spore-laden dust)

cutaneous
via lesion from handling infected meat/contaminated materials

gastrointestinal
(infected meat, contaminated water/vegetables)

Cycle of infection in anthrax

death, if possible. Any equipment used should be sterilized. The carcasses should not be burned on open fields. Any soil that may have been infected by the carcasses should be treated with anhydrous calcium oxide (quicklime).

8. The effluents and trade wastes of rendering plants handling potentially infected animals should be controlled. Likewise, the wastes from factories that manufacture products from hair, wool, bones or hides that may be infected.

9. All animals at risk should be promptly immunized and the immunization repeated annually. Animals displaying symptoms should be treated with penicillin or tetracyclines and then immunized after the cessation of therapy. These animals should not be used as a food source for several months.

Primary contacts (those in contact with the original animal source) should have daily medical surveillance for one week. Contacts of human cases do not require such medical surveillance. Close cooperation between health and local authorities together with the veterinary services is necessary when cases or outbreaks occur.

14

Rabies

Rabies is an acute infection caused by a virus. It is usually transmitted via the bite of a rabid animal. The illness that results inspires
dread, not only because it is almost always fatal but also because
of the symptoms themselves, which include the well-known foaming
at the mouth and the extreme reaction to water (hydrophobia).

Rabies was recognized as a disease as long ago as 2300 BC in
ancient Babylon, where dog owners were fined if their rabid animals
bit anyone. Ancient Greek philosophers such as Democitrus and
Aristotle also described the disease. Transmission of the disease via
the saliva of rabid animals was recognized in the first century AD.

Rabies in animals occurs in all continents except Australia and
Antarctica. Canine rabies is endemic throughout most of Asia, Africa
and Latin America. In Europe, foxes are the predominant host, but
many other animals can become infected, including dogs, cats, cattle,
horses, badgers, martens and deer. In the USA, racoons and bats
account for 85 per cent of animal cases of rabies, but it has also
been found in skunks and foxes. The United Kingdom has been free
of indigenous animal rabies since 1922, except for a single rabid
bat that was found on the Sussex coast in 1996.

Humans are occasionally infected by wild animals, but domestic
dogs and cats are responsible for more than 90 per cent of human
cases worldwide. In western Europe, although 86 per cent of rabies
is found in the fox population, about 75 per cent of all cases of
human exposure result from dog bites, reflecting the close relationship between humans and dogs.

Incidence of human rabies

The World Health Organization reports that deaths from rabies amount to fewer than 2,000 cases each year. This is considered as a gross underestimate of the true figure. In India alone, it is estimated that there were 30,000 deaths from rabies in 1992, and in Bangladesh approximately 2,000 deaths in the same year. In the United States there were more than 25 human deaths each year in the 1940s, but since 1960 this figure has declined to about six a year. There have been no indigenous cases of human rabies reported in the United Kingdom since 1902. In the 15 years prior to that, 173 people died from rabies in England and Wales. Since then there have been a number of deaths from rabies but these have all been acquired abroad, mainly in the Indian subcontinent. In continental Europe only a few cases are reported each year.

Transmission

Transmission cannot occur across intact skin, but the rabies virus can penetrate through wounds and mucous membranes. Humans are usually infected when the saliva containing the virus is introduced through the skin by the bite of a rabid dog or other mammal. Saliva can also infect if the skin is already broken, for example, by the animal's claws. Animals can also be infected via the gastrointestinal tract, but this mode of transmission has never been recorded in humans. The inhalation of the rabies virus was thought to be responsible for the deaths of two men in Mexico. They were thought to have inhaled an aerosol of bats' infected nasal secretions while visiting caves inhabited by thousands of the Mexican free-tailed bat.

Person to person spread of the disease has not been documented, except in six cases of patients who had received infected corneal grafts. The three donors of the corneas had died of undiagnosed neurological diseases. Twenty-two to 39 days after transplantation, the recipients began to display symptoms of rabies and died shortly afterwards. A seventh recipient was prevented from developing rabies by rigorous treatment.

Symptoms in humans

The incubation period for rabies can range from four days to over two years, although in three-quarters of cases it is between 20 and 90 days. The incubation period is shortest for bites on the face – on average 35 days. For bites on the limbs the average incubation period is 52 days.

In most patients early symptoms of rabies include itching and pain at the site of the wound. There may also be fever, headache, general malaise, sensitivity to light, anxiety, irritability and, in some cases, symptoms of upper respiratory tract and gastrointestinal infections.

As the disease progresses it may present in two different forms: furious rabies and paralytic or dumb rabies.

Furious rabies is more common. In this form the most common diagnostic symptom is the known hydrophobia, which consists of spasm in the throat and respiratory muscles, which is associated with terror. This symptom is initially provoked by attempts to drink water, but eventually even the sight, sound or even mention of water can provoke the symptom. Patients may also display general arousal and maniacal, sometimes aggressive, behaviour and may suffer from hallucinations. This behaviour usually alternates with lucid intervals. Disturbances in the autonomic nervous system result in the well-reported 'foaming at the mouth', which is in fact caused by an excess production of saliva. Usually about one-third of patients die during a hydrophobic spasm within the first few days unless given supportive treatment. The remainder lapse into coma and generalized flaccid paralysis and rarely survive for more than a week without intensive care.

Paralytic or dumb rabies is the clinical presentation in fewer than a fifth of human cases but is always the form displayed if vampire bats have been the source of infection. Initial symptoms are similar to furious rabies, but in this form flaccid paralysis develops, usually in the bitten limb, which then ascends symmetrically or asymmetrically with pain and brief, rhythmic twitching in the affected muscles. Paralysis of all four limbs usually ensues, followed by the final fatal involvement of the respiratory muscles. Hydrophobia is unusual in this form of the disease. Even without intensive care, some patients have survived for up to 30 days.

Treatment

Very few people have survived rabies, but there are now four documented cases of recovery. One of these was a Mexican boy with severe dog bites who was given a post-exposure vaccine. Patients should be heavily sedated and given analgesia to relieve their pain and terror. Intensive care can also prevent the onset of complications.

It is important to try to neutralize the virus before it enters the nervous system. Cleaning the wound with soap or a detergent and treatment with a viricidal agent, such as alcohol or iodine, can be effective in reducing the risk of rabies developing, as can the use of post-exposure immunization.

A number of vaccines, both pre- and post-exposure, have been developed which can protect against rabies. The earliest of these was developed over a hundred years ago by Louis Pasteur.

15

The Worldwide Picture

This chapter contains a tabular presentation of data concerning over 200 countries and states. A number of prevalent diseases and parasites are covered and a rough guide to the risk of malaria is given. In addition, the possibility of an HIV test being required, water quality, and so on, are included. This is merely a quick summary of the countries where certain diseases and conditions are common and is not meant as a comprehensive guide for the traveller.

Before the tables, a number of the abbreviations and symbols used are explained, but before turning to them, some aspects of the diseases mentioned will be considered. Both meningitis and hepatitis are covered fully earlier in the book. We shall therefore turn our attention here to:

> malaria
> yellow fever
> Japanese encephalitis
> tetanus
> dengue fever
> Chagas' disease
> cholera
> typhus

We then consider the growing threat of haemorrhagic fever viruses, which are becoming more numerous and, consequently, more dangerous year by year.

Malaria

Malaria is an infection caused by minute parasites in the blood and is characterized by recurring bouts of fever. It cannot be contracted in the United Kingdom, but infection can be acquired by those travelling abroad and then brought back. The disease affects the red blood corpuscles or cells, liver and central nervous system.

The cause of malaria is infection by any one of four types of single-celled protozoan organisms. These belong to the genus *Plasmodium* and are *P. falciparum*, *P. malariae*, *P. vivax* and *P. ovale*. The most dangerous of these is *P. falciparum*, which is responsible for around three-quarters of infections in sub-Saharan Africa and a significant proportion in South America. This is the organism that causes malignant malaria, and it can kill within 48 hours if left unchecked. About two to three million people are infected by *P. falciparum* every year and as many as 10 per cent may die.

These organisms complete some stage of their life cycle within female *Anopheles* mosquitoes. The mosquito is the carrier and acquires the organisms when it sucks blood from an infected person. It passes them on in its saliva when it bites an uninfected person. The parasite passes in the blood circulation to the liver and multiplies there. Eventually they return to the blood and occupy red blood cells, further enlarging and multiplying in the process. Finally, they rupture and destroy the red blood cells. The bouts of fever correspond with the rupturing of the red blood cells and the parasites that are released go on to invade new cells. In some types of malaria (*P. vivax* and *P. ovale*) the parasite persists within the liver.

A person may die as a result of the high fever that can occur during a malarial attack. Also, the parasites may be so numerous that they block small blood vessels in the brain, which again can be fatal (cerebral malaria). A very dangerous complication is blackwater fever, characterized by high fever, severe anaemia, great destruction of red blood cells and the presence of haemoglobin (the red blood pigment) in the urine. Malaria is likely to be more dangerous if treatment is inadequate and does not eradicate the organisms. Also, people who are poorly nourished or otherwise ill or run-down from some other cause will tend to suffer more.

The symptoms depend on the type of malarial parasite but usually develop from about one to four weeks after a bite from an infected mosquito. The person may feel somewhat unwell for one or two days before the onset of an attack, which typically passes through three stages, although these are not always apparent. The first stage (cold stage) is marked by extreme shivering and feeling very cold although the person has a high temperature. After about one hour, this is followed by the hot stage. The person is burning with fever, has a very high temperature, a headache, nausea and giddiness, and pain, and may become delirious. The final, sweating stage is marked by profuse perspiration and a fall in temperature. The aches and pains subside and the person, although weak, feels better. Depending on the type of parasite, there is a gap of two or three days or a few hours before the next attack. There may be widespread destruction of red blood cells, especially with recurrent attacks, and if the disease becomes chronic the person may become severely anaemic. The liver and spleen are enlarged, and the person becomes jaundiced. Usually over a few weeks, even without treatment, the number of parasites in the blood drops to a low level and no more attacks occur. However, they can become active again and multiply to produce further bouts of fever. Any person returning from a country where malaria occurs who develops these symptoms should seek immediate medical treatment.

Treatment for malaria consists of complete bed rest, and the adequate intake of fluids is important. There are various drugs used for the prevention of malaria, and it is necessary to consult a doctor to obtain a course of these before travelling to a country where the disease occurs. The drugs afford some degree of protection but are not totally effective, and infection may still occur. Treatment involves the taking of various antimalarial drugs, especially chloroquine, but may vary according to the area in which the infection was acquired. Treatment is normally effective for most forms of malaria. However, life-threatening complications can arise and some people may require intensive treatment in hospital.

As with many other infections, the drugs are becoming less effective against the infecting organism. There are a number of strains of *Plasmodium* that are now resistant to chloroquine, and across the world there is a greater area containing resistant forms than organisms susceptible to this drug. As a result, the treatment has been enhanced with an additional drug, proguanil. The course of drugs should be started before going to an infected area, and although there are likely to be side effects, it is important to continue with and complete the treatment. Unfortunately, resistance eventually develops whenever a drug is introduced, and in some regions yet more, different, drugs are being used. Mefloquine is a third type of drug being used, but there are doubts about its side effects.

The situation concerning drug resistance is changing constantly, and the race is on to find new treatments and, it is hoped, an effective prophylaxis (a treatment to prevent the disease). It does seem that, with the experience of hindsight, the bugs responsible will not take long before they build up resistance. However, a very recent development from Australia brings some hope regarding cerebral malaria. Researchers in Melbourne have identified the protein produced by *P. falciparum* that causes the clogging of blood capillaries in the brain.

Tetanus

Tetanus is a very serious and sometimes fatal disease caused by bacteria that enter through a wound. The motor nerves, spinal cord and muscles are all affected The cause of tetanus is a bacterium called *Clostridium tetani*. It is found in soil, especially that which has been treated with manure, but also may occur in other circumstances. People engaged in any outdoor sporting activity, farming, gardening, forestry, etc, should take care to keep tetanus immunizations up-to-date.

Symptoms usually appear about two or three weeks after the person has received a wound, often after it has healed. In the early stages there is a stiffening and rigidity of muscles near the site of the wound. Later, there is rigidity and spasm of muscles in other parts of the body, which causes extreme agony. Characteristically, the muscles of the face and jaw are affected. The person is unable to open the mouth, hence the alternative name of lockjaw, and finds it very difficult to swallow. The spasms in the muscles of the face give a characteristic appearance, exposing the teeth, and this is called risus sardonicus.

The muscular seizures occur at the slightest stimulus and may cause extreme pain. Since the muscles involved in breathing and respiration may be very severely affected, it is possible that the person will die from asphyxia and exhaustion. Frequently, there is an accompanying high fever and profuse sweating, and the person experiences great anxiety as the symptoms are painful and frightening. A person with symptoms of tetanus requires immediate emergency medical treatment. Also, anyone who receives a wound, especially while outdoors, when it may be contaminated with soil or manure, and who is unsure about his or her state of immunity, should seek medical advice. A person who has a wound requiring medical attention is usually given tetanus antitoxin as a precaution unless it is certain that immunization is up-to-date.

If hospitalization is necessary, the treatment will involve bed rest in a quiet and darkened room. Tetanus antitoxin is given by means of injection, and muscle relaxants and sedatives may also be needed. Other antibiotics may be prescribed. The outcome depends on the severity of the symptoms, the patient's age and state of immunity, and how soon treatment begins. Tetanus can be successfully cured in most cases, and the incidence of the disease and numbers of deaths have been greatly reduced by immunization. Preventative measures, including routine immunization of children, is by means of a course of three anti-tetanus injections with a booster every ten years.

Dengue

Dengue is a tropical fever, also known as breakbone fever or dandy-fever, that affects the joints and skin. It is caused by a virus carried by the mosquito *Aedes* and transmitted in its bite. It is common in Asia, and in 1996 an outbreak in Delhi struck 10,000 people and there were 400 fatalities.

Symptoms appear usually within five to eight days of infection, although it may take up to 15 days. There is then a quick appearance of a headache with chills, pain in the eyes and back, and extreme aching in the legs and joints, contributing to a weakness approaching collapse. The temperature rises and a rash may appear, particularly on the face. The fever may last from two to four days and is then followed by a day or two of remission. A second rise in temperature follows, with a nasty rash, often over much of the body except the face. The rash, fever and headache with other pains are often called the dengue triad. The good thing about dengue is that it is not fatal, unlike its nasty cousin, dengue haemorrhagic fever (*see* page 126).

Treatment involves treating the symptoms. The joint pains can usually be relieved with codeine but aspirin is not usually recommended. In severe cases, pethidine may be used. Calamine lotion eases the rash to some extent, and bed rest is essential. It is also vital that fluid intake is maintained. In some cases, the fever may return more than once, and the weakness and joint pains may take months to disappear. In areas where there is a risk of being bitten by these mosquitoes, the use of an insect repellent and mosquito nets should help to reduce the risk. Also, to break the chain of events and prevent more mosquitoes taking up the virus, anyone infected should remain under a mosquito net until the second episode of fever has gone away.

Yellow fever

Yellow fever is an acute viral infection, again carried by the mosquito *Aedes*, with the specific name *aegypti*. It can be fatal and is so in a little under 10 per cent of cases, but there is a very effective immunization which confers protection for ten years.

After infection is passed on by the mosquito, the symptoms appear suddenly after incubation. A fever is accompanied initially by a rapid pulse which then slows, the face is flushed and there is a headache. In addition there can be vomiting, nausea, constipation, stomach and muscle pains. In mild cases, the disease runs its course at this point, after between one and three days. In more severe cases, a period of remission is followed by a 'period of intoxication' in which the fever returns and it may be accompanied by jaundice, vomiting of blood (which usually appears black), haemorrhaging and, in its later stages, delirium, convulsions and coma.

Treatment attends to the symptoms, with complete bed rest and restoration of the body's fluid and electrolyte levels. Drugs are used to combat the tendency to haemorrhage and to treat the aches and vomiting. To prevent ongoing transmission, patients should be kept in mosquito-free rooms.

Yellow fever is, in the main, confined to Africa and South America, but there are now fears that it will spread to Asia where the mosquito carrier is common and the population is not vaccinated. India, in particular, is at risk because of trading links with other countries, especially through expatriates. The rate of infection worldwide is increasing, with over 23,000 cases reported in the decade up to 1995, compared with 4,200 in the previous decade. The figure is certain to be greater, possibly by a factor of eight or ten. Although there are suggestions that yellow fever in Asia would be less of a problem than in Africa, because some resistance may be conferred by antibodies to dengue (another flavivirus), the situation nevertheless gives great cause for concern.

Chagas' disease

This is a disease found in South and Central America, called South American trypanosomiasis, a version of sleeping sickness. It is caused by the protozoan *Trypansoma cruzi* and is spread by a bug called, alternatively, the kissing bug or assassin bug. Scientifically these are known as triatomid bugs. The disease is passed to the host by contamination of the bite by infected faeces from the bug being rubbed into the wound.

In addition to the swelling around the bite wound, there is fever, facial swelling and other complications, including the possibility of convulsions which may result in mental defects or death. However, a much more common condition caused by this disease is acute myocarditis, that is, inflammation of the heart, which may cause death. Chagas' disease is more common in young children, and, unfortunately, there is no effective therapy for it and serious organ damage appears to be irreversible.

The primary weapon in the armoury against this disease is prevention. The bugs responsible inhabit poorly made housing, such as mud huts. Preventative measures are therefore relatively straightforward and involve improvement of such accommodation and the use of nets and insecticides.

Japanese encephalitis

This is a viral disease spread, as with many others, by the mosquito (but a different species, *Culex*). The disease is prevalent in Southeast Asia, Japan, Korea, China, India, the Philippines and the eastern states of the CIS.

The virus may be carried by many people who show no symptoms of the disease, but when it is manifested it is extremely nasty. The fatality rate is very high, about 30 per cent, and of those who survive, about three-quarters suffer neurological damage that may result in a condition similar to a needles and pins feeling or, more seriously, paralysis.

The mosquitoes are particularly active in areas of paddy fields and during the monsoons in Nepal, India and Thailand. Prevention is the best cure, so repellents and mosquito nets are vital.

Cholera

Cholera is a severe bacterial infection of the small intestine. It remains a serious killer disease in many countries, especially in conditions of overcrowding and poor sanitation (for example, in refugee camps). During epidemics, the death rate exceeds 50 per cent, with children and elderly persons being at particular risk. The disease is rare in the United Kingdom, and such cases that occur are contracted abroad. Strict standards of hygiene, sanitation and nursing ensure that the infection does not spread and prevents an epidemic. Early and prompt detection and treatment enable most patients to make a full recovery. This vigilance remains necessary because cholera caused thousands of deaths in the nineteenth century during widespread epidemics in many countries. Cholera is endemic in parts of Africa, the Middle East, Asia and the Gulf Coast of the United States.

The disease is caused by the bacterium *Vibrio cholerae*. It is spread by contamination of drinking water by the faeces of those affected by the disease and also by flies landing on infected material and then crawling on food. In countries where cholera is present, drinking water must be treated or boiled and strict standards of hygiene used in food preparation. Efforts should be made to eliminate flies from houses and to ensure that they do not come into contact with food. Risks remain wherever there are conditions of overcrowding, poverty and poor sanitation. The incubation period is one to three days.

There is considerable variation in the severity of symptoms and in the manner in which they present themselves. In mild cases, the patient may hardly feel ill whereas in those severely affected during epidemics, death may occur very rapidly, within a few hours.

In most cases, three stages of cholera are recognized. During the first stage, there is copious diarrhoea and vomiting, with the production of characteristic 'rice water stools' containing flakes of fibrin (a protein substance formed in the blood during blood clotting). There are severe pains and cramps, extreme thirst and increasing signs of dehydration. In the second stage, death may occur as a result of dehydration and collapse. The person's skin is cold and wrinkled, the eyes are sunken, the pulse becomes imperceptible and the voice is a hoarse whisper (called vox cholerica). During the third stage, the person starts to recover and gradually improve and the symptoms subside. Relapse is still possible at this stage, particularly in the form of a fever. A person who has travelled abroad and has any signs of illness should seek medical advice.

Uncomplicated cholera is self-limited and recovery occurs within three to six days. However, the death rate can be greater than 50 per cent in untreated severe cases. If treatment is available quickly, then the death rate falls dramatically to under 1 per cent. The majority of sufferers are free of *Vibrio cholerae* in about two weeks.

Treatment involves isolation of the patient and scrupulous attention to hygiene during nursing. This includes treatment and very careful disposal of the body waste of the infected person to prevent the spread of the disease. Treatment also involves bed rest and the use of drugs such as tetracycline or other sulphonamides to kill the bacteria. The patient requires salt solutions to counteract the dehydration that occurs, and these are taken by mouth and/or given intravenously. Prevention of cholera is by means of vaccination, but this is effective for only about six months.

Typhus

Typhus is an infectious disease that is found in several forms throughout the world. It is carried by insects such as ticks, lice and fleas and belongs to the genus *Rickettsia*. The infecting organism has some characteristics of both bacteria and viruses, and there are essentially four types of the disease:

epidemic typhus (also classic, European or louse-borne typhus, jail fever)
endemic typhus (also murine, rat flea and urban typhus of Malaya)
scrub typhus (also tropical, mite-borne typhus, Tsutsugamushi disease)
Brill-Zinsser disease

The first three are worthy of a brief mention.

Epidemic typhus

This is transmitted by the human body louse, *Pediculus humanus*. In its faeces is contained the organism *Rickettsia prowazekii*, which enters a bite wound upon scratching. The organism can survive in the dried faeces of lice for up to 60 days. The organism is passed on to lice biting infected patients in the fever stage of the disease. This disease is found worldwide but mainly in Africa, although outbreaks occur elsewhere. For example, in the United States a form was found that came from parasites on the bodies of flying squirrels.

Incubation takes from seven to 14 days, and then there follows a fever, intense headache and weakness with pains in the limbs. A rash appears after a few days, and in worsening cases the headache intensifies further and delirium may follow. Death usually occurs because of heart failure after about two weeks. The death rate varies enormously. In groups of refugees who are already at a low ebb, it can approach 100 per cent; in untreated cases where individuals are over 50 years old, it can reach 60 per cent.

Endemic typhus

Endemic typhus is similar to the epidemic form but is milder and carried by rat fleas. The organism responsible is *R. typhi*, and it is found in fleas on wild mice, rats and other rodents, but overall the occurrence is low. Symptoms include a headache, fever and chills, which may last for up to 12 days. Deaths tend to occur only in elderly patients.

Scrub typhus

Scrub typhus occurs in areas of Australia, Japan and India. It is carried by a mite on rodents, and infection is transferred by a bite from the larva of the mite. There is an incubation period of between six and 21 days, after which a fever, headache and chills set in very quickly. A body rash then develops after a few days, and a cough in the early days can progress to inflammation of the lungs in the later stages. More severe symptoms are sometimes met, but, overall, recovery is prompt with effective treatment. Insecticides and repellents are the best means of overcoming the likelihood of contracting this disease.

Treatment

Treatment for these forms of typhus is essentially very similar. Prophylactic measures should always be taken, and insecticides such as DDT have proved to be very effective. Controlling the carrier is also good policy, for example, reducing rat populations. Antibiotic treatment is, currently, very effective in defeating the disease, the commonest one used being a tetracycline.

Haemorrhagic viruses

Of all the illnesses to strike humans, probably the most virulent of recent times are the haemorrhagic fever viruses. These are among the most dangerous biological agents known, and the rate at which new ones are being identified is almost as frightening as the diseases themselves. There are a number of classes, split as follows, and within some are diseases already mentioned in the text:

Group:	Flaviviruses
Examples:	yellow fever (Amaril virus)
	dengue haemorrhagic fever
	tick-borne encephalitis
Group:	Arenaviruses
Examples:	Lassa fever (Nigeria)
	Machupo (Bolivia)
	Guanarito (Venezuela)
	Junín (Argentina)
	Sabià (Brazil)
Group:	Bunyaviruses
Subgroup:	Hantaviruses
Examples:	Rift Valley fever (Africa)
	Crimean-Congo fever
	Sin Nombre (Mexico)
	Hantaan (Korea)
	Puumala (NW Europe)

Group:	Filoviruses
Examples:	Ebola (Congo, formerly Zaire)
	Marburg (Germany)

The reason for these new 'discoveries' is simply that the analytical tools employed nowadays are far better than they were in the past. These viruses have been around for some time, a long time in many cases, but only over the past 10 to 15 years have they been noticed, isolated and identified. As the above list shows, the viruses are usually given the names of places – the locations where they first caused a recognized outbreak of the disease.

The arenaviruses and bunyaviruses are found naturally in animal populations and transmission between people is uncommon. Animals hold the viruses and act as vectors (carriers) in passing them on to people. It is, as yet, not known how the filoviruses are spread.

The viruses seem to have emerged because there have been changes in environmental conditions, which are often caused by human intervention. This may be the clearing of a forest, farming crops where dust is generated, or similar activities. In all cases, the host animal is thrust into contact with a burgeoning human population, resulting in a greater possibility of the disease being transmitted. Nature may also take a hand. If, for example, climatic conditions are particularly suited to a certain rodent and the animal population explodes, then the risk of transmission is increased. Some of the bunyaviruses are carried by mosquitoes, for example, Rift Valley fever.

In addition to 'natural' causes, accidents are very likely to spread these diseases. Lax practices in hospitals can spread the virus, and inadequate safeguards in the biomedical industry can have disastrous consequences. This is what happened in Marburg, where vaccines were being prepared from animals. In this case, the monkeys from Uganda passed on the infection and seven laboratory workers died.

Hantaviruses

Sin Nombre (Spanish for 'no name') was first identified in 1994 when an outbreak of 24 cases in New Mexico, Colorado and Nevada resulted in 11 deaths. The symptoms start with a fever, followed by bleeding at numerous sites. The complications that follow are numerous and affect the cardiovascular, neurological and digestive systems. Death can be the result of the failure of many organs or massive haemorrhaging.

Arenaviruses

Sabià first appeared in 1990 in São Paulo, Brazil, although the initial diagnosis was of yellow fever. Only one fatality has occurred, but there have in all likelihood been more – they simply would not have been identified correctly. The symptoms and progress of the disease are very similar to those of Sin Nombre.

Junín or Argentinian haemorrhagic fever is a threat for agricultural workers. Large tracts of land are cultivated for maize, and this has led to an increase in a species of mouse that carries the organism. There is therefore a greater risk of contact, but, in addition, harvesting the crop creates vast clouds of dust which is infected (from the faeces of the mice), and any animals slaughtered by the machinery are instantly ground up and their blood sprayed about – blood that is also infected.

Filoviruses

This group of haemorrhagic fever viruses, including Marburg (*see* above), is extremely frightening. Perhaps one of the best known examples is Ebola, which, although it is virulent in the extreme, is nevertheless self-limiting. Ebola kills very quickly, and the fatality rate is over 90 per cent, in about two weeks. This means, paradoxically, that in killing its victims rapidly the virus is not passed on easily, unless it is helped inadvertently, often by people. In the last 20 years there have been four known outbreaks, and in all cases the virus was 'helped' by people. Quite often customs lead to spreading the virus – touching a body, removing organs and similar practices will rapidly infect other people. In another instance, people were injected for malaria with reused, unsterilized syringes, and when an Ebola sufferer mistakenly received the same injection, the infected needle spread the disease very efficiently indeed.

It is all too easy for the disease to be spread when the cause of the illness is unknown. One such episode happened in Kikwit, Democratic Republic of Congo (formerly Zaire), where a laboratory technician became infected, unknowingly, with Ebola. After falling ill, he suffered fever and a bloated stomach. He was operated on, firstly, to remove his appendix. Then followed a second operation that was believed to be for internal repair, but when the abdomen was opened, the operating staff were drenched with blood. The bleeding could not be stopped and the patient died very quickly – and those contaminated with the blood contracted Ebola.

Major factors in the spread of these diseases are poverty and very poor medical facilities. However, it is not known what happens to the virus between epidemics and what the limiting factors are on its transmission. All outbreaks have been transmitted by fluids, and once ritualistic post-mortem practices were curbed, the incidence of Ebola dropped. The direct link is the key to transmission, but should Ebola ever mutate and become an airborne virus, then the consequences would be very grave indeed.

Ebola was actually identified and named following epidemics in the Democratic Republic of Congo (formerly Zaire), near the Ebola river. Out of 318 cases, 280 resulted in death.

Nature of haemorrhagic fever viruses

The genetic make-up of these viruses is the reason behind their variability and the speed with which they evolve. The genes in these viruses have a type of RNA (ribonucleic acid) rather than the DNA of most cells. The RNA needs a particular component before it can make viral proteins in an infected cell, and these components cause errors that result in a mixed population of viruses, allowing rapid adaptation to changed environmental conditions.

Understanding of how these viruses cause disease is very limited. Unfortunately, they are so very dangerous that they can only be studied in laboratories that have exceedingly safe and specialized equipment and conditions. Because the common laboratory rat does not become ill when infected, monkeys have to be used, and that is the dangerous aspect – a scratch can be fatal.

The viruses have certain similar effects in the body, resulting in a reduction in the number of platelets, although not enough to explain the massive haemorrhaging common to these diseases. There may also be destruction of cells or a disruption of the immune system altogether. The bunyaviruses have a short incubation period. The liver is the object of attack and often a large part of it is destroyed. This causes a reduction in the production of compounds that coagulate blood, a situation exacerbated by platelets sticking to blood vessels, as a result of a further effect of the virus. Arenaviruses take longer to incubate and inhibit the immune system and also cause neurological problems. Hantaviruses also take longer to incubate, from 12 to 21 days, and they attack the cells lining the walls of the capillary vessels. Some attack these vessels in the kidneys while others target the lungs, causing death by oedema.

The Tables

The data presented in the following pages of tables is a guide to the countries and states of the world and the prevalent diseases. It indicates, for example, which immunizations would be a good idea if travelling to that country and also mentions parasitic infections that may be present.

Malaria is a potential problem in many countries, but the categorization of risk is again only a guide. It does, however, show the spread of the problem.

Abbreviations or symbols used in the tables are as follows:

✓	=	immunization recommended
(✓)	=	a good idea
[✓]	=	rarely needed
✓ (underlined)	=	a wise precaution if an extended stay is likely
✗	=	present
c	=	certificate needed – applies particularly to yellow fever if coming from an infected area
(✓)	=	(for yellow fever) required for onward travel
(✓)	=	(with HIV) needed in certain circumstances, such as for long stays (for example, students). It is important to check with the appropriate authorities
Diphth & TB	=	ideally get a booster for diphtheria and a check for TB
TBE	=	tick-borne encephalitis

JE   = Japanese encephalitis
Onch   = onchocerciasis (known as river blindness – caused
              by a parasitic worm)
DF   = Dengue fever (not haemorrhagic form)
Msf   = Mediterranean spotted fever

Water quality is put into one of three categories:
1   = safe
2   = chlorinated in the main centres but unsafe else-
              where
3   = unsafe
This means that travellers' diarrhoea is more of a risk within category 3 than 2, and in 2 compared to 1.

COUNTRY	Cholera	Echinococcosis	Filariasis	Hepatitis A	Hepatitis B	Leishmaniasis	Meningitis	Polio	Rabies	Schistosomiasis
Afghanistan				✓	(✓)	✗		✓	(✓)	
Albania				✓	(✓)			✓	(✓)	
Algeria				✓	(✓)	✗		✓	(✓)	✗
American Samoa			✗	✓	(✓)			✓		
Andora										
Angola	c		✗	✓	(✓)		(✓)	✓	(✓)	✗
Anguilla				[✓]				✓		
Antigua & Barbuda				[✓]				✓		
Argentina				✓	[✓]	✗		✓	(✓)	
Armenia				(✓)	[✓]			✓	(✓)	
Aruba				(✓)				✓		
Australia										
Austria										
Azerbaijan				(✓)	(✓)			✓	(✓)	
Bahamas				(✓)				✓		
Bahrain				✓	(✓)			✓		
Bangladesh			✗	✓	(✓)	✗	(✓)	✓	(✓)	
Barbados				(✓)	(✓)			✓		
Belarus				(✓)				✓	(✓)	

Tetanus	Typhoid	Yellow Fever	HIV Test	Water Quality	Malaria Risk	COMMENTS
✓	✓	c		3	high	Hep. E in contaminated water
✓	✓	c		2	none	Diphtheria present
✓	✓	c	✓	2	little	Diphtheria present; parasitic worms
✓	✓	c		3	none	JE present; DF present
(✓)				2	none	No health precautions recommended
✓	✓	✓c		3	high	parasitic worm infections – wear shoes
✓	[✓]			2	none	
✓	[✓]	c	(✓)	2	none	
✓	✓	(✓)		2	low	Chagas' disease in rural north
✓	(✓)			3	none	Diphtheria and TB present
✓	(✓)	c		2	none	Some DF
		c	✓	1	none	No immunizations recommended
				1	none	TBE in some areas; no other immunizations required
✓	(✓)			3	none	Diphtheria boost; also TB and TBE
✓	(✓)	c		2	none	
✓	✓	c		2	none	
✓	✓	c		3	high	JE for rural travel; DF present
✓	(✓)	c		1	none	
✓	(✓)			2		Diphtheria, TB and Hep. boosters; TBE in forests; several tick-borne diseases

COUNTRY	Cholera	Echinococcosis	Filariasis	Hepatitis A	Hepatitis B	Leishmaniasis	Meningitis	Polio	Rabies	Schistosomiasis
Belgium										
Belize				✓	(✓)			✓		
Benin				✓	(✓)		(✓)	✓	(✓)	✗
Bhutan	(✓)			✓	(✓)		(✓)	✓	(✓)	
Bolivia				✓	(✓)			✓	(✓)	
Bonaire				(✓)				✓		
Bosnia Herzegovina				(✓)		✗		✓		
Botswana				✓	(✓)			✓	(✓)	
Brazil			✗	✓	(✓)			✓	(✓)	✗
Brunei				✓	(✓)			✓	[✓]	
Bulgaria				(✓)	(✓)			✓	(✓)	
Burkina Faso			✗	✓	(✓)		(✓)	✓	(✓)	✗
Burma (Myanmar)			✗	✓	(✓)			✓	(✓)	
Burundi				✓	(✓)		(✓)	✓	(✓)	
Cambodia				✓	(✓)			✓	(✓)	✗
Cameroon	(c)			✓	(✓)		(✓)	✓	(✓)	✗
Canada										
Cape Verde Islands			✗	✓	(✓)	✗		✓	(✓)	
Cayman Islands				(✓)				✓		

Tetanus	Typhoid	Yellow Fever	HIV Test	Water Quality	Malaria Risk	COMMENTS
(✓)			✓	1	none	No immunizations recommended
✓	✓	(✓)c	✓	2	moderate	DF present
✓	✓	✓c		3	high	
✓	✓	c		3	moderate	JE in some areas; Hep. E
✓	✓	✓c	✓	3	moderate	
✓	(✓)	c		2	none	Some DF
✓	(✓)			2	none	TBE, Lyme disease
✓	✓	(c)		3	high	TBE, tick typhus present
✓	✓	✓c		3	high	Chagas' disease, DF present, HIV high
✓	✓	c	✓	2	none	JE in rural areas; DF from mosquitoes
✓			✓	2	moderate	TBE; tick-borne diseases
✓	✓	✓c		3	high	DF; sleeping sickness and others present
✓	✓	c		3	high	JE, DF and various parasites present
✓	✓	✓c		3	high	
✓	✓	c		3	high	JE in rural areas; DF present
✓	✓	✓c		3	high	Parasistes common
				1	none	No immunizations recommended
✓	✓	c		3	low	DF present
✓	[✓]		✓	2	none	DF present

COUNTRY	Cholera	Echinococcosis	Filariasis	Hepatitis A	Hepatitis B	Leishmaniasis	Meningitis	Polio	Rabies	Schistosomiasis
Central African Republic			✗	✓	(✓)		(✓)	✓	(✓)	✗
Chad			✗	✓	(✓)		(✓)	✓	(✓)	✗
Chile				✓	[✓]			✓	[✓]	
China			✗	✓	(✓)	✗		✓	(✓)	✗
Columbia				✓	(✓)			✓	(✓)	
Comoros Islands				✓	(✓)			✓	(✓)	
Congo				✓	(✓)		(✓)	✓	(✓)	
Congo (Zaire)	(c)			✓	(✓)		(✓)	✓	(✓)	
Cook Islands			✗	✓	(✓)			✓		
Costa Rica				✓	[✓]	✗		✓	(✓)	
Côte d'Ivoire				✓	(✓)		(✓)	✓	(✓)	✗
Croatia				(✓)		✗		✓	(✓)	
Cuba				✓	(✓)			✓	(✓)	
Curacao				(✓)				✓		
Cyprus								(✓)		
Czech Republic								(✓)		
Denmark										
Djibouti				✓	(✓)		(✓)	✓	(✓)	
Dominica				(✓)				✓		✗
Dominican Republic				✓	(✓)			✓		✗
Ecuador				✓	(✓)			✓	(✓)	
Egypt	✗			✓	(✓)		[✓]	✓	(✓)	
El Salvador				✓	(✓)			✓	(✓)	
Equatorial Guinea				✓	(✓)		(✓)	✓	(✓)	
Eritrea				✓	(✓)	✗	(✓)	✓	(✓)	✗

Tetanus	Typhoid	Yellow Fever	HIV Test	Water Quality	Malaria Risk	COMMENTS
✓	✓	✓c		3	high	Many parasites endemic
✓	✓	✓c		3	high	Some parasites
✓	✓			3	none	Chagas' disease rurally
✓	✓	c		2	moderate	JE in rural/suburban areas; DF
✓	✓	✓	✓	3	high	DF; Chagas' disease present regionally
✓	✓			2	high	DF present
✓	✓	✓c		3	high	Many parasites endemic
✓	✓	✓c		3	high	Orch. plague and other diseases
✓	✓			2	none	JE in rural areas, also DF
✓	✓	c	✓	2	high	DF on coasts
✓	✓	✓c		3	high	
✓	(✓)			2	none	TBE, Lyme disease present
	✓	✓	(✓)	2	none	Some DF
✓	(✓)	c		2	low	Some DF
(✓)			✓	1	none	
✓			(✓)	2	none	TBE and Lyme disease present
				1	none	Some Lyme disease in forests
✓	✓	✓c		3	moderate	
✓	✓	c		2	none	Some DF
✓	(✓)			2	moderate	Some DF
✓	✓	✓c	(✓)	3	moderate	Diphtheria, some DF
✓	✓	c	✓	2	moderate	Parasites common – wear shoes
✓	✓	(✓)c		3	high	DF present
✓	✓	✓c		3	high	
✓	✓	✓c		3	high	Wear shoes

COUNTRY	Cholera	Echinococcosis	Filariasis	Hepatitis A	Hepatitis B	Leishmaniasis	Meningitis	Polio	Rabies	Schistosomiasis
Estonia				(✓)	(✓)			✓	(✓)	
Ethiopia				✓	(✓)	✗	(✓)	✓	(✓)	✗
Falkland Islands										
Fiji			✗	✓	(✓)			✓		
Finland										
France						✗				
French Guiana				✓	(✓)	✗		✓	(✓)	
French Polynesia			✗	✓	(✓)			✓		
Gabon				✓	(✓)		(✓)	✓	(✓)	
Gambia			✗	✓	(✓)		(✓)	✓	(✓)	✗
Georgia				(✓)	(✓)	✗		✓	(✓)	
Germany										
Ghana				✓	(✓)		(✓)	✓		
Gibraltar										
Greece						✗				
Grenada				(✓)				✓	(✓)	✗
Guadeloupe				(✓)	(✓)	✗		✓		✗
Guam			✗	✓	(✓)			✓		
Guatemala				✓	(✓)			✓	(✓)	
Guinea	(c)		✗	✓	(✓)		(✓)	✓	(✓)	
Guinea-Bissau				✓	(✓)		(✓)	✓	(✓)	
Guyana			✗	✓	(✓)			✓	(✓)	✗
Haiti			✗	✓	(✓)			✓		
Honduras				✓	(✓)			✓	(✓)	
Hong Kong				✓	(✓)			✓		

Tetanus	Typhoid	Yellow Fever	HIV Test	Water Quality	Malaria Risk	COMMENTS
✓	(✓)			2	none	Diphtheria, TB for long stays
✓	✓	✓c		3	moderate	
				1	none	Nothing required
✓	✓	c		2	none	DF
			(✓)	1	none	TBE, Lyme disease present in forests
				1	none	Some Lyme disease
✓	✓	✓c		2	high	HIV risk; DF (coastal)
✓	✓	c		2	none	DF present
✓	✓	✓c		3	high	Orch. and African tick typhus present
✓	✓	✓c		3	high	
✓	(✓)			2	none	Diphtheria and TBE present
			✓	1*	none	*2 in East; TBE and Lyme disease in forests
✓	✓	✓c		3	high	
				1	none	No requirements
		c	(✓)	2	none	
✓	(✓)	c		2	none	
✓	✓	c		2	none	Some DF
✓	✓			2	none	Some DF, JE
✓	✓	(✓)c		3	high	Several local diseases
✓	✓	✓c		3	high	Avoid insect bites
✓	✓	✓c		3	high	Several insect-borne diseases
✓	✓	✓c		2	high	DF present
✓	✓	c		3	high	DF present
✓	✓	(✓)c		3	high	DF present
✓	✓			1	none	Some JE, DF

COUNTRY	Cholera	Echinococcosis	Filariasis	Hepatitis A	Hepatitis B	Leishmaniasis	Meningitis	Polio	Rabies	Schistosomiasis
Hungary				[✓]	(✓)			✓		
Iceland										
India	✓		✗	✓	(✓)	✗	(✓)	✓	(✓)	
Indonesia	(c)		✗	✓	(✓)			✓	(✓)	✗
Iran			✗	✓	(✓)	✗		✓	(✓)	✗
Iraq				✓	(✓)	✗		✓	(✓)	✗
Ireland										
Israel				✓	(✓)	✗		✓	(✓)	
Italy						✗				
Jamaica				(✓)				✓		
Japan					(✓)			(✓)		
Jordan				✓	(✓)	✗		✓	(✓)	✗
Kazakhstan	(✓)			(✓)	(✓)	✗		✓	(✓)	
Kenya		✗		✓	(✓)		(✓)	✓	(✓)	
Kiribati			✗	✓	(✓)			✓		
Korea			✗	✓	(✓)			✓	(✓)	
Kuwait				✓	(✓)			✓	(✓)	
Kyrgyzstan				(✓)	(✓)			✓	(✓)	
Laos			✗	✓	(✓)			✓	(✓)	✗
Latvia				(✓)	(✓)			✓	(✓)	

Tetanus	Typhoid	Yellow Fever	HIV Test	Water Quality	Malaria Risk	COMMENTS
✓			(✓)	1	none	TBE and Lyme disease in forests
				1	none	Nothing required
✓	✓	c	✓	3	moderate	JE rurally; Hep. E and DF present; many parasites in rural areas
✓	✓	c		2	moderate	DF and JE present; also Dengue haemorrhagic fever; avoid bites
✓	✓	c	(✓)	2	moderate	
✓	✓	c	✓	3	moderate	
				1	none	Nothing required
✓	✓	(✓)	(✓)	2	none	Care required in rural areas
				1	none	Some TBE and Lyme disease
✓	(✓)	c		2	none	
	(✓)			1	none	Some JE; parasite risk in raw or undercooked fish
✓	✓	c	(✓)	3	none	Some typhus
✓	(✓)			3	low	Diphtheria and TB
✓	✓	✓c		2	moderate	
✓	✓	c		3	none	Some DF
✓	✓		(✓)	2	none	JE rurally; some DF
✓	✓		(✓)	2	none	
✓	(✓)			2	none	Diphtheria and TB if working; TBE
✓	✓	c		3	moderate	JE in rural areas; DF present
✓	(✓)			3	none	Diphtheria and TB if working; TBE

COUNTRY	Cholera	Echinococcosis	Filariasis	Hepatitis A	Hepatitis B	Leishmaniasis	Meningitis	Polio	Rabies	Schistosomiasis
Lebanon				✓	(✓)	✗		✓	(✓)	✗
Liberia	(c)			✓	(✓)		(✓)	✓	(✓)	
Libya				✓	(✓)			✓	(✓)	
Liechtenstein										
Lithuania				(✓)	(✓)			✓	(✓)	
Luxembourg										
Macau				✓	(✓)			✓		
Macedonia				(✓)				✓	(✓)	
Madagascar				✓	(✓)			✓	(✓)	✗
Malawi	(c)			✓	(✓)	✗	(✓)	✓	(✓)	✗
Malaysia	(c)		✗	✓	(✓)			✓	(✓)	✗
Maldives			✗	✓	(✓)			✓	(✓)	
Mali				✓	(✓)		(✓)	✓	(✓)	
Malta				(✓)	(✓)	✗		✓		
Marshall Islands				✓	(✓)			✓		
Martinique				(✓)		✗		✓		✗
Mauritania				✓	(✓)	✗	(✓)	✓	(✓)	✗
Mauritius				✓	(✓)			✓	(✓)	
Mexico				✓	(✓)			✓	(✓)	
Micronesia				✓	(✓)			✓		
Moldova				(✓)	(✓)			✓	(✓)	
Monaco										
Mongolia				✓	(✓)			✓	(✓)	
Montserrat				(✓)				✓		✗

Tetanus	Typhoid	Yellow Fever	HIV Test	Water Quality	Malaria Risk	COMMENTS
✓	✓	c		2	none	Tick-borne diseases, e.g. MSF
✓	✓	✓c		3	high	Avoid raw shellfish
✓	✓	c	(✓)	3	low	
				1	none	Nothing required
✓	(✓)			2	none	Diphtheria and TB if working; TBE in forests
				1	none	Nothing required
✓	✓			2	none	JE present
✓	(✓)			2	none	
✓	✓	c		2	low	
✓	✓	✓c		3	high	Tick typhus present
✓	✓	c		2	moderate	JE and leptospirosis in rural areas; DF present
✓	✓	c		2	none	Some DF
✓	✓	✓c		3	high	Orch. and other parasites present
✓	(✓)	c		1	none	
✓	✓			1	none	
✓	(✓)	c		2	none	DF present
✓	✓	✓c		3	low	
✓	✓	c	(✓)	2	low	
✓	✓	c	(✓)	2	low	
✓	✓		(✓)	2	low	
✓	(✓)			2	low	Diphtheria and TB if working; TBE in forests
				1	none	Nothing required
✓	✓		(✓)	3	none	Meningitis B present
✓	(✓)		(✓)	2	none	DF present

COUNTRY	Cholera	Echinococcosis	Filariasis	Hepatitis A	Hepatitis B	Leishmaniasis	Meningitis	Polio	Rabies	Schistosomiasis
Morocco				✓	(✓)	✗		✓	(✓)	✗
Mozambique				✓	(✓)		(✓)	✓	(✓)	
Namibia				✓	(✓)	✗	(✓)	✓	(✓)	
Nauru			✗	✓	(✓)			✓		
Nepal			✗	✓	(✓)	✗	(✓)	✓	(✓)	
Netherlands										
New Caledonia			✗	✓	(✓)			✓		
New Zealand										
Nicaragua				✓	(✓)			✓	(✓)	
Niger			✗	✓	(✓)		(✓)	✓	(✓)	✗
Nigeria			✗	✓	(✓)		(✓)	✓	(✓)	
Niue			✗	✓	(✓)			✓		
North Korea	(✓)			✓	(✓)			✓	(✓)	
Northern Mariana Islands			✗	✓	(✓)			✓		
Norway										
Oman				✓	(✓)	✗		✓	(✓)	✗
Pakistan	(✓)			✓	(✓)	✗		✓	(✓)	
Palau			✗	✓	(✓)			✓		
Panama				✓	(✓)			✓	(✓)	
Papua New Guinea			✗	✓	(✓)			✓		
Paraguay				✓	(✓)	✗		✓	(✓)	
Peru				✓	(✓)	✗		✓	(✓)	
Philippines			✗	✓	(✓)			✓	(✓)	✗

Tetanus	Typhoid	Yellow Fever	HIV Test	Water Quality	Malaria Risk	COMMENTS
✓	✓			2	low	Avoid bites
✓	✓	c		3	high	
✓	✓	c		2	high	Avoid bites
✓	✓	c		2	none	JE present, as is DF
✓	✓	c		2	moderate	JE present; some DF
				1	none	Nothing required
✓	✓	c		2	none	DF present
				1	none	Nothing required
✓	✓	(✓)c		3	high	DF active
✓	✓	✓c		3	high	Orch. and tick typhus present
✓	✓	✓c		3	high	Many parasites; DF present
✓	✓	c		2	none	DF present
✓	✓			3	none	JE present, as is DF
✓	✓			2	none	Some JE, DF
				1	none	Some Lyme disease; avoid tick bites
✓	✓	c		3	high	Several parasites
✓	✓	c	(✓)	3	high	Some JE; take care with everything
✓	✓			2	none	DF and JE present
✓	✓	(✓)c	(✓)	2	high	
✓	✓	c	(✓)	2	high	JE present, as is DF; many parasites
✓	✓	c		2	moderate	DF present
✓	✓	✓c		3	moderate	Some DF
✓	✓	c	(✓)	2	moderate	JE for rural areas; some DF and many parasites

COUNTRY	Cholera	Echinococcosis	Filariasis	Hepatitis A	Hepatitis B	Leishmaniasis	Meningitis	Polio	Rabies	Schistosomiasis
Pitcairn Island				✓	(✓)			✓		
Poland				(✓)	(✓)			✓		
Portugal						✗				
Puerto Rico				(✓)				✓		
Qatar				✓	(✓c)			✓	(✓)	
Reunion				✓	(✓)			✓		
Romania	(✓)			(✓)	(✓)			✓		
Russia				(✓)	(✓)			✓	(✓)	
Rwanda				✓	(✓)		(✓)	✓	(✓)	
São Tomé & Principe			✗	✓	(✓)		(✓)	✓	(✓)	✗
Saudi Arabia		✗		✓	(✓)	✗	(✓)	✓	(✓)	✗
Senegal				✓	(✓)		(✓)	✓	(✓)	✗
Serbia/ Montenegro				(✓)				✓	(✓)	
Seychelles				✓	(✓)			✓	(✓)	
Sierra Leone				✓	(✓)		(✓)	✓	(✓)	
Singapore				✓	(✓)			✓		
Slovak Republic										
Slovenia				(✓)				✓	(✓)	
Solomon Islands				✓	(✓)			✓		
Somalia			✗	✓	(✓)		(✓)	✓	(✓)	✗
South Africa				✓	(✓)			✓	(✓)	
Spain				(✓)		✗				

Tetanus	Typhoid	Yellow Fever	HIV Test	Water Quality	Malaria Risk	COMMENTS
✓	✓	c		1	none	Some DF
✓			(✓)	2	none	TBE is working; Lyme disease
		(c)		2	none	Nothing required
✓	(✓)			2	none	Avoid insect bites
✓	✓	c	(✓)	2	none	TB, leprosy, syphilis certificates may be needed
✓	✓	c		3	none	
✓	(✓)			3	none	Diphtheria and TB present; TBE and Lyme disease present
✓	(✓)		(✓)	2	none	Diphtheria and TB present; some TBE and Lyme disease
✓	✓	✓c		3	high	Many local diseases
✓	✓	✓c		3	high	
✓	✓	c		2	moderate	DF and parasites present
✓	✓	✓c		3	high	Many regional diseases
✓	(✓)			2	none	Some TBE
✓	✓	c	(✓)	2	none	
✓	✓	✓c		3	high	Lassa fever rurally
✓	✓	c	(✓)	2	none	Some DF
			(✓)	2	none	TBE minor risk
✓	(✓)			2	none	TBE in some areas
✓	✓	c		3	moderate	JE rurally; soil parasites
✓	✓	✓c		3	high	
✓	✓	c		2	moderate	
	(✓)			2	none	Some MSF and Lyme disease

COUNTRY	Cholera	Echinococcosis	Filariasis	Hepatitis A	Hepatitis B	Leishmaniasis	Meningitis	Polio	Rabies	Schistosomiasis
Sri Lanka			✗	✓	(✓)			✓	(✓)	
St Kitts & Nevis				(✓)				✓		
St Lucia				(✓)				✓		
St Vincent & the Grenadines			✗	(✓)				✓		
Sudan				✓	(✓)	✗	(✓)	✓	(✓)	
Suriname			✗	✓	(✓)	✗		✓	(✓)	✗
Swaziland				✓	(✓)			✓	(✓)	✗
Sweden										
Switzerland										
Syria				✓	(✓)	✗		✓	(✓)	✗
Taiwan				✓	(✓)			✓	(✓)	
Tajikistan	(✓)			(✓)			✗	✓	(✓)	
Tanzania	(✓)			✓	(✓)		(✓)	✓	(✓)	✗
Thailand				✓	(✓)			✓	(✓)	
Togo				✓				✓		
Tokelau			✗	✓	(✓)			✓		
Tonga			✗	✓	(✓)			✓		
Trinidad & Tobago				(✓)				✓	[✓]	
Tunisia				✓	(✓)	✗		✓	(✓)	
Turkey				✓	(✓)	✗	[✓]	✓	(✓)	✗

Tetanus	Typhoid	Yellow Fever	HIV Test	Water Quality	Malaria Risk	COMMENTS
✓	✓	c		2	moderate	JE for rural stays; DF and haemorrhagic form present; soil-borne parasites
✓	(✓)	c		2	none	Some DF
✓	(✓)	c		2	none	
✓	(✓)	c		2	none	Some DF
✓	✓	✓c		3	high	Regional diseases
✓	✓	✓c		3	high	DF present
✓	✓	c		3	high	Avoid tick bites
				1	none	Nothing required; some tick-borne diseases rurally
				1	none	Avoid tick bites; nothing required
✓	✓	c	(✓)	2	moderate	
✓	✓	c		2	none	JE rurally; some DF; parasites in uncooked food
✓	(✓)			3	moderate	Diphtheria and TB; TBE in forests
✓	✓	✓c		3	high	Orch. and tick typhus present
✓	✓	c		2	moderate	JE rurally and some DF
✓	✓	✓c		3	high	Lassa fever rurally
✓	✓			2	none	Some JE and DF
✓	✓	c		2	none	Some JE and DF
✓	(✓)	(✓)c		2	low	Some DF present
✓	✓	c		2	low	Parasites common
✓	(✓)			2	moderate	Tick-borne diseases

COUNTRY	Cholera	Echinococcosis	Filariasis	Hepatitis A	Hepatitis B	Leishmaniasis	Meningitis	Polio	Rabies	Schistosomiasis
Turkmenistan				(✓)	(✓)			✓	(✓)	
Turks & Caicos				(✓)				✓		
Tuvalu			✗	✓	(✓)			✓		
Uganda	(c)			✓	(✓)		(✓)	✓	(✓)	
Ukraine				(✓)	(✓)	✗		✓	(✓)	
United Arab Emirates				✓	(✓)	✗		✓	(✓)	
Uruguay				✓	[✓]			✓	(✓)	
USA										
Uzbekistan	(✓)			✓	(✓)	✗		✓	(✓)	
Vanuatu			✗	✓	(✓)			✓		
Venezuela				✓	(✓)			✓	(✓)	✗
Vietnam				✓	(✓)			✓	(✓)	✗
Virgin Islands								(✓)		✗
Wallis & Futuna			✗	✓	(✓)			✓		
Western Samoa			✗	✓	(✓)			✓		
Yemen				✓	(✓)	✗		✓	(✓)	✗
Zaire *see* Congo (Zaire)										
Zambia				✓	(✓)		(✓)	✓	(✓)	
Zimbabwe				✓	(✓)		(✓)	✓	(✓)	

Tetanus	Typhoid	Yellow Fever	HIV Test	Water Quality	Malaria Risk	COMMENTS
✓	(✓)			3	none	Diphtheria and TB; tick-borne diseases
✓	(✓)	c		2	none	
✓	✓	c		2	none	Some JE and DF
✓	✓	✓c		3	high	Many other diseases
✓	(✓)		(✓)	3	none	Diphtheria and TB; TBE in forests; also Lyme disease
✓	✓		(✓)	2	low	Tick typhus present
✓	✓			2	none	Chagas' disease rurally
				1	none	Nothing required
✓	✓		✓	2	low	Diphtheria and TB; TBE in forests
✓	✓			2	high	JE and DF in some areas
✓	✓	✓		2	high	DF quite common
✓	✓	c		3	low	JE rurally; DF present; many parasites
(✓)				2	none	Some DF
✓	✓			2	none	JE for long stay; DF and River Ross fever present
✓	✓	c		2	none	DF present
✓	✓	c		2	moderate	Orch. and other parasites present
✓	✓	c		3	high	Worm parasites common rurally
✓	✓	c		3	moderate	Hookworm common

A–Z of Medical Terms

A

abdomen the region of the body that lies below the THORAX, being divided from it by the DIAPHRAGM, and above the PELVIS. The abdominal cavity contains the DIGESTIVE ORGANS (e.g. the STOMACH and INTESTINES), the EXCRETORY ORGANS (BLADDER and KIDNEYS) and, in females, the REPRODUCTIVE ORGANS (UTERUS and OVARIES).

abortion the removal of an EMBRYO or FOETUS from the UTERUS, either by natural expulsion or by human intervention, before it is considered to be viable at the 24th week of PREGNANCY. An abortion may be spontaneous, and this is commonest during the first three months of pregnancy and is thought to be most often associated with abnormalities in the foetus. Or an abortion may be induced, when it is also descvribed as therapeutic, or termination of pregnancy, and is carried out for medical or social reasons.

abscess a collection of pus at a localized site anywhere in the body resulting from an infection caused by bacteria. Treatment is by the surgical opening of the abscess and by the administration of ANTIBIOTICS.

acetabulum *see* HIP JOINT.

acetonuria *see* KETONURIA.

acetylcholine an important organic chemical substance that is present in the body and is known as a NEUROTRANSMITTER. It is involved in the transmission of electrical impulses along nerves.

acetylsalicylic acid the chemical name for ASPIRIN.

achalasia a failure to relax, usually referring to a condition called achalasia of the cardia. It describes the situation where the muscle fibres surrounding the opening of the OESOPHAGUS (gullet) into the stomach do not relax properly and hinder the passage of swallowed food.

Achilles tendon a large, thick TENDON present in the lower leg that attaches the calf muscles to the heel bone, enabling this to be moved. It is prone to damage during the playing of sport.

achondroplasia the commonest cause of DWARFISM, in which the long bones of the limbs are abnormally short. It is inherited as a dominant characteristic in both sexes.

acidosis a condition in which the acidity of the BLOOD and body fluids rises to an abnormally high level as a result of a failure in the mechanisms that regulate the acid/base balance in the body. It is commonly caused by a faulty METABOLISM, as in DIABETES MELLITUS, or during starvation and excessive vomiting.

acini (*sing* **acinus**) *see* PANCREAS.

acquired a term used to describe a condition or malady that is not CONGENITAL but arises after birth.

acromegaly an abnormal growth of BONES and tissues in the hands, head, feet and chest, caused by excessive secretion of GROWTH HORMONE by the PITUITARY GLAND.

acrosome *see* SPERM.

ACTH *see* ADRENOCORTICOTROPHIC HORMONE.

action potential *see* NERVE IMPULSE.

acute a term used to describe a disease or condition that is short-lived and starts rapidly with severe symptoms.

Addison's disease a disease caused by the failure of the ADRENAL GLANDS to secrete the adrenocortical hormones, because the adrenal cortex has been damaged. It most frequently results from disturbances in the immune system. The symptoms are wasting, weakness, low blood pressure and dark pigmentation of the skin.

adenine *see* NUCLEOTIDE.

adenitis inflammation of one or more GLANDS or LYMPH NODES.

adenoids a clump of lymphoid tissue situated at the back of the nose (in the nasopharynx). The adenoids may become swollen as a result of persistent throat infections and obstruct breathing.

adenohypophysis *see* PITUITARY GLAND.

adenosine triphosphate *see* ATP.

adhesion the joining together of two surfaces that should normally be separate as a result of severe INFLAMMATION. Bands of FIBROUS TISSUE are formed that join the structures together. Adhesions may form within a damaged joint or following abdominal surgery, when they may form between loops of the intestine, etc. Adhesions at a JOINT restrict its movement (ANKYLOSIS) and can sometimes be resolved by manipulation. Adhesions within the abdomen or involving the lungs (in PLEURISY) may require surgery.

adipose tissue a type of loose, fibrous CONNECTIVE TISSUE containing a mass of fat cells. It is a reserve energy store and has an insulating function.

adrenal gland *or* **suprarenal gland** each of the two KIDNEYs within the body bears an adrenal GLAND on its upper surface. The adrenal glands are important ENDOCRINE organs, producing HORMONES that regulate various body functions. Each adrenal gland has two parts, an outer CORTEX and an inner MEDULLA, which secrete a variety of hormones, two of the most important being ADRENALINE and CORTISONE.

adrenaline *or* **epinephrine** a very important HORMONE produced by the MEDULLA of the ADRENAL GLANDS, which, when released, prepares the body for 'fright, flight or fight' by increasing the depth and rate of RESPIRATION, raising the heartbeat rate and improving MUSCLE performance. It also has an inhibitive effect on the processes of DIGESTION and EXCRETION. It can be used medically in a variety of ways, for instance in the treatment of bronchial ASTHMA, where it relaxes the airways, and also to stimulate the heart when there is cardiac arrest. *See* ADDISON'S DISEASE.

adrenocorticotrophic hormone (ACTH) an important substance produced and stored by the anterior PITUITARY GLAND. It regulates the release of CORTICOS-TEROID hormones from the ADRENAL GLANDS and is used medically, by INJECTION, to test their function. It is also used in the treatment of ASTHMA and rheumatic disorders.

adult respiratory distress syndrome a condition of severe respiratory failure brought about by a number of different disorders. There is a lack of oxygen in the blood, which exhibits itself by imparting a blue tinge to the skin (CYANOSIS) and rapid breathing and pulse rate. The syndrome may be caused by physical damage to the LUNGS, by INFECTION or by an adverse reaction following surgery or transfusion. It is often fatal.

afferent a term meaning 'inwards to an organ, etc', especially the BRAIN or SPINAL CORD, e.g. an afferent NERVE. *Compare* EFFERENT.

African trypanosomiasis *see* SLEEPING SICKNESS.

afterbirth a mass of tissue that consists of the PLACENTA, UMBILICAL CORD and membranes, detached and expelled from the womb (URERUS) during the third stage of LABOUR following a birth.

agglutinin, agglutinogen *see* BLOOD GROUPS.

agonist *see* FLEXOR.

Aids the acronym for Acquired Immune Deficiency Syndrome. *See* page 61.

albinism an inherited disorder in which there is a lack of pigmentation in the SKIN, HAIR and EYES. The PIGMENT involved is MELANIN.

albino an individual affected by ALBINISM who typically has pink skin and eyes and white hair. The pink colour is imparted by blood in the blood vessels in the skin, which, in a normal person, is masked by the presence of the pigment MELANIN.

albumin a water-soluble PROTEIN that coagulates when heated and is found in PLASMA, egg white, etc.

alimentary canal the whole of the passage along which food is passed, starting at the MOUTH and ending at the ANUS.

alkalosis an abnormal rise in the alkalinity (a decrease in pH) of the blood and body fluids because of a failure or swamping of the mechanisms that regulate the acid-base balance in the body. It may arise through acid loss following prolonged vomiting or occur in a patient who has been treated for a gastric ulcer with a large amount of alkalis. Respiratory alkalosis may arise if breathing is too deep for the amount of physical exertion being undertaken. The symptoms of alkalosis include muscular cramps and fatigue.

allotransplant *see* TRANSPLANTATION.

allele one of several forms of a GENE at a given place on the CHROMOSOME. They are usually present on different chromosomes and are responsible for certain characteristics of the PHENOTYPE. It is the dominance of one allele over another that determines the phenotype of the individual.

allergen any substance, usually a PROTEIN, that causes a hypersensitive (allergic) reaction in a person who is exposed to the allergen. There is a great variety of allergens, which cause reactions in different tissues and body functions.

allergy a state of hypersensitivity in an affected individual to a particular ALLERGEN, which produces a characteristic response whenever the person is exposed to the substance. In an unaffected person, ANTIBODIES present in the bloodstream destroy their particular antigens (allergens). However, in an affected individual this reaction causes some cell damage and there is a release of substances, such as HISTAMINE, which cause the allergic reaction. Examples of allergies are dermatitis, hay fever, asthma and the severe response known as ANAPHYLAXIS.

alopecia *see* BALDNESS.

alpha fetoprotein a type of PROTEIN formed in the liver and gut of the FOETUS, detectable in the AMNIOTIC FLUID and maternal blood. It is normally present in small amounts, but when the foetus has a neural tube defect (SPINA BIFIDA and ANENCEPHALY) this level rises higher in the first six months of pregnancy. *See* AMNIOCENTESIS.

alveolus (*pl* **alveoli**) a small sac or cavity that in numbers forms the alveolar sacs at the end of the BRONCHIOLES in the lungs. Each alveolus is fed by a rich blood supply via capillaries (*see* CAPILLARY) and is lined with a moist membrane where oxygen and carbon dioxide, the respiratory gases, are exchanged. The alveolar sacs provide an enormous surface area for efficient respiration.

Alzheimer's disease the commonest cause of DEMENTIA, afflicting those in middle or old age, and a degenerative disease of the CEREBRAL CORTEX for which there is no cure. Symptoms include progressive loss of memory and speech and paralysis. The cause is not understood but is the subject of ongoing research.

amines naturally occurring compounds found in the body which have an important role in a variety of functions. They are derived from AMINO ACIDS and ammonia and include such substances as ADRENALINE and HISTAMINE.

amino acids the end products of the digestion of PROTEIN foods and the building blocks from which all the protein components of the body are built up. They all contain an acidic carboxyl group (-COOH) and an amino group (-NH$_2$), which are both bonded to the same central carbon atom. Some can be manufactured within the body whereas others, the ESSENTIAL AMINO ACIDS, must be derived from protein sources in the diet.

amnesia loss of memory, which may be partial or total. Anterograde amnesia is the loss of memory of recent events following a trauma of some kind. Retrograde amnesia is the inability to remember events that preceded a trauma. Other types of amnesia are post-traumatic and hysterical and more than one kind may be experienced by an individual.

amniocentesis a procedure carried out to sample the AMNIOTIC FLUID surrounding a FOETUS. A fine needle is inserted through the abdominal wall of the mother and the amniotic sac is pierced so that a small quantity of fluid can be drawn off. The amniotic fluid contains ALPHA FETOPROTEIN and cells from the embryo, and various disorders such as DOWN'S SYNDROME and SPINA BIFIDA can be detected. It is usually carried out between the 16th and 20th week of pregnancy if a foetal abnormality is suspected.

amnion a fibrous, tough membranous sac that lines the womb and encloses the FOETUS floating within it surrounded by AMNIOTIC FLUID. A CAUL is a piece of the amnion.

amniotic fluid the liquid in the AMNIOTIC CAVITY, which is clear and composed mainly of water containing foetal cells, lipids and urine from the FOETUS. At first it is produced by the AMNION, but its volume is supplemented by urine from the kidneys of the foetus. It is circulated by being swallowed by the foetus and excreted by the kidneys back into the cavity and has an important protective function. The amniotic fluid ('waters') is released when the membranes rupture during LABOUR.

amoeba (*pl* **amoebae**) a microscopic invertebrate that consists of a gelatinous mass which constantly alters its state. It is found in freshwater ponds and ditches and in soil. It is parasitic in humans and animals and can cause amoebic DYSENTERY and amoebiasis.

amoebiasis an intestinal INFECTION caused by AMOEBae.

amphetamines a group of drugs that are chemically similar to ADRENALINE and have a stimulating effect on the CENTRAL NERVOUS SYSTEM. They act on the SYMPATHETIC NERVOUS SYSTEM and produce feelings of mental alertness and wellbeing, eliminating tiredness. They are highly addictive and dangerous, and their medical use is very strictly controlled.

ampullae (*sing* **ampulla**) *see* BREAST.

amylase *see* DIASTASE; ENZYME; PANCREAS.

anabolic steroid a synthetic male sex HORMONE (that mimicks ANDROGEN) used to enhance tissue growth by promoting the build-up of PROTEIN, e.g. to enhance MUSCLE bulk. Anabolic steroids are used medically to aid weight gain after wasting illnesses and to promote growth in children with certain types of DWARFISM. They may also be used in the treatment of OSTEOPOROSIS. They should not be taken by healthy people as they have serious SIDE EFFECTS, especially after prolonged use, and have been misused by athletes.

anabolism *see* CATABOLISM; METABOLISM.

anaemia a decrease in the ability of the BLOOD to carry oxygen because of a reduction in the number of red blood cells (ERYTHROCYTES) or in the amount of HAEMOGLOBIN that they contain. There are a number of different types of anaemia and a variety of reasons for it, and treatment depends on the underlying cause.

anaesthesia a loss of sensation or feeling in the whole or part of the body, usually relating to the administration of ANAESTHETIC drugs so that surgery can be performed without pain. *See also* EPIDURAL ANAESTHESIA; SPINAL ANAESTHESIA.

anaesthetic a substance that, when administered, produces a loss of sensation in the whole body (general anaesthetic) or part of it (local anaesthetic). A general anaesthetic results in a loss of consciousness, and usually a combination of drugs is used to achieve an optimum effect. These drugs act to depress the activity of the CENTRAL NERVOUS SYSTEM, have an ANALGESIC effect and relax MUSCLES, enabling surgical procedures to be carried out with no awareness on the part of the patient. A local anaesthetic blocks the transmission of NERVE IMPULSES in the area where it is applied so that no pain is felt.

analgesic a drug or substance that relieves pain, varying in potency from mild, such as PARACETAMOL and ASPIRIN, to very strong, e.g. MORPHINE.

anaphylaxis a response exhibited by a hypersensitive individual when confronted with a particular ANTIGEN. It results from the release of HISTAMINE in body tissues following the antigen-antibody reaction within CELLS. An allergic reaction is an example of mild anaphylaxis. Anaphylatic shock is a much rarer and more serious condition that can follow the injection of drugs or VACCINES, or a bee sting, to which the individual is hypersensitive.

anaplasia the condition in which cells and tissues become less differentiated and distinctive and revert to a more primitive form. This state is typical in TUMOURS that are MALIGNANT and growing very rapidly.

androgen one of a group of HORMONES that is responsible for the development of the sex organs and also the SECONDARY SEXUAL CHARACTERISTICS in the male. Androgens are steroid HORMONES, and the best-known example is TESTOSTERONE. They are mainly secreted by the testes (*see* TESTICLE) in the male but are also produced by the adrenal cortex and by the ovaries of females in small amounts.

aneurysm a balloon-like swelling in the wall of an artery that occurs when it becomes weakened or damaged in some way. There may be a congenital weakness in the muscular wall of the artery involved, as is often the case within the brain. Damage may also be the result of infection, particularly SYPHILIS, or degenerative conditions, e.g. ATHEROMA.

angina a suffocating, choking pain, usually used in reference to angina pectoris, which is felt in the chest. The pain is felt or brought on by exercise and relieved by rest, and occurs when the blood supply to the heart muscle is inadequate. During exercise the demand for blood (supplied by the coronary arteries) is increased and if the supply is insufficient, because the arteries are damaged, chest pain results. The coronary arteries may be damaged by ATHEROMA, the most common cause. Angina pectoris is usually first treated with drugs but if the condition worsens, coronary-artery bypass surgery may need to be performed.

angioma a clump of distended BLOOD VESSELS pushing onto the surface of the BRAIN. It may cause EPILEPSY and occasionally a vessel may burst to cause a SUBARACHNOID HAEMORRHAGE.

angitis *or* **vasculitis** a condition in which there is inflammation of the walls of small blood vessels, usually in patches.

animal starch *see* GLYCOGEN.

anorexia literally, a loss of appetite. Anorexia nervosa is a psychological disorder in which a person has a false image of himself or herself as being fat and a develops a fear or phobia relating to obesity and becomes unable to eat. He or she may take laxatives and induce vomiting, as well as starving, in order to lose weight. Accompanying symptoms include AMENORRHEA, low BLOOD PRESSURE, ANAEMIA and a risk of sudden death from heart damage.

anoxia the condition in which the body tissues do not receive sufficient oxygen. It may be caused by high altitudes (and thus lower atmospheric pressure), a lack of red blood cells, or a disease such as PNEUMONIA in which the amount of oxygen reaching the lung surfaces is limited and therefore that available for transfer to the blood is reduced.

antacid a substance that neutralizes acidity, usually hydrochloric acid in the digestive juices of the stomach.

antagonistic action an action in which systems or processes act against each other so that the activity of one reduces that of the other. Two MUSCLES may operate in this way, the contraction of one necessitating the relaxation of the other, as in the movement of a limb (*see* VOLUNTARY MUSCLE). Hormones and drugs also act antagonistically, the release of one limiting the effect of the other.

antenatal before birth. Pregnant women attend antenatal clinics, which monitor the health of mothers and their unborn babies.

anterior a term meaning 'situated towards the front or at the front', the opposite of POSTERIOR.

anthracosis *see* PNEUMOCONIOSIS.

anthrax *see* page 103.

antibiotic a substance, derived from a microorganism, that kills or inhibits the multiplication of other microorganisms, usually BACTERIA or fungi. Examples are PENICILLIN and STREPTOMYCIN.

antibodies PROTEIN substances of the GLOBULIN type that are produced by lymphoid tissue and circulate in the blood. They react with their corresponding ANTIGENS, neutralize them and render them harmless. They are produced against a wide variety of antigens and these reactions are responsible for IMMUNITY and ALLERGY.

anticoagulant a drug that delays or tends to prevent blood clotting, examples of which are warfarin and heparin. These are used in the treatment of EMBOLISM and THROMBOSIS to disperse blood clots in vessels.

anticonvulsant a drug that is used to reduce the severity of epileptic fits (CONVULSIONS) or to prevent them from occurring.

antidepressant a drug that is administered in order to alleviate depression and its accompanying symptoms.

antidiuretic hormone *see* VASOPRESSIN.

antidote a substance that counteracts the effect of a poison.

antiemetic a drug taken to prevent VOMITING.

antigen any substance that causes the formation by the body of ANTIBODIES to neutralize their effect. Antigens are often PROTEIN substances, regarded as 'foreign' and 'invading' by the body, and elicit the production of antibodies against them. *See* ALLERGEN; ALLERGY; ANAPHYLAXIS.

antihaemophilic factor *see* FACTOR VIII.

antihistamines drugs that counteract the effects of HISTAMINE release in the body.

They are widely used to treat allergic reactions of various sorts, particularly to relieve skin conditions. Those taken by mouth have a sedative effect and so care must be taken.

anti-inflammatory anything that reduces INFLAMMATION. Typical anti-inflammatory drugs are the ANTIHISTAMINES and NON-STEROIDAL ANTI-INFLAMMATORY DRUGS.

antimetabolite one of a group of drugs, used in the treatment of certain cancers, that mimic substances (metabolites) present in the cells. They combine with ENZYMES that would otherwise use the metabolites for cell growth. Hence they reduce the growth of cancer cells but also have attendant SIDE EFFECTS, which can be severe.

antiseptic a substance that prevents the growth of disease-causing microorganisms, such as BACTERIA, and is applied to the skin to prevent infection and to cleanse wounds.

antiserum a SERUM, usually prepared from horses, that contains a high concentration of ANTIBODIES against a particular ANTIGEN. It is injected to give IMMUNITY against a particular disease or TOXIN.

antitoxin *see* TOXIN; TOXOID.

antrum (*pl* **antra**) a natural CAVITY or SINUS, particularly in a BONE.

anuria a failure of the KIDNEYS to produce URINE, which may result from a disorder that causes a prolonged drop in BLOOD PRESSURE. Anuria is typical of increasing URAEMIA, and HAEMODIALYSIS may be necessary.

anus the opening of the ALIMENTARY CANAL, at the opposite end from the MOUTH, through which FAECES are voided. The anus is at the lower end of the bowel and its opening is controlled by two MUSCLES, the internal and external SPHINCTERS.

aorta the major large ARTERY of the body, which arises from the left VENTRICLE of the HEART and which carries BLOOD to all areas. The other arteries of the body are all derived from the aorta.

aortic having to do with the AORTA, e.g. the aortic VALVE.

aortic stenosis a narrowing of the opening of the aortic VALVE, resulting in the obstruction of BLOOD flow from the left VENTRICLE to the AORTA. A common cause of this is calcium deposits formed on the valve, associated with ATHEROMA, or damage may have been caused by previous RHEUMATIC FEVER. It may also be CONGENITAL. The effect is that the left ventricle muscle has to work harder to try to maintain the blood flow and becomes thicker as a result.

aphasia speechlessness caused by disease or injury to those parts of the brain that govern the activities involved in speech-making. It is caused by THROMBOSIS, EMBOLISM or HAEMORRHAGE of a blood vessel within the brain, as in a STROKE, or by a TUMOUR.

aplasia a complete or partial failure in the correct development of an organ or tissue.

apnoea a temporary halt in breathing, which may result from a number of different causes. Apnoea is quite common in newborn infants and can be registered by an apnoea monitor, which sounds an alarm if the baby ceases to breathe.

apocrine the term for SWEAT GLANDS that occur in hairy parts of the body. The odours associated with sweating are the result of bacterial action on the sweat produced. *See also* PERSPIRATION.

apoplexy *see* STROKE.

appendicitis INFLAMMATION of the vermiform APPENDIX, which, in its acute form, is the most common abdominal emergency in the western world, usually requiring treatment by surgical removal.

appendix a blind-ended tube that is an appendage of various organs within the body. It normally refers to the vermiform appendix, which projects from the CAECUM of the large INTESTINE. It has no known function and can become the site of infection.

aqueous humour *see* EYE and GLAUCOMA.

arachidonic *see* ESSENTIAL FATTY ACID.

arachnodactyly *see* MARFAN'S SYNDROME.

arachnoid mater the enveloping MEMBRANE of the BRAIN and SPINAL CORD, between the dura mater and the pia mater. *See* MENINGES.

arenavirus a HAEMORRHAGIC FEVER virus. *See* page 128.

Argentinian *or* **Junín haemorrhagic virus** *see* page 126.

arginine *see* ESSENTIAL AMINO ACID.

arrhythmia any disturbance in the normal rhythm of heartbeat. The built-in PACE-MAKER of the HEART is the SINOATRIAL NODE situated in the wall of the right ATRIUM, which itself is regulated by the AUTONOMIC NERVOUS SYSTEM. The electrical impulses produced by the pacemaker control the rate and rhythm of heartbeat. Arrhythmias occur when these electrical impulses are disturbed.

arteriole a small branch of an ARTERY leading to a CAPILLARY.

arteriosclerosis a vague term used to describe several degenerative conditions affecting the arteries. *See also* ATHEROMA, ATHEROSCLEROSIS and HYPERTEN-SION.

arteritis INFLAMMATION of an ARTERY.

artery a BLOOD VESSEL that carries blood away from the HEART. Oxygenated (bright red) blood is carried by the arteries to all parts of the body. However, the pulmonary arteries carry dark, unoxygenated blood from the heart to the LUNGS. An artery has thick, elastic walls that are able to expand and contract and contain smooth MUSCLE fibres under the control of the SYMPATHETIC NERVOUS SYSTEM.

arthritis INFLAMMATION of the JOINTS or SPINAL COLUMN, the symptoms of which are pain and swelling, restriction of movement, redness and warmth of the skin. There are many different causes, including OSTEOARTHRITIS, RHEUMATOID ARTHRITIS, TUBERCULOSIS and RHEUMATIC FEVER.

artificial insemination SEMEN collected from a donor that is inserted by means of an instrument into the VAGINA of a woman in the hope that she will conceive.

artificial respiration an emergency procedure carried out when normal respiration has ceased in order to ventilate the lungs artificially, usually referred to as 'mouth-to-mouth resuscitation'. In hospital, where a seriously ill person is unable to breathe unaided, artificial respiration is achieved by a machine called a ventilator.

asbestosis a disease of the lungs caused by the inhalation of asbestos dust. Asbestos dust causes scarring of the lungs. There is a serious risk of MESOTHE-LIOMA or cancer of the lung.

ascorbic acid *see* VITAMIN C.

asphyxia the state of suffocation during which breathing eventually stops and oxygen fails to reach tissues and organs. It occurs as a result of drowning, strangulation and inhaling poisonous fumes. It can also result from obstruction of the air passages either by a foreign body lodged at the opening (e.g. a piece of food) or swelling as a result of a wound or infection.

aspiration the process of removing fluid or gases from cavities in the body by means of suction, using an aspirator.

aspirin *or* **acetylsalicylic** a drug in widespread use for relieving mild pain, e.g. headache, neuralgia and that associated with RHEUMATOID ARTHRITIS. It is used to combat fever and is also helpful in the prevention of CORONARY THROMBOSIS. In susceptible individuals it may cause irritation and bleeding of the stomach lining and is not normally given to children under the age of 12.

asthma a condition characterized by breathing difficulties caused by narrowing of the airways (BRONCHI) of the lung. It may occur at any age but usually begins in early childhood and is a hypersensitive response that can be brought on by exposure to a variety of ALLERGENS, exercise, stress or INFECTIONS. An sufferer may have other hypersensitive conditions, such as ECZEMA and HAY FEVER.

astigmatism a defect in VISION that results in sight being blurred and distorted. It is caused by abnormal curvature of the CORNEA.

ataxia a loss of coordination in the limbs because of a disorder of the CENTRAL NERVOUS SYSTEM. There may be a disease of the SENSORY nerves (sensory ataxia) or of the CEREBELLUM (cerebellar ataxia). An ataxic person has clumsy movements and lacks fine control.

atheroma a degenerative condition of the arteries (*see* ARTERY). The inner and middle coats of the arterial walls become scarred, and fatty deposits (CHOLESTEROL) are built up at these sites. Blood CIRCULATION is impaired, and it may lead to such problems as ANGINA pectoris, stroke and MYOCARDIAL INFARCTION.

atherosclerosis similar to ATHEROMA, being a degenerative disease of the arteries (*see* ARTERY) associated with fatty deposits on the inner walls, leading to reduced blood flow.

athetosis *see* CEREBRAL PALSY.

athlete's foot a fungal infection of the skin, particularly between the toes and often caused by RINGWORM.

atlas the first cervical VERTEBRA of the SPINAL COLUMN, which articulates with the OCCIPITAL BONE.

ATP (adenosine triphosphate) an important molecule, found in MITOCHONDRION, that is synthesized or broken down to produce energy to drive metabolic processes.

atrial the term used to describe anything relating to the ATRIUM.

atrium (*pl* **atria**) **1.** one of the two thin-walled, upper chambers of the HEART, which receive BLOOD from major VEINS. The right atrium receives (deoxygenated) blood from the venae cavae (*see* VENA CAVA) and the left atrium is supplied with (oxygenated) blood from the PULMONARY vein. **2.** a chamber in various other parts of the body.

atrophy the wasting of a body part because of lack of use, malnutrition or as a result of ageing.

aural a term used to describe anything relating to the ear.

auricle 1. the external part of the EAR flap, the pinna. **2.** an ear-shaped appendage of the ATRIUM of the heart.

autoantibody an antibody produced by the body against one of its own tissues, a feature of AUTOIMMUNE DISEASE.

autograft a graft of skin or tissue taken from one part of a person's body and transferred to another region. The graft is 'self' and is therefore not rejected by the body's IMMUNE system.

autoimmune disease one of a number of conditions resulting from the production of antibodies by the body that attack its own tissues. For reasons that are not yet understood the immune system loses the ability to distinguish between 'self' and 'non-self'. Autoimmune disease is currently thought to be the cause of a number of disorders, including acquired haemolytic ANAEMIA.

autoimmunity a failure of the immune system in which the body develops ANTI-BODIES that attack components or substances belonging to itself. *See* AUTOANTIBODY, AUTOIMMUNE DISEASE.

autonomic nervous system the part of the nervous system that controls body functions that are not under conscious control, e.g. the heartbeat and other smooth muscles and glands. It is divided into the SYMPATHETIC and PARASYM-PATHETIC NERVOUS SYSTEMS.

autotransplant *see* TRANSPLANTATION.

avidin *see* BIOTIN.

axon one of numerous long threadlike extensions of a NERVE cell that conduct NERVE IMPULSES from the CELL body. *See also* MOTOR NEURON; NEURON.

B

bacillus (*pl* **bacilli**) **1.** a bacterium (*see* BACTERIA) that is rod-shaped. **2.** a genus of Gram-positive (*see* GRAM'S STAIN) bacteria that includes *B. anthracis*, the cause of ANTHRAX.

Bacillus Calmette-Guérin vaccine *see* BCG VACCINE.

backache pain in the back, which may vary in intensity, sharpness and cause. Much back pain is the result of mechanical/structural problems, including FRACTURES, MUSCLE strain or pressure on a NERVE. Other causes may include tumours, BONE disease (such as OSTEOPOROSIS) referred pain from an ULCER or INFLAMMATIONS, e.g. SPONDYLITIS. Treatment is varied and may be surgical, by heat, ULTRASOUND, medication, etc.

backbone *see* SPINAL COLUMN.

bacteria (*sing* **bacterium**) single-celled organisms that underpin all life-sustaining processes. GRAM'S STAIN is a test used to distinguish between the two types. They are also identified by shape: spiral, (spirilli), rod-like (bacilli), spherical (cocci), comma-shaped (vibrios) and the spirochaetal, which are corkscrew-like. They are the key agents in the chemical cycles of carbon, oxygen, nitrogen and sulphur.

bactericide something that kills bacteria, used especially when referring to drugs and antiseptics.

bacteriophage *or* **phage** a VIRUS that attacks BACTERIA. They replicate in the host, which is ultimately destroyed as new phages are released. Each phage is specific to a certain bacterium and uses are found in genetic engineering, in cloning and manufacturing.

baldness the gradual depletion of HAIR on the head, which is, to a great extent, hereditary but may also be caused by disease. Alopecia is a patchy baldness of the scalp.

barbiturate a drug that has ANAESTHETIC, hypnotic or SEDATIVE effects. Barbiturates reduce BLOOD PRESSURE and body TEMPERATURE and depress the CENTRAL NERVOUS SYSTEM and RESPIRATION. TRANQUILLIZERS are replacing barbiturates to lessen drug abuse.

barium sulphate a chemical powder used in X-RAY examinations. Because of its opaque nature (to X-rays), it forms a shadow in whatever cavity it lies. It is used in the examination of the STOMACH and INTESTINES and to trace a meal through the digestive tract.

bartonellosis *see* SANDFLY FEVER.

basal ganglion (*pl* **basal glanglia**) GREY MATTER at the base of the CEREBRUM that is involved in the subconscious control of voluntary movement.

B-cell *see* LYMPHOCYTE.

BCG vaccine *or* **Bacillus Calmette-Guérin vaccine** a VACCINE against TUBERCULOSIS, usually administered intradermally.

bed sores *or* **pressure sores** *or* **decubitus ulcers** sore and ulcerated skin caused by constant pressure on an area of the body. Bedridden, particularly unconscious, patients are at risk, and their position has to be changed to relieve the prone areas: heels, buttocks, elbows, lower back, etc. The best action is preventative because healing may be slowed by reduced blood supply.

Bell's palsy a PARALYSIS of the facial MUSCLES on either or both sides of the FACE, caused by INFECTION or INFLAMMATION, when it may be temporary. Permanent paralysis may result from a basal skull fracture, stroke, etc. It results in an inability to open and close the eye or to smile or close the mouth on the side that is affected.

B endorphin a painkiller released by the PITUITARY in response to pain and stress.

bends *or* **compressed air illness** *or* **caisson disease** a condition that may affect workers operating in high pressure in diving bells or at depth underwater if they surface too rapidly. Pain in the joints (the bends), headache and dizziness (decompression sickness) and paralysis may be caused by the formation of nitrogen bubbles in the blood, which then accumulate in different parts of the body. Death may occur.

benign a term used most frequently to refer to TUMOURS, meaning not harmful, the opposite of MALIGNANT.

beriberi a disease that causes INFLAMMATION of the NERVES because of a dietary lack of VITAMIN B1 (thiamine) and results in fever, paralysis, palpitations and occasionally HEART FAILURE. It occurs mainly in countries where the staple diet is polished rice.

beta-blocker a drug used to treat ANGINA, reduce high BLOOD PRESSURE and manage abnormal HEART rhythms. Certain receptors of nerves in the SYMPATHETIC NERVOUS SYSTEM are blocked, reducing heart activity. A notable SIDE EFFECT is constriction of bronchial passages, which may adversely affect some patients.

biceps a MUSCLE that is said to have two heads, e.g. the biceps of the upper arm (biceps brachii).

bile a viscous, bitter fluid produced by the LIVER and stored in the GALL BLADDER. It is an alkaline solution of bile salts, pigments, some mineral salts and CHOLESTEROL, which aids in fat digestion and absorption of nutrients. Discharge of bile into the intestine is increased after food, and of the amount secreted each day (up to one litre), most is reabsorbed with the food, passing into the blood to circulate back to the liver. If the flow of bile into the intestine is restricted, it stays in the blood, resulting in JAUNDICE.

bile duct a duct that carries BILE from the liver. The main duct is the hepatic, which joins the cystic duct from the GALL BLADDER to form the common bile duct, which drains into the small INTESTINE.

bilharziasis *see* SCHISTOSOMIASIS.

bilirubin one of the two important BILE pigments, formed primarily from the breakdown of HAEMOGLOBIN from red blood cells. It is orange-yellow in colour while its oxidized form, biliverdin, is green. The majority of bile produced daily is eventually excreted and confers colour to the stools.

biliverdin *see* BILIRUBIN; JAUNDICE.

biopsy the removal of a small sample of living tissue from the body for examination under the microscope. It is particularly important in differentiating between benign and malignant TUMOURS.

biotin a B-complex VITAMIN that is synthesized by BACTERIA in the INTESTINE. A deficiency can occur only if large amounts of ALBUMIN are ingested because a constituent, avidin, binds to the biotin.

birthmark *or* **naevus** an agglomeration of dilated BLOOD VESSELS that creates a malformation of the skin and is present at birth. It may occur as a large port-wine stain, which can now be treated by laser, or a strawberry mark, which commonly fades in early life.

blackwater fever a severe and sometimes fatal form of MALARIA. *See* page 116.

bladder a SAC of fibrous and muscular tissue that contains secretions and can increase and decrease in capacity. Discharge of the contents is through a narrow opening (*see also* GALL BLADDER; URINARY ORGANS).

blindness the inability to see, a condition that may vary from a complete lack of light perception (total blindness) through degrees of visual impairment. The commonest causes are GLAUCOMA, senile CATARACT, VITAMIN A deficiency (night blindness) and DIABETES MELLITUS.

blister a thin VESICLE on the skin containing watery matter or SERUM.

blood a suspension of red blood cells (or corpuscles) called ERYTHROCYTES, white blood cells (LEUCOCYTES) and platelets (small disc-shaped cells involved in BLOOD CLOTting) in a liquid medium, blood PLASMA. The circulation of blood through the body provides a mechanism for transporting substances. Its functions include:

1 carrying oxygenated blood from the HEART to all tissues via the arteries while the veins return deoxygenated blood to the heart.

2 carrying essential nutrients, e.g. glucose, fats and AMINO ACIDS to all parts of the body.

3 removing the waste products of METABOLISM – ammonia and carbon dioxide – to the liver, where UREA is formed and then transported by the blood to the KIDNEYs for excretion.

4 carrying important molecules, e.g. HORMONES, to their target cells.

The red blood cells, produced in the BONE MARROW, are HAEMOGLOBIN-containing discs, while the white varieties vary in shape and are produced in the marrow and lymphoid tissue. The plasma comprises water, proteins and ELECTROLYTES and forms approximately half the blood volume.

blood clot a hard mass of blood PLATELETs, trapped red blood cells and FIBRIN. After tissue damage, blood vessels in the area are constricted and a plug forms to seal the damaged area. The plug formation is initiated by an ENZYME released by the damaged blood vessels and platelets.

blood groups the division and classification of people into one of four main groups based on the presence of ANTIGENS on the surface of the red blood cells (corpuscles). The classifying reaction depends on the SERUM of one person's blood agglutinating (clumping together) the red blood cells of someone else. The antigens, known as agglutinogens, react with ANTIBODIES (agglutinins) in the serum. There are two agglutinogens termed A and B and two agglutinins called anti-A and anti-B. This gives rise to four groups: corpuscles with no agglutinogens, group O; with A; with B; with both A and B (hence blood group AB). The agglutinin groups match those of the agglutinogens. thus a person of blood group B has anti-A serum in his or her blood. It is vital that blood groups are matched for transfusion because incompatibility will produce blood clotting. The rhesus factor or Rh factor is another antigen (named after the rhesus monkey, which has a similar antigen), those with it being Rh-positive and those without Rh-negative. About 85 per cent of people are Rh-positive. If a Rh-negative person receives Rh-positive blood, or if a Rh-positive FOETUS is exposed to antibodies to the factor in the blood of the Rh-negative mother, then HAEMOLYSIS occurs in the foetus and newborn child. This may cause the stillbirth of the child or jaundice after birth. Testing of pregnant women is thus essential.

blood poisoning *see* SEPTICAEMIA.

blood pressure the pressure of the blood on the HEART and BLOOD VESSELS in the system of CIRCULATION. Also, the pressure that has to be applied to an ARTERY to stop the PULSE beyond the pressure point. Blood pressure peaks at a heart beat (SYSTOLE) and falls in between (DIASTOLE). The systolic pressure in young adults is equivalent to approximately 120 mm mercury (and 70 mm in diastole). The pressure also depends on the hardness and thickness of vessel walls and tends to increase with age as arteries thicken and harden. A temporary rise in blood pressure may be precipitated by exposure to cold; a permanent rise by kidney disease and other disorders. A lower blood pressure can be induced by a hot bath or caused by exhaustion.

blood sugar glucose concentration in the BLOOD for which the typical value is 3.5 to 5.5 mmol/l (millimoles per litre). *See also* HYPOGLYCAEMIA and HYPER-GLYCAEMIA.

blood transfusion the replacement of BLOOD lost because of injury, surgery, etc. A patient may receive whole blood or a component, e.g. packed red cells (red blood cells separated from the PLASMA, used to counteract ANAEMIA and restore HAEMOGLOBIN levels). Blood from donors is matched to the recipient for BLOOD GROUP and haemoglobin.

blood vessel the VEINS and arteries (*see* ARTERY) and their smaller branchings, venules and arterioles, through which blood is carried to and from the HEART.

boil *or* **furuncle** a SKIN infection in a HAIR follicle or gland that produces INFLAMMATION and PUS. It is often caused by the bacterium *Staphylococcus*, but healing is generally quick upon release of the pus or administration of ANTIBIOTICS.

bone the hard connective tissue that, with CARTILAGE, forms the SKELETON. Bone has a matrix of COLLAGEN fibres with bone salts, in which are the bone cells, OSTEOBLASTS and OSTEOCYTES. The bone cells form the matrix. There are two types: compact or dense, forming the shafts of long bones, and spongy or cancellous, which occurs on the inside and at the ends of long bones and also forms the short bones. Compact bone is a hard tube covered by the periosteum (a membrane) and enclosing the BONE MARROW and contains very fine canals around which the bone is structured in circular plates. *See also* SKULL.

bone marrow a soft tissue found in the spaces of BONES. In young animals, all bone marrow, the red marrow, produces blood cells. In older animals the marrow in long bones is replaced by yellow marrow, which contains a large amount of fat and does not produce blood cells. In mature animals, the red marrow occurs in the ribs, sternum, vertebrae and the ends of the long bones (e.g. the femur). The red marrow contains MYELOID tissue with ERYTHROBLASTS from which red blood cells develop. LEUCOCYTES also form from the myeloid tissue and themselves give rise to other cell types.

botulism *see* page 75.

bovine spongiform encephalopathy (BSE) a disease of cattle that proves fatal and is similar to scrapie in sheep and CREUTZFELDT-JAKOB DISEASE in humans. *See* page 12.

bowel the large INTESTINE.

brachial relating to the upper arm, hence brachial artery, etc.

brachiocephalic trunk *see* INNOMINATE ARTERY.

bradycardia slowness of the heartbeat and pulse to below 60 per minute.

bradykinesia the condition in which there is abnormally slow movement of the body and limbs and slowness of speech, as may be caused by PARKINSONISM.

brain the part of the CENTRAL NERVOUS SYSTEM contained within the CRANIUM that is connected via the SPINAL CORD to the remainder of the nervous system. It interprets information received from SENSE ORGANS and emits signals to control MUSCLES. It comprises distinct areas: the CEREBRUM, CEREBELLUM, PONS, MEDULLA OBLONGATA and mid-brain or MESENCEPHALON. GREY MATTER and WHITE MATTER make up the brain, in different arrangements, and a dense network of BLOOD VESSELS supplies the grey matter, and both blood vessels and nerve cells are supported by a fibrous network, the NEUROGLIA. Three membranes (the MENINGES) separate the brain from the skull, and between each pair is a fluid-filled space to cushion the brain. There are 12 nerves connected to the brain, mainly in the region of the brain stem, and four arteries carrying blood to the brain. Two veins drain the central portion and many small veins open into venous SINUSes that connect with the internal jugular vein.

brain-stem death *or* **brain death** a complete and continuous absence of the vital reflexes controlled by centres in the brain stem (breathing, pupillary responses, etc). Tests are performed by independent doctors, repeated after an interval, before death is formally confirmed.

breast the MAMMARY GLAND that produces milk. Each breast has a number of compartments with lobules surrounded by fatty tissue and muscle fibres. Milk formed in the lobules gathers in branching tubes or ducts that together form lactiferous ducts. Near the nipple the ducts form ampullae (small 'reservoirs') from which the ducts discharge through the nipple.

breastbone *see* STERNUM.

breast cancer a CARCINOMA or SARCOMA, which is the commonest cancer in women. Incidence is low in countries where breast-feeding persists and animal fat intake in the diet is low. The first sign may be a lump in the breast or armpit (the latter being caused by spread to the LYMPH NODES). A localized TUMOUR may be removed surgically and, in addition, radiotherapy, chemotherapy and hormone therapy can form part of the treatment.

breathlessness a depletion in blood oxygen resulting in excessive and/or laboured breathing to gain more air. The causes are numerous, ranging from lung diseases or conditions (PNEUMONIA, EMPHYSEMA, BRONCHITIS) to heart conditions and obesity. In children, narrowing of the air passages is a cause, as is ASTHMA.

breech presentation the position of a baby in the UTERUS whereby it would be delivered buttocks first instead of the usual head-first delivery. The baby, and possibly the mother, may be at risk.

brittle bone disease *see* OSTEOGENESIS IMPERFECTA.

bronchi (*sing* **bronchus**) air passages supported by rings of CARTILAGE. Two bronchi branch off from the TRACHEA, and these split into further bronchi. The two main bronchi branch to form five lobar bronchi, then twenty segmental bronchi, and so on.

bronchial the term used to describe the BRONCHI and BRONCHIOLES.

bronchiectasis *see* CYSTIC FIBROSIS.

bronchioles very fine tubes occurring as branches of the BRONCHI. The bronchioles end in alveoli (*see* ALVEOLUS) where carbon dioxide and oxygen are exchanged.

bronchitis INFLAMMATION of the BRONCHI, which occurs in two forms, acute and chronic. BACTERIA or VIRUSES cause the acute form, which is initially typified by the symptoms of the common COLD but develops, with painful coughing, wheezing, throat and chest pains and the production of purulent (PUS-containing) MUCUS. If the infection spreads to the BRONCHIOLES (bronchiolitis) the consequences are more serious as the body is deprived of oxygen. Antibiotics and expectorants can relieve the symptoms. It is a common cause of death among the elderly, and there are several parameters of direct consequence to its cause: excessive smoking of cigarettes; cold, damp climate; obesity; respiratory infections. Damage to the bronchi and other complications may occur, giving rise to constant BREATHLESSNESS.

bronchodilator a drug used to relax the smooth MUSCLE of the BRONCHIOLES, thus increasing their diameter and the air supply to the LUNGS. They are used in the treatment of ASTHMA.

bronchopneumonia *see* PNEUMONIA.

brucellosis a disease of farm animals (pigs, cattle, goats) caused by a species of a Gram-negative bacillus, *Brucella* (*see* GRAM'S STAIN). It may be passed to humans through contact with an infected animal or by drinking contaminated, untreated, milk. It is characterized by fever, sweats, joint pains, backache and headache.

BSE the abbreviation of BOVINE SPONGIFORM ENCEPHALOPATHY.

bubonic plague *see* PLAGUE.

buccal a term used generally to pertain to the mouth, specifically the inside of the cheek or the gum next to the cheek.

bulimia nervosa an overwhelming desire to eat a lot of food, followed by misuse of LAXATIVES or induced VOMITING to avoid weight gain. There are some similarities with ANOREXIA nervosa.

bunion *see* CORN.

burns burns and scalds show similar symptoms and require similar treatment, the former being caused by dry heat, the latter by moist heat. Burns may also be caused by electric currents and chemicals. They are categorized as being either superficial, where sufficient tissue remains to ensure skin regrows, or deep, where GRAFTing will be necessary. Severe injuries can prove dangerous because of SHOCK as a result of fluid loss at the burn. For minor burns and scalds, treatment involves holding the affected area under cold water. In more severe cases, ANTISEPTIC dressings are normally applied, and in very severe cases hospitalization is required.

bursa (*pl* **bursae**) a small fluid-filled fibrous SAC that reduces friction between parts of the body, especially at the JOINTS.

bursitis HOUSEMAID'S KNEE.

C

caecum (*pl* **caeca**) an expanded, blind-ended SAC at the start of the large INTESTINE between the small intestine and COLON. The small intestine and vermiform APPENDIX open into the caecum.

Caesarean section a surgical operation to deliver a baby by means of an INCISION through the ABDOMEN and UTERUS. It is performed when there is a risk to the health of the baby or mother in normal delivery, both as a planned and as an emergency procedure.

caisson disease *see* BENDS.

calcaneus (*pl* **calcanei**) *see* TALUS.

calciferol a form of VITAMIN D that is manufactured in the SKIN in the presence of sunlight or derived from certain foods (e.g. liver and fish oils). Its main role is in calcium METABOLISM, enabling calcium to be absorbed from the gut and laid down in BONE. A deficiency leads to the bone disease OSTEOLAMACIA and also RICKETS.

calcification the deposition of calcium salts, which is normal in the formation of BONE but may occur at other sites in the body. *See* OSSIFICATION.

calcitonin *see* PAGET'S DISEASE OF BONE.

calcium a metallic element that is essential for normal growth and functioning of body processes. It is an important component of BONES and teeth and has a role in vital metabolic processes, e.g. muscle contraction, passage of nerve impulses and blood clotting. Its concentration in the blood is regulated by thyroid HORMONES.

calcium-channel blocker *or* **calcium antagonist** a drug that inhibits the movement of calcium ions into smooth MUSCLE and cardiac muscle cells. Their effect is to relax the muscle and reduce the strength of contraction and to cause VASODILATION. They are used in the treatment of high BLOOD PRESSURE and ANGINA.

calculi *see* CONCRETIONS.

cancer a widely used term for any form of malignant TUMOUR. It is characterized by an uncontrolled and abnormal growth of cancer cells, which invade surrounding tissues and destroy them. Cancer cells may spread throughout the body via the bloodstream or LYMPHATIC SYSTEM, a process known as METASTASIS, and set up secondary growths elsewhere. There are known to be a number of different causes, including smoking, radiation, ultraviolet light, some viruses and possibly the presence of cancer GENES (oncogenes). Treatment depends on the site of the cancer but involves radiotherapy, chemotherapy and surgery, and survival rates in affected people are showing encouraging improvements.

candidiasis *see* THRUSH.

Canicola fever *see* page 100.

canine *see* TOOTH.

capillary a fine BLOOD VESSEL that communicates with an ARTERIOLE or VENULE. They form networks in most tissues and have walls that are only one cell thick. There is a constant exchange of substances (oxygen, carbon dioxide, nutrients, etc) between the capillaries, arterioles and venules, supplying the needs of surrounding tissues.

capsule 1. a sheath of CONNECTIVE TISSUE or MEMBRANE surrounding an organ. The ADRENAL GLAND, KIDNEY and SPLEEN are all housed within a capsule. **2.** a FIBROUS TISSUE sheath surrounding various JOINTS. **3.** a small, gelatinous pouch containing a drug, which can be swallowed.

carbohydrates organic compounds, which include sugars and starch and contain carbon, hydrogen and oxygen. They are the most important source of energy available to the body and are an essential part of the diet. They are eventually broken down in the body to the simple sugar, glucose, which can be used by cells in numerous metabolic processes.

carbon dioxide *or* **carbonic acid** (formula CO_2) a gas formed in the tissues as a result of metabolic processes within the body. Medically, it is used combined with oxygen during ANAESTHESIA.

carbon monoxide (formula CO) an odourless and colourless gas that is highly dangerous when inhaled, leading to carbon monoxide poisoning. In the BLOOD it has a very great affinity for oxygen and converts HAEMOGLOBIN into carboxyhaemoglobin. The tissues of the body are quickly deprived of oxygen because there is no free haemoglobin left to pick it up in the LUNGS. Carbon monoxide is present in coal gas fumes and vehicle exhaust emissions. The symptoms of poisoning include giddiness, flushing of the skin (because of carboxyhaemoglobin in the blood, which is bright red), nausea, headache, raised respiratory and pulse rate and eventual coma, respiratory failure and death.

carboxyhaemoglobin *see* CARBON MONOXIDE.

carcinogen any substance that causes damage to tissue cells likely to result in CANCER. Various substances are known to be carcinogenic, including tobacco smoke, asbestos and ionizing radiation.

carcinoma a CANCER of the EPITHELIUM, i.e. the tissue that lines the body's internal organs and skin.

cardia the opening of the OESOPHAGUS into the STOMACH.

cardiac arrest the cessation of the pumping action of the HEART. There is a loss of consciousness and breathing and the PULSE ceases. Death follows very rapidly unless the heartbeat can be restored, and methods of achieving this include external or direct CARDIAC MASSAGE, ARTIFICIAL RESPIRATION and DEFIB-RILLATION.

cardiac cycle the whole sequence of events that produces a heartbeat and normally takes place in less than one second. The atria (*see* ATRIUM) contract together and force the BLOOD into the VENTRICLES (DIASTOLE). These then also contract (SYSTOLE), and blood exits the HEART and is pumped around the body. As the ventricles are contracting, the atria relax and fill up with blood once again.

cardiac massage a means of restoring the heartbeat if this has suddenly ceased. Direct cardiac massage, which is only feasible if the person is in hospital, involves massaging the HEART by hand through an INCISION in the chest wall. Another method, used in conjunction with ARTIFICIAL RESPIRATION, is by rhythmic compression of the chest wall while the person is laid on his or her back.

cardiac muscle specialized MUSCLE unique to the HEART, consisting of branching, elongated fibres possessing the ability to contract and relax continuously.

cardiac pacemaker *see* PACEMAKER; SINOATRIAL NODE.

cardiomyopathy any disease or disorder of the CARDIAC MUSCLE that may arise from a number of different causes, including viral infections, congenital abnormalities and chronic alcoholism.

cardiovascular system the HEART and the whole of the circulatory system, which is divided into the systemic (arteries and veins of the body) and pulmonary (arteries and veins of the lungs). It is responsible for the transport of oxygen and nutrients to the tissues, and for removing waste products and carbon dioxide from them, taking these to the organs from which they are eliminated.

carditis INFLAMMATION of the HEART.

carotid artery either of the two large arteries (*see* ARTERY) in the neck that branch and provide the BLOOD supply to the head and neck. The paired common carotid arteries arise from the AORTA on the left side of the HEART and from the innominate artery on the right. These continue up on either side of the neck and branch into the internal CAROTID BODY and the external carotid body.

carotid body a small area of specialized reddish-coloured tissue situated one on either side of the neck where the common CAROTID ARTERY branches to form the internal and external carotids. It is sensitive to chemical changes in the blood, containing CHEMORECEPTORS that respond to oxygen, carbon dioxide and hydrogen levels. If the oxygen level falls, impulses are transmitted to the respiratory centres in the brain, resulting in an increase in the rate of respiration and heartbeat.

carpus the Latin word for the WRIST, which consists of eight small bones that articulate with the ULNA and RADIUS of the forearm on one side and with the METACARPAL BONES (of the hand) on the other.

cartilage a type of firm CONNECTIVE TISSUE that is pliable and forms part of the SKELETON. There are three different kinds: hyaline cartilage, which is found at the JOINTS of movable BONES and in the TRACHEA, NOSE, BRONCHI and as costal cartilage joining the RIBS to the STERNUM; fibrocartilage, which is found in the INTERVERTEBRAL DISCS of the SPINAL COLUMN and in TENDONS; and elastic cartilage, which is found in the external part of the EAR (pinna).

catabolism the biochemical processes within the body (METABOLISM) are divided into two different sorts – those that build up or produce (synthesize) substances, which is anabolism, and those that break down material (LYSIS), known as catabolism. In catabolism, more complex materials are broken down into simpler ones with a release of energy, as occurs during the DIGESTION of food.

cataract a condition in which the LENS of the EYE becomes opaque, which results in a blurring of VISION. It may arise from a number of different causes, including injury to the eye, as a CONGENITAL condition or as a result of certain diseases, such as DIABETES. However, the commonest cause is advancing age, during which changes naturally take place in the lens involving the PROTEIN components.

catecholamine *see* DOPAMINE.

catheter a fine flexible tube that is passed into various organs of the body either for diagnostic purposes or to administer some kind of treatment.

caul a piece of MEMBRANE (part of the AMNION) that sometimes partly covers a newborn baby.

cavernous sinus one of a pair of cavities located on either side of the SPHENOID BONE behind the eye sockets at the base of the SKULL. Venous blood drains into it from the brain, part of the cheek, eye and nose and leaves through the facial veins and internal jugular.

cavity a hollow space within the body, e.g. the abdominal cavity.

cell the basic building block of all life and the smallest structural unit in the body. Human body cells vary in size and function and number several billion. Each cell consists of a cell body surrounded by a membrane. The cell body consists of a substance known as cytoplasm, containing various organelles and also a nucleus. The nucleus contains the CHROMOSOMES, composed of the genetic material, the DNA. Most human body cells contain 46 chromosomes (23 pairs), half being derived from the individual's father and half from the mother. Cells are able to make exact copies of themselves by a process known as mitosis, and a full complement of chromosomes is received by each daughter cell. However, the human sex cells (sperm and ova) differ in always containing half the number of chromosomes. At FERTILIZATION, a sperm and ovum combine and a complete set of chromosomes is received by the new embryo.

central nervous system the BRAIN and the SPINAL CORD, which receive and integrate all the nervous information from the PERIPHERAL NERVOUS SYSTEM.

cephalosporin one of a group of semi-synthetic ANTIBIOTICS that are effective against a broad spectrum of microorganism and are used to treat a variety of infections. They are sometimes able to destroy organisms that have become resistant to penicillin.

cerebellum the largest part of the hind brain, consisting of a pair of joined hemispheres. It has an outer grey cortex, which is a much folded layer of GREY

MATTER, and an inner core of WHITE MATTER. The cerebellum coordinates the activity of various groups of voluntary muscles and maintains posture and balance.

cerebral cortex the outer layer of GREY MATTER of the cerebral hemispheres of the CEREBRUM. It is highly folded, contains many millions of nerve cells and makes up about 40 per cent of the brain by weight. It controls intellectual processes such as thought, perception, memory and intellect, and is also involved in the senses of sight, touch and hearing. It also controls the voluntary movement of muscles and is connected with all the different parts of the body.

cerebral palsy an abnormality of the BRAIN that usually occurs before or during birth. It may arise as a development defect in the FOETUS because of genetic factors, as the result of a (viral) INFECTION during PREGNANCY or a lack of oxygen during a difficult LABOUR. After birth, the condition can result from HAEMOLYTIC DISEASE OF THE NEWBORN or infection of the brain, e.g. MENINGITIS. It can also be caused by cerebral THROMBOSIS or trauma. The condition is characterized by spastic PARALYSIS of the limbs, the severity of which is variable. Also, there may be involuntary writhing movements (athetosis) and balance and posture are also affected.

cerebrospinal fluid a clear, colourless fluid with a similar composition to LYMPH. It fills the ventricles and cavities in the CENTRAL NERVOUS SYSTEM and bathes all the surfaces of the brain and spinal cord. The BRAIN floats in it, and it has a protective function, acting as a shock absorber and helping to prevent mechanical injury to the central nervous system. The cerebrospinal fluid is secreted by the CHOROID PLEXUSES in the ventricles of the brain, and it contains some white blood cells (but no red), salts, glucose and enzymes. It is reabsorbed by veins back into the bloodstream.

cerebrovascular accident see STROKE.

cerebrum the largest and most highly developed part of the BRAIN, consisting of a pair of cerebral hemispheres divided from each other by a longitudinal fissure. The hemispheres are covered by the CEREBRAL CORTEX, below which lies WHITE MATTER in which the BASAL GANGLIA are situated. The cerebrum controls complex intellectual activities and also all the voluntary responses of the body.

cervical a term meaning relating to the neck and often used in connection with the CERVIX, the neck of the womb (UTERUS).

cervical cancer cancer of the neck or CERVIX. In the precancerous stage, readily detectable changes occur in the cells lining the surface of the cervix. These can be identified by a CERVICAL SMEAR test and, if treated at this stage, the prevention and cure rates of the cancer are high. The sexual behaviour of a woman influences her risk of contracting cervical cancer. Early sexual intercourse and many different partners are now recognized to increase the risk.

cervical smear a simple test, involving scraping off some CELLS from the CERVIX and examining them microscopically. The test is carried out every three years to detect early indications of cancer and is a form of PREVENTIVE MEDICINE.

cervix a neck-like structure, especially the cervix uteri or neck of the UTERUS. It is partly above and partly within the VAGINA, projecting into it and linking it with the cavity of the UTERUS via the cervical canal.

Chagas' disease a form of SLEEPING SICKNESS that is found in South and Central America. See page 122.

cheloid see KELOID.

chemoreceptor a CELL (present in the NOSE and TASTE BUDS) that detects the presence of specific chemical compounds. An electrical impulse is then sent to the BRAIN. See also CAROTID BODY.

chemotherapy the treatment of disease by the administration of chemical substances or drugs. It includes the treatment of infectious diseases with ANTIBIOTICS and other drugs. Also, the treatment and control of various tropical diseases and, especially in recent years, many different forms of CANCER with ANTIMETABOLITE drugs.

chest *or* **thorax** the upper part of the body cavity, separated from the lower abdomen by the DIAPHRAGM. The chest cavity is enclosed within the rib cage. The thoracic skeleton consists of the RIBS and COSTAL CARTILAGES attached to the STERNUM (breastbone) at the front. At the back, the ribs join the thoracic VERTEBRAe of the spine. The thorax contains the LUNGS, HEART and OESOPHAGUS and above it lie the neck and head.

chickenpox a highly infectious disease that mainly affects children and is caused by the *Varicella zoster* VIRUS. There is an INCUBATION period of two to three weeks and then usually a child becomes slightly feverish and unwell. Within 24 hours an itchy rash appears on the skin, which consists of fluid-filled blisters. Eventually these form scabs that fall off after about one week. The treatment consists of the application of lotion to reduce the itching and isolation from other children. The disease is uncommon in adults as a childhood attack gives lifelong IMMUNITY and most children are exposed to it at some stage. However, the virus may remain within the system and become active later as shingles (HERPES zoster).

choking violent coughing and interference in breathing caused by an obstruction in the airway in the region of the LARYNX. If the obstruction is large, there is a danger of suffocation.

cholecalciferol *see* VITAMIN D.

cholera *see* page 123.

cholesterol a fatty insoluble molecule (sterol) that is widely found in the body and is synthesized from saturated FATTY ACIDS in the LIVER. It is an important substance in the body, being a component of CELL membranes and a precursor in the production of STEROID hormones (SEX HORMONES) and BILE salts. An elevated level of BLOOD cholesterol is associated with ATHEROMA, which may result in high BLOOD PRESSURE and CORONARY THROMBOSIS, and this is seen in the disease DIABETES MELLITUS. It is recommended that people should reduce their consumption of saturated fat and look for an alternative in the form of unsaturated fat, found in vegetable oils.

choluria BILE in the URINE, which occurs when there is an elevated level of bile in the BLOOD. This may result from the condition known as obstructive JAUNDICE, when the bile ducts become obstructed so that bile manufactured in the liver fails to reach the intestine. The urine is dark coloured and contains bile salts.

chondromalacia patellae *see* CREPITUS.

chorda tympani *see* EAR.

chorea a disorder of the NERVOUS SYSTEM, characterized by involuntary jerky movements of the MUSCLES, mainly of the face, shoulders and hips. Sydenham's chorea (or Saint Vitus' Dance) is a disease that mainly affects children and is associated with acute RHEUMATISM. About one-third of affected children develop rheumatism elsewhere in the body, often involving the heart, and the disease is more common in girls than in boys. If the heart is affected, there may be problems in later life but treatment consists of rest and the giving of mild sedatives. The condition usually recovers over a period of a few months. Huntington's chorea is an inherited condition that does not appear until after the age of 40 and is accompanied by DEMENTIA. Senile chorea afflicts some elderly people but there is no dementia. *See also* RHEUMATIC FEVER.

chorionic gonadotrophic hormone *or* **human chorionic gonadotrophin (HCG)** a HORMONE produced during PREGNANCY by the PLACENTA, large amounts of which are present in the URINE of a pregnant woman. Its presence is the basis of most PREGNANCY TESTS. It is given by injection to treat cases of delayed PUBERTY and, with another hormone, called follicle-stimulating hormone, to women who are sterile because of a failure in ovulation. It may also be used to treat PREMENSTRUAL TENSION.

choroid *see* RETINA; DETACHED RETINA.

choroid plexus an extensive network of BLOOD VESSELS present in the VENTRICLES of the brain and responsible for the production of the CEREBROSPINAL FLUID.

Christmas factor *see* HAEMOPHILIA.

chromatin *see* NUCLEUS.

chromosomes the rod-like structures, present in the nucleus of every body CELL, that carry the genetic information or GENES. Each human body cell contains 23 pairs of chromosomes, apart from the SPERM and ova (*see* OVUM), half derived from the mother and half from the father. Each chromosome consists of a coiled double filament (double helix) of DNA, with genes carrying the genetic information arranged linearly along its length. The genes determine all the characteristics of each individual. Of the pairs of chromosomes, 22 are the same in males and females. The 23rd pair are the SEX CHROMOSOMES. *See also* SEX-LINKED INHERITANCE.

chyle *see* DIGESTION; LACTEAL VESSELS.

chyme the partly digested food that passes from the STOMACH into the INTESTINE. It is produced by the mechanical movements of the stomach and the acid secretions present in the GASTRIC JUICE.

chymotrypsin *see* PANCREAS.

cilia (*sing* **cilium**) fine hair-like projections found lining the EPITHELIUM of the upper respiratory tract. These beat and help to maintain the flow of air and remove and trap particles of dust.

ciliary body *see* EYE.

circulation of the blood all the BLOOD from the body returns to the HEART via the VEINS, eventually entering the right ATRIUM through the inferior and superior venae cavae (*see* VENA CAVA). The atrium contracts and forces the blood into the right VENTRICLE, from where it is driven to the LUNGS via the pulmonary ARTERY. In the lungs, oxygen is taken up and carbon dioxide released, and the blood then passes into the pulmonary veins and is returned to the left atrium of the heart. Blood is forced from there into the left ventricle and from there into the AORTA. The aorta branches, giving off the various arteries that carry the blood to all the different parts of the body. The blood eventually enters the fine network of arterioles and capillaries and supplies all the tissues and organs with oxygen and nutrients. It passes into the venules and veins, eventually returning to the right atrium through the vena cavae.

circumcision a surgical removal of the FORESKIN of the PENIS in males and part or all of the external GENITALIA in females. In females, and usually in males, the procedure is carried out for religious reasons. Male circumcision may be required in the medical conditions known as PHIMOSIS and PARAPHIMOSIS. Female circumcision is damaging and not beneficial to a woman's health.

cirrhosis a disease of the LIVER in which FIBROUS TISSUE resembling SCAR tissue is produced as a result of damage and death to the CELLS. The LIVER becomes yellow-coloured and nodular in appearance, and there are various types of the disease, including alcoholic cirrhosis and postnecrotic cirrhosis caused by viral HEPATITIS. The cause of the cirrhosis is not always found (cryptogenic cirrhosis), but the progress of the condition can be halted if this can be identified and removed. This particularly is applicable in alcoholic cirrhosis where the consumption of alcohol has to cease.

CJD the abbreviation of CREUTZFELD-JAKOB DISEASE, *see* page 12.

clavicle the collar BONE, forming a part of the shoulder girdle of the SKELETON. It is the most commonly fractured bone in the body.

cleft palate a developmental defect in which a fissure is left in the midline of the PALATE as the two sides fail to fuse. It may also involve the lip (HARELIP), and the condition is corrected by surgery.

climacteric *see* MENOPAUSE.

clitoris a small organ present in females, situated where the labial folds meet below the pubic bone. It contains erectile tissue that enlarges and hardens with sexual stimulation.

clone a group of CELLs that are derived from one cell (by asexual division) and are genetically identical.

clostridium one of a group of BACTERIA that are present in the INTESTINES of humans and animals. Some species are responsible for diseases such as BOTULISM, TETANUS and GAS GANGRENE.

clot *see* BLOOD CLOT; COAGULATION.

coagulation the natural process in which BLOOD is converted from a liquid to a semi-solid state to arrest bleeding (HAEMORRHAGE). A substance known as prothrombin and calcium are normally present in the blood, and the ENZYME thromboplastin is present in the PLATELETs. When bleeding occurs, thromboplastin is released and prothrombin and calcium are converted by the enzyme into thrombin. FIBRINOGEN is always present in the blood and is converted by thrombin into FIBRIN, the final stage in the coagulation process. A fibrous meshwork or BLOOD CLOT is produced, consisting of fibrin and blood cells, which seals off the damaged blood vessel. Normally, thromboplastin is not released and so a clot cannot form. The coagulation or clotting time is the time taken for blood to clot and is normally between three and eight minutes.

coagulation factors substances present in plasma that are involved in the process of blood COAGULATION. They are designated by a set of Roman numerals, e.g. factor VIII, and a lack of any of them means that the blood is unable to clot. *See* HAEMOPHILIA.

coccyx the end of the backbone (SPINAL COLUMN), which consists of four fused and reduced VERTEBRAe and corresponds to the tail of other mammals. It is surrounded by muscle and joins with the SACRUM, a further group of fused vertebrae, which is part of the PELVIS.

cochlea a spiral-shaped organ, resembling a snail shell, forming a part of the inner EAR and concerned with hearing. It consists of three fluid-filled canals with receptors that detect pressure changes caused by sound waves. NERVE IMPULSES are sent to the brain where the information is received and decoded.

coeliac pertaining to the CAVITY of the ABDOMEN.

coeliac disease *or* **gluten enteropathy** a wasting disease of childhood in which the INTESTINES are unable to absorb fat. The intestinal lining is damaged because of a sensitivity to the protein gluten, which is found in wheat and rye flour. An excess of fat is excreted, and the child fails to grow and thrive. Successful treatment is by adhering strictly to a gluten-free diet throughout life.

cold a widespread and mild infection of the upper RESPIRATORY TRACT caused by a VIRUS. There is INFLAMMATION of the MUCOUS MEMBRANES, and symptoms include feverishness, coughing, sneezing, runny nose, sore throat, headache and sometimes face ache as a result of CATARRH in the SINUSES. The disease is spread by coughing and sneezing, and treatment is by means of bed rest and the taking of mild ANALGESICS.

cold sore *see* HERPES.

colic spasmodic, severe abdominal pain that occurs in waves with brief interludes in between. Intestinal colic is usually the result of the presence of some indigestible food, which causes contraction of the intestinal muscles. Infantile colic, common in young babies, is caused by wind associated with feeding. An attack of colic is generally not serious but can result in a twisting of the bowel, which must receive immediate medical attention. Colic-type pain may also be caused by an obstruction in the bowel, such as a tumour, which again requires early medical treatment.

colitis INFLAMMATION of the COLON, the symptoms of which include abdominal pain and diarrhoea, sometimes bloodstained. Ulcerative colitis tends to affect young adults and usually occurs periodically over a number of years. There is abdominal discomfort, fever, frequent watery diarrhoea containing mucus and blood, and anaemia. It can be fatal but usually there is a gradual recovery. Treatment is by means of bed rest, drug treatment with CORTICOSTEROIDS and iron supplements, and a bland, low roughage diet.

collagen a PROTEIN substance that is widely found in the body in CONNECTIVE TISSUE, TENDONS, SKIN, CARTILAGE, BONE and LIGAMENTS. It plays a major part in conferring tensile strength to various body structures.

collar bone *see* CLAVICLE.

colon the main part of the large INTESTINE, which removes water and salts from the undigested food passed into it from the small intestine. When water has been extracted, the remains of the food (FAECES) are passed on to the RECTUM.

colostomy a surgical operation to produce an artificial opening of the COLON through the abdominal wall. It may just be temporary, as part of the management of a patient's condition, e.g. to treat an obstruction in the colon or RECTUM. However, if the rectum or part of the colon has been removed because of cancer, the colostomy is permanent and functions as the ANUS.

colostrum the first fluid produced by the MAMMARY GLANDS. It is a fairly clear fluid containing ANTIBODIES, serum and white blood cells and is produced during the first two or three days prior to the production of milk.

colour blindness any of a number of conditions in which there is a failure to distinguish certain colours. It is more prevalent in males than in females and is usually inherited. The most common form is Daltonism, in which reds and greens are confused. This is a SEX-LINKED DISORDER, the recessive gene responsible being carried on the X-chromosome and hence more likely to be present in males. The cause of colour blindness is thought to be a failure in the operation of the CONES, which detect colours.

coma a state of deep unconsciousness from which a person cannot be roused. There may be an absence of pupillary and corneal reflexes and no movements of withdrawal when painful stimuli are applied. It may be accompanied by deep, noisy breathing and strong heart action, and is caused by a number of conditions, including apoplexy, high fever, brain injury, diabetes mellitus, carbon monoxide poisoning and drug overdose. A comatose person may eventually die but can recover, depending on the nature of the coma and its cause.

comminuted fracture a serious injury to a BONE in which more than one break occurs accompanied by splintering and damage to the surrounding tissues. It usually results from a crushing force, with damage to nerves, muscles and blood vessels, and the bone is difficult to set.

commissure a joining or connection of two similar structures on either side of a midline, usually applied to bundles of NERVE fibres connecting the right and left side of the BRAIN and SPINAL CORD.

compressed air illness *see* BENDS.

concretions *or* **calculi** (*sing* **calculus**) hard, stony masses of various sizes formed within the body.

concussion a loss of consciousness caused by a blow to the head. The sudden knock causes a compression wave, which momentarily interrupts blood supply to the brain. The unconsciousness may last for seconds or hours, and when the person comes round there may be some headache and irritability, which can last for some time. A mild case may not involve complete loss of consciousness but be marked by giddiness, confusion and headache. In all cases, the person needs to rest and remain under observation.

conduction anaesthesia *see* NERVE BLOCK.

condyle a rounded knob at the ends of some BONES, e.g. the FEMUR and HUMERUS, that articulates with an adjacent bone.

cone a type of photoreceptor (light-sensitive cell) found in the RETINA of the eye, which detects colour. Cones contain the PIGMENT retinene and the protein opsin, and there are three different types which react to light of differing wavelengths (blue, green and red).

congenital a term used to describe a disease or condition that is present at birth, the opposite of ACQUIRED.

conjunctivitis inflammation of the MUCOUS MEMBRANE (conjunctiva) that lines the inside of the eyelid and covers the front of the EYE. The eyes become pink and watery, and the condition is usually caused by an infection that may be bacterial, viral or caused by the microorganism *Chlamydia*. Treatment depends on the cause, but a number of drugs are used, often in the form of eyedrops.

connective tissue supporting or packing tissue within the body that holds or separates other tissues and organs. It consists of a ground material composed of substances called mucopolysaccharides. In this, certain fibres such as yellow elastic, white collagenous and reticular fibres are embedded along with a variety of other cells, e.g MAST CELLS, MACROPHAGES, fibroblasts and fat cells. The constituents vary in proportions in different kinds of connective tissue to produce a number of distinct types. Examples are ADIPOSE TISSUE, CARTILAGE, BONE, TENDONS and LIGAMENTS.

constipation the condition in which the bowels are opened too infrequently and the FAECES become dry and hard and difficult and painful to pass. The frequency of normal bowel opening varies from person to person but when constipation becomes a problem, it is usually a result of inattention to this habit or to the diet. To correct the condition, a change of lifestyle may be needed, including taking more exercise and increasing fluids and roughage in the diet. LAXATIVES and ENEMAS are also used to alleviate the condition. Constipation is also a symptom of the more serious condition of blockage of the bowel (by a TUMOUR), but this is less common.

consumption *see* TUBERCULOSIS.

contraception prevention of pregnancy by various means. It can be prevented by barrier methods, in which there is a physical barrier to prevent the sperm from entering the cervix: the condom (sheath) and diaphragm (cap). As well as being a contraceptive, the sheath reduces the risk of either partner contracting a VENEREAL DISEASE, including HIV infection. Non-barrier methods include the INTRAUTERINE CONTRACEPTIVE DEVICE (coil) and oral contraceptives (the Pill), which are hormonal preparations. STERILIZATION of either a man or a woman provides a means of permanent contraception. It is also possible to give a high dose of oral contraceptives within 72 hours of unprotected intercourse, but this is usually regarded as an emergency method. The rhythm method of contraception involves restricting sexual intercourse to certain days of a woman's monthly cycle when conception is least likely to occur.

convulsions *or* **fits** involuntary, alternate, rapid, muscular contractions and relaxations that throw the body and limbs into contortions. They are caused by a disturbance of BRAIN function, and in adults usually result from EPILEPSY. In babies and young children they occur quite commonly but, although alarming, are generally not serious. Causes include a high fever because of infection, brain diseases such as MENINGITIS, and breath-holding, which is quite common in infants and very young children. They are thought to be more common in the very young because the nervous system is immature. Unless they are caused by a disease or infection that requires treatment, they are rarely life-threatening.

Cooley's anaemia *see* THALASSAEMIA.

corn *and* **bunion** a corn is a small, localized cone-shaped portion of hardened, thickened skin occurring on or between the toes. The point of the cone, known as 'the eye', points inwards and causes pain. It is caused by pressure from poorly-fitting shoes. A bunion is found over the joint at the base of the largest toe and is also caused by tight-fitting footwear. With a bunion, the joint between the toe and the first metatarsal bone becomes swollen and forms a lump beneath the thickened skin because of bending caused by the shoe. A hammer toe is similar but involves the second toe, which becomes bent at the joint to resemble a hammer because shoes or boots are too tight or pointed.

cornea the outermost, exposed layer of the EYE, which is transparent and lies over the IRIS and LENS. It refracts light entering the eye, directing the rays to the lens and thus acting as a coarse focus. It is a layer of CONNECTIVE TISSUE that has no blood supply of its own but is supplied with nutrients from the aqueous HUMOUR within the eye. It is highly sensitive to pain, and presence or absence of response if the cornea is touched is used as an indicator of a person's condition, e.g. in a comatose patient.

coronary arteries the arteries (*see* ARTERY) that supply blood to the HEART and arise from the AORTA.

coronary artery disease any abnormal condition that affects the arteries (*see* ARTERY) of the heart. The commonest disease is coronary ATHEROSCLEROSIS, which is more prevalent in those populations with high fat, saturated fat, refined carbohydrates, etc, in their diet. ANGINA is a common symptom of such diseases.

coronary bypass graft a surgical operation that is carried out when one or more of the coronary arteries have become narrowed by disease (ATHEROMA). A section of vein from a leg is grafted in to bypass the obstruction, and this major operation is usually successful and greatly improves a person's quality of life.

coronary thrombosis a sudden blockage of one of the coronary arteries by a BLOOD CLOT or THROMBUS that interrupts the blood supply to the heart. The victim collapses with severe and agonizing chest pain, often accompanied by vomiting and nausea. The skin becomes pale and clammy, the temperature rises and there is difficulty in breathing. Coronary thrombosis generally results from ATHEROMA, and the part of the heart muscle that has its blood supply disrupted dies, a condition known as MYOCARDIAL INFARCTION. Treatment consists of giving strong pain-relieving drugs, e.g. morphine. Specialist care in a coronary care unit is also usually required to deal with ARRHYTHMIA, heart failure and CARDIAC ARREST, which are the potentially fatal results of coronary thrombosis.

corpuscle *see* BLOOD.

corpus luteum the tissue that forms within the ovary after a Graafian FOLLICLE ruptures and releases an OVUM. It consists of a mass of cells containing yellow, fatty substances and secretes the hormone PROGESTERONE, which prepares the UTERUS to receive a fertilized egg. If the egg is not fertilized and no implantation of an embryo takes place, it degenerates. However, if a pregnancy ensues, the it expands and secretes progesterone until this function is taken over by the PLACENTA at the fourth month of PREGNANCY.

cortex (*pl* **cortices**) the outer part of an organ situated beneath its enclosing CAPSULES or outer MEMBRANE. Examples are the adrenal cortex of the ADRENAL GLANDS, renal cortex of the KIDNEYS and CEREBRAL CORTEX of the BRAIN.

corticosteroid any STEROID hormone manufactured by the adrenal cortex, of which there are two main types. Glucocorticosteroids, such as CORTISONE, are required by the body mainly for glucose metabolism and for responding to stress. Mineralocorticosteroids regulate the salt and water balance. Both groups are manufactured synthetically and used in the treatment of various disorders.

cortisone a glucoCORTICOSTEROID produced by the adrenal cortex. It is used medically to treat deficiency of corticosteroid HORMONES. Deficiency occurs in ADDISON'S DISEASE and if the adrenal glands have had to be surgically removed for some reason. Its use is restricted because it causes severe SIDE EFFECTS, including damage to the muscle and bone, eye changes, stomach ulcers and bleeding.

cosmetic surgery *see* PLASTIC SURGERY.

costal cartilage a type of CARTILAGE connecting a rib to the STERNUM.

cot death *see* SUDDEN INFANT DEATH SYNDROME.

cough a deep inspiration of air followed by a spasmodic and noisy expiration, caused by some irritation in the air passages (dry cough) or to expel MUCUS (wet cough). *See also* EXPECTORANT.

Coxsackie virus *see* ENTEROVIRUS.

cramp a prolonged and painful spasmodic muscular contraction that often occurs in the limbs but can affect certain internal organs (*see* COLIC and GASTRALGIA). Cramp may result from a salt imbalance, as in heat cramp. Working in high temperatures causes excessive sweating and consequent loss of salt. It can be corrected and prevented by an increase of the salt intake. Occupational cramp results from continual repetitive use of particular muscles, e.g. WRITER'S CRAMP. Night cramp occurs during sleep and is especially common among elderly people, diabetics and pregnant women.

cranial nerves 12 pairs of NERVES that arise directly from the BRAIN, each with dorsal and ventral branches known as roots. Each root remains separate and is assigned a Roman numeral as well as a name. Some are mainly SENSORY while others are largely MOTOR, and they leave the SKULL through separate apertures. The cranial and spinal nerves (*see* SPINAL CORD) are an important part of the PERIPHERAL NERVOUS SYSTEM.

cranium the part of the skull that encloses the BRAIN, formed from eight fused and flattened bones that are joined by immovable SUTURE joints.

creatinine *see* URINE.

crepitus 1. the grating sound heard when the ends of fractured bones rub together and also from arthritic joints. **2.** the grating sound and pain in chondromalacia patellae, which is a roughening of the inner surface of the kneecap. **3.**

the sound heard by means of a from an inflamed lung when there is fluid in the alveoli (*see* ALVEOLUS).

Creutzfeldt-Jakob disease (CJD) *or* **spongiform encephalopathy** *see* page 12.

Crohn's disease chronic INFLAMMATION of the bowel, especially the ILEUM. *See also* ILEITIS.

croup a group of diseases characterized by a swelling, partial obstruction and INFLAMMATION of the entrance to the LARYNX, occurring in young children. The breathing is harsh and strained, producing a typical crowing sound, accompanied by coughing and feverishness. DIPHTHERIA used to be the most common cause, but it now usually results from a LARYNGOTRACHEOBRONCHITIS. It is relieved by inhaling steam (a soothing preparation such as tincture of benzoin is sometimes added to the hot water) and also by mild sedatives and/or pain killers. Rarely, the obstruction becomes dangerous and completely blocks the larynx, in which case emergency TRACHEOSTOMY or nasotracheal INTUBATION may be required.

crown *see* TOOTH.

culture BACTERIA, VIRUSES or other microorganisms or cells grown in the laboratory on a nutrient base known as a culture medium.

Cushing's syndrome a metabolic disorder that results from excessive amounts of CORTICOSTEROIDS in the body because of an inability to regulate cortisol or ADRENOCORTICOTROPIC HORMONE (ACTH). The commonest cause is a TUMOUR of the PITUITARY GLAND (producing secretion of ACTH) or a malignancy elsewhere, e.g. in the lung or adrenal gland, requiring extensive therapy with corticosteroid drugs.

cutaneous a term used to describe anything belonging to the SKIN or existing on or affecting the skin.

cuticle 1. a name for the outer layer or EPIDERMIS of the SKIN. **2.** the outer layer of CELLS covering a HAIR.

cyanocobalamin *see* VITAMIN B12.

cyanosis a blue appearance of the SKIN because of insufficient oxygen within the BLOOD. It is first noticeable on the lips, tips of the ears, cheeks and nails and occurs in HEART FAILURE, lung diseases and ASPHYXIA.

cyst a small, usually benign, TUMOUR containing fluid (or soft secretions) within a membranous sac. Examples are SEBACEOUS CYSTS, cysts in the breasts (caused by blocked milk ducts), and ovarian cysts, which may be large and contain a clear, thick liquid. Dermoid cysts are CONGENITAL and occur at sites in the body where embryonic clefts have closed up before birth. Hydatid cysts are a stage in the life cycle of certain parasites (tapeworm) and may be found in humans, especially in the liver.

cystic fibrosis a genetic disease, the defective gene responsible for it being located on human CHROMOSOME no. 7. It affects all the MUCUS-secreting GLANDS of the LUNGS, PANCREAS, MOUTH and gastrointestinal tract and also the SWEAT GLANDS of the skin. A thick mucus is produced, which affects the production of pancreatic ENZYMES and causes the BRONCHI to widen (bronchiectasis) and become clogged. Respiratory infections are common, and the sweat contains abnormally high levels of sodium and chloride. The FAECES also contain a lot of mucus and have a foul smell. The disease is incurable and cannot be diagnosed by before birth.

cystitis INFLAMMATION of the bladder, normally caused by bacterial infection, the causal organism usually being ESCHERICHIA coli. It is marked by the need to pass URINE frequently, accompanied by a burning sensation. It is common in females and is usually not serious but there is a danger that the infection may spread to the kidneys. The prevalence in women is because the URETHRA is much shorter than in men and the bacteria (which are present and harmless in the bowel) are more likely to gain access to both the urinary tract and the VAGINA. Treatment is by means of antibiotics and also by drinking a lot of fluid.

cytokine *see* INTERLEUKIN.

cytoplasm the substance within the CELL wall that surrounds the NUCLEUS and contains a number of ORGANELLES. *See also* MAST CELL.

cytosine *see* NUCLEOTIDE.

cytotoxic a term used to describe a substance that damages or destroys CELLS. Cytotoxic drugs are used in the treatment of various forms of CANCER and act by inhibiting cell division. They also damage normal cells and have to be carefully regulated. They may be used in combination with RADIOTHERAPY or on their own.

D

Daltonism *see* COLOUR BLINDNESS.

D and C *see* DILATATION AND CURETTAGE.

deafness a partial or complete loss of hearing. It may be temporary or permanent, conductive or sensory, congenital or acquired. Congenital hearing loss is not a common cause. In many cases, the loss is because of a problem in the COCHLEA. This is a common condition in the elderly although no particular cause can be identified. Other causes include exposure to industrial noise or explosions. Conductive hearing loss is the result of poor transmission of sound waves to the inner EAR, possibly because of OTITIS, which can cause middle ear inflammation and perforation of the eardrum. This can be treated by surgery or helped by the use of a hearing aid.

decidua the soft epithelial tissue that forms a lining to the UTERUS during PREGNANCY and is shed in birthing. *See also* EPITHELIUM.

decubitus ulcers *see* BED SORES.

deficiency disease a disease that is caused by a lack of VITAMINS or other essential dietary items, e.g. BERIBERI, PELLAGRA and SCURVY.

degeneration deterioration over time of body tissues or an organ, resulting in a lessening of function. The changes may be structural or chemical, and there are a number of types: fatty, FIBROID, calcareous (as with CONCRETIONS), mucoid, etc. Degeneration may the result of ageing, heredity or poor nutrition. Poisons such as alcohol also contribute to degeneration, as with CIRRHOSIS.

dehydration the removal of water. More specifically, the loss of water from the body through DIURESIS, sweating, etc, or a reduction in water content because of a low intake. Essential body ELECTROLYTES (such as sodium chloride and potassium) are disrupted, and after the first symptom, thirst, irritability and confusion follow.

delirium a mental disorder typified by confusion, agitation, fear, anxiety, illusions and sometimes hallucinations. The causal cerebral dysfunction may be deficient nutrition, stress, toxic poisoning or mental shock.

delirium tremens a form of DELIRIUM, often caused by partial or total withdrawal of alcohol after a period of excessive intake. Symptoms are varied and include insomnia, agitation, confusion and fever, often with vivid hallucinations. The treatment involves lessening and removing the dependence on alcohol.

deltoid the MUSCLE, triangular in shape, that covers the shoulder and is attached to the CLAVICLE, shoulder blade and HUMERUS. It enables the arm to be raised from the side.

dementia a mental disorder typified by confusion, disorientation, memory loss, personality changes and a lessening of intellectual capacity. It occurs in several forms: SENILE DEMENTIA, ALZHEIMER'S DISEASE and multi-infarct dementia. The causes are various and include vascular disease, brain tumour, SUBDURAL HAEMATOMA, HYDROCEPHALUS and HYPERTHYROIDISM.

dendrite one of numerous thin branching extensions of a NERVE cell. The dendrites are at the 'receiving end' of the nerve cell (NEURON), and they form a network that increases the area for receiving impulses from the terminals of AXONS of other neurons at the SYNAPSE.

dengue fever *see* page 120.

dentine the material that forms the bulk of a TOOTH, lying between the pulp cavity and the enamel. It is similar to BONE in composition but contains blood capillaries, nerve fibres and extensions of odontoblasts (cells producing the dentine).

deoxyribonucleic acid *see* DNA.

depressant a drug that is used to reduce the functioning of a system of the body, e.g. a respiratory depressant. Drugs such as opiates, general anaesthetics, etc, are depressants.

depression a mental state of extreme sadness dominated by pessimism, in which normal behaviour patterns (sleep, appetite, etc) are disturbed. Causes are varied: upsetting events, loss, etc, and treatment involves the use of therapy and drugs.

dermatitis an INFLAMMATION of the SKIN that is similar in many respects to, and often interchanged with, ECZEMA. It is characterized by ERYTHEMA, pain and PRURITIS. Several forms can be identified: contact dermatitis is caused by the skin coming into contact with a substance to which it is sensitive. Light dermatitis manifests itself as a reddening and blistering of skin exposed to sunlight, and this occurs on hands, face and neck, usually during the summer. Some individuals become sensitized by drugs or perfumes in cosmetics, while others have an innate sensitivity. Erythroderma or exfoliative dermatitis involves patches of reddened skin that thicken and peel off. It is often associated with other skin conditions, e.g. PSORIASIS. CORTICOSTEROIDS form a central part of the treatment.

dermis *see* EPIDERMIS; SKIN.

detached retina the condition when the RETINA of the EYE becomes detached from the choroid (a layer of the eyeball with blood vessels and pigment that absorbs excess light, preventing blurred VISION). The detachment may be caused by a TUMOUR or INFLAMMATION or by the leaking of vitreous HUMOUR through holes in the retina to fill the space between the retina and choroid, thus disrupting the fine attachments. It can be corrected by surgery, whereby heat binds the retina and choroid together using scarred tissue.

dhobi itch *see* RINGWORM.

diabetes insipidus a rare condition that is completely different from DIABETES MELLITUS and is characterized by excessive thirst (*see* POLYDIPSIA) and POLYURIA. It is caused by a lack of antidiuretic hormone or the inability of the kidney to respond to the hormone.

diabetes mellitus a complex metabolic disorder involving carbohydrate, fat and protein. It results in an accumulation of sugar in the blood and urine and is the result of a lack of INSULIN produced by the PANCREAS, so that sugars are not broken down to release energy. Fats are thus used as an alternative energy source. Symptoms include thirst, POLYURIA and loss of weight, and the use of fats can produce KETOSIS and KETONURIA. In its severest form, CONVULSIONS are followed by a diabetic COMA. Treatment relies on dietary control with doses of insulin or drugs. Long-term effects include thickening of the arteries, and in some cases, the eyes, kidneys, nervous system, skin and circulation may be affected (*see also* HYPOGLYCAEMIA and HYPERGLYCAEMIA).

diagnosis (*pl* **diagnoses**) the process whereby a particular disease or condition is identified after consideration of the relevant parameters, i.e. symptoms, physical manifestations, results of laboratory tests, etc. It often requires greater skills than does the treatment.

dialysis (*pl* **dialyses**) the use of a semipermeable MEMBRANE to separate large and small molecules by selective diffusion. Starch and PROTEINS are large molecules while salts, glucose and AMINO ACIDS are small molecules. If a mixture of large and small molecules is separated from distilled water by a semipermeable membrane, the smaller molecules diffuse into the water, which is itself replenished. This principle is the basis of the artificial KIDNEY, which, because a patient's blood is processed, is known as HAEMODIALYSIS.

diaphragm 1. a MEMBRANE of MUSCLE and TENDON that separates the chest and abdominal cavities. It is covered by a SEROUS MEMBRANE and attached at the lower RIBS, breastbone (STERNUM) and backbone (SPINAL COLUMN). The diaphragm is important in breathing, when it bulges up to its resting position during exhalation. It flattens during inhalation and in so doing it reduces pressure in the thoracic cavity and helps to draw air into the lungs. **2.** a rubber bowl-shaped cap used as a contraceptive with spermicidal cream. It fits inside the VAGINA over the neck of the UTERUS.

diaphysis (*pl* **diaphyses**) the central part or shaft of a long BONE.

diarrhoea increased frequency and looseness of bowel movement, involving the passage of unusually soft FAECES. Diarrhoea can be caused by food poisoning, COLITIS, IRRITABLE BOWEL SYNDROME, DYSENTERY, etc. A severe case will result in the loss of water and salts, which must be replaced.

diastase (amylases) ENZYMES that break down starch into sugar. It is used to help in the digestion of starch in some digestive disorders.

diastole the point at which the HEART relaxes between contractions, when the VENTRICLES fill with blood. It lasts about half a second, at the end of which the ventricles are about three-quarters full.

diazepam *see* TRANQUILLIZER.

digestion the process of breaking down food into substances that can be absorbed and used by the body. It begins with the chewing and grinding of food, at which point it is mixed with SALIVA to commence the process of breakdown. Most digestion occurs in the STOMACH and small INTESTINE. In the stomach the food is subjected to GASTRIC JUICE, which contains PEPSINS, to break down PROTEINS, and hydrochloric acid. The food is mixed and becomes totally soluble before passing into the small intestine as CHYME, where it is acted on by pancreatic juice, BILE, BACTERIA and succus entericus (intestinal juices). Water is absorbed in the intestine in a very short time, while the bulk of the food may take several hours to be processed. The chyme forms chyle because of the action of bile and pancreatic juice. Fats are removed from this in emulsion form into the lymph vessels (*see* LACTEAL VESSELS) and then into the blood. Sugars, salts and AMINO ACIDS move directly into the small blood vessels in the intestine, and the whole process is promoted by microfolding of the intestine wall producing finger-like projections (villi). The food passes down the intestine as a result of muscular contractions of the intestine wall (PERISTALSIS), and ultimately the residue and waste are excreted.

digitalis a powder derived from the leaf of the wild foxglove (*Digitalis purpurea*), which is used in cases of HEART disease. It acts to strengthen each heartbeat and increase each pause (DIASTOLE) so that damaged heart muscle has longer to rest. It also has a diuretic effect. Poisoning may occur with prolonged use or an overdose.

dilatation and curettage (D and C) the technique whereby the CERVIX is opened and then the lining is scraped. Such sampling is performed for the removal of incomplete ABORTIONS and TUMOURS, to diagnose disease of the uterus or to correct bleeding, etc.

dipeptide *see* PEPTIDE.

diphtheria an infectious disease caused by the bacterium *Corynebacterium diphtheriae* and commonest in children. The infection causes a membranous lining on the throat, which can interfere with breathing and eating. The toxin produced by the bacterium damages HEART tissue and the CENTRAL NERVOUS SYSTEM and can be fatal if not treated. The infection is countered by injection of antitoxin with PENICILLIN or ERYTHROMYCIN given to kill the bacterium. It can be prevented by VACCINATION.

diplegia PARALYSIS on both sides of the body.

disc a flattened circular structure, such as the CARTILAGE between VERTEBRAe. *See also* INTERVERTEBRAL DISC.

disinfection the process of killing PATHOGENIC organisms (not spores) to prevent the spread of infection. Different compounds are used, appropriate to the surface being disinfected.

dislocation an injury to a JOINT in which BONES are displaced from their normal, respective positions. Associated effects include bruising of the surrounding tissues and tearing of the LIGAMENTs. Most dislocations are simple rather than compound (when the bone punctures the skin) and ACQUIRED rather than CONGENITAL. Immediate treatment involves application of a splint or bandage to render the joint stable. Repositioning the bone (REDUCTION) requires skill, after which the limb must be fixed to avoid a repetition. Even after time, care is necessary when using the limb.

diuresis an increase in urine production as a result of disease, drugs, HORMONE imbalance or increased fluid intake.

diuretic a substance that increases URINE formation and excretion and may work specifically within the KIDNEY, e.g. by prevention of sodium, and therefore water, reabsorption or outside the kidney.

diverticulitis INFLAMMATION of diverticula (*see* DIVERTICULUM) in the large INTESTINE. There are cramp-like pains in the left side of the abdomen, possibly with constipation and fever. Treatment normally involves complete rest with no solid food, and antibiotics.

diverticulosis the condition in which there are diverticula (*see* DIVERTICULUM) in the large INTESTINE, occurring primarily in the lower COLON. They are caused by the muscles of the bowel forcing the bowel out through weak points in the wall. It is thought that it may be related to diet but symptoms are not always produced.

diverticulum (*pl* **diverticula**) in general, a pouch extending from a main cavity. Specifically, in the INTESTINE, a SAC-like protrusion through the wall, many of which usually develop later in life and are thought to be related to dietary factors. The formation of diverticula is called DIVERTICULOSIS, and their INFLAMMATION (causing pain, pyrexia and constipation) is called DIVERTICULITIS.

DNA (deoxyribonucleic acid) a nucleic acid and the primary constituent of CHROMOSOMES. It transmits genetic information from parents to offspring in the form of GENES. It is a very large molecule comprising two twisted nucleotide chains that can store enormous amounts of information in a stable but not rigid way, i.e. parental traits and characteristics are passed on but evolutionary changes are allowed to occur.

dopa an AMINO ACID compound that is formed from tyrosine (an amino acid synthesized in the body) and is a precursor of DOPAMINE and NORADRENALINE. A drug form, levodopa or l-dopa, is used to treat PARKINSONISM, as it can increase the concentration of dopamine in the BASAL GANGLIA.

dopamine a catecholamine derived from DOPA and an intermediate in the synthesis of NORADRENALINE. (Catecholamines comprise benzene, hydroxyl groups and an amine group and are physiologically important in the functioning of the NERVOUS SYSTEM, mainly as NEUROTRANSMITTERS.) It is found mainly in the BASAL GANGLIA of the BRAIN and a deficiency is typical in PARKINSONISM.

dorsal the term used to describe anything relating to the back or SPINAL COLUMN or the posterior part of an organ.

Down's syndrome a syndrome created by a CONGENITAL chromosome disorder that occurs as an extra CHROMOSOME 21, producing 47 in each body cell. Characteristic facial features are produced – a shorter, broader face with slanted eyes. It also results in a shorter stature, weak muscles and the possibility of heart defects and respiratory problems. The syndrome also confers mental retardation. It occurs once in approximately 600 to 700 live births, and although individuals may live beyond middle age, life expectancy is reduced and many die in infancy. The incidence increases with the age of the mother, so pregnant women over 35 are offered an AMNIOCENTESIS test.

drug any substance, vegetable, animal or mineral, used in the composition or preparation of medicine.

drug metabolism the process by which a drug is altered by the body into a metabolite (i.e. necessary for metabolic action), which may be the active agent. It is the process that ultimately results in the removal of the drug and thus determines the length of time during which it is active.

duct a narrow tube-like structure joining a GLAND with an organ or the body surface, through which a secretion passes, e.g. sweat ducts opening on to the skin.

ductless gland a GLAND that releases its secretion directly into the blood for transport around the body, e.g. the PITUITARY and THYROID. Some glands, such as the PANCREAS, operate as a ductless gland (for INSULIN) but secrete a digestive juice via ducts into the small INTESTINE.

dullness *see* RESONANCE.

duodenal ulcer the commonest type of PEPTIC ULCER. They may occur after the age of 20 and are more common in men. The cause is open to debate but probably results from an abrasion or break in the DUODENUM lining, which is then exacerbated by GASTRIC JUICE. Smoking seems to be a contributory but not a causal factor. The ulcer manifests itself as an upper abdominal pain roughly two hours after a meal and also occurs during the night. Food (e.g. milk) relieves the symptom, and a regime of frequent meals and milky snacks, with little or no fried food and spices and a minimum of strong tea and coffee, is usually adopted. Recent drug treatments enable the acid secretion to be reduced, thus allowing the ulcer to heal. Surgery is required only if there is no response to treatment, if the PYLORUS is obstructed or if the ulcer becomes perforated. The last is treated as an emergency.

duodenum the first part of the small INTESTINE where food (CHYME) from the stomach is subject to action by BILE and pancreatic ENZYMES. The duodenum also secretes a HORMONE secretion that contributes to the breakdown of fats, proteins and carbohydrates. In the duodenum, the acid conditions pertaining from the stomach are neutralized and rendered alkaline for the intestinal enzymes to operate.

dura mater *see* BRAIN; MENINGES.

dwarfism an abnormal underdevelopment of the body manifested by small stature. There are several causes, including incorrect functioning of the PITUITARY or THYROID GLANDs. Pituitary dwarfism produces a small but correctly proportioned body and, if diagnosed sufficiently early, treatment with growth hormone can help.

dysentery an INFECTION and ulceration of the lower part of the bowels that causes severe diarrhoea with the passage of mucus and blood. There are two forms of dysentery caused by different organisms. Amoebic dysentery is caused by *Entamoeba histolytica*, which is spread via infected food or water and occurs mainly in the tropics and subtropics. The appearance of symptoms may be delayed, but in addition to diarrhoea there is indigestion, anaemia and weight loss. Drugs are used in treatment. Bacillary dysentery is caused by the bacterium *Shigella* and spreads by contact with a carrier or contaminated food. Symptoms appear from one to six days after infection and include diarrhoea, cramp, nausea aned fever. The severity of the attack varies.

dyslexia a disorder that renders reading or learning to read difficult. There is usually an associated problem in writing and spelling correctly. A very small number of children are affected severely, and boys are more prone to it than girls by a factor of three.

dyspepsia *or* **indigestion** discomfort in the upper ABDOMEN or lower chest after eating, with HEARTBURN, NAUSEA and FLATULENCE accompanying a feeling of fullness. The causes are numerous and include GALLSTONES, PEPTIC ULCER, HIATUS HERNIA and diseases of the liver or pancreas.

dysphasia a general term for an impairment of speech, whether it is manifested as a difficulty in understanding language or in self-expression. There is a range of conditions with varying degrees of severity. Global aphasia is a total inability to communicate, but some individuals partially understand what is said to them. Dysphasia is when thoughts can be expressed up to a point. Non-fluent dysphasia represents poor self-expression but good understanding while the reverse is called fluent dysphasia. The condition may be caused by a STROKE or other BRAIN damage and can be temporary or permanent.

E

ear the SENSE ORGAN used for detection of sound and maintenance of balance. It comprises three parts: the external or outer, the middle and the inner ear, the first two acting to collect sound waves and transmit them to the inner ear, where the hearing and balance mechanisms are situated. The outer ear (auricle or pinna) is a CARTILAGE and skin structure that is not actually essential to hearing in humans. The middle ear is an air-filled cavity that is linked to the PHARYNX via the EUSTACHIAN TUBE. Within the middle ear are the ear (or auditory) ossicles, three bones called the incus, malleus and stapes (anvil, hammer and stirrup). Two small muscles control the bones and the associated nerve (the chorda tympani). The ossicles bridge the middle ear, connecting the eardrum with the inner ear and, in so doing, convert sound (air waves) into mechanical movements that then impinge on the fluid of the inner ear. The inner ear lies within the temporal bone of the skull and contains the apparatus for hearing and balance. The COCHLEA is responsible for hearing, and balance is maintained by the semicircular canals. These are made up of three loops positioned mutually at right angles, and in each is the fluid endolymph. When the head is moved, the fluid moves accordingly, and sensory cells produce impulses that are transmitted to the brain.

eating disorders *see* ANOREXIA; BULIMIA NERVOSA.

ECG *see* ELECTROCARDIOGRAM.

echinococcosis the condition created when CYSTS from the larval stages of a tapeworm create malignant TUMOURS in the BRAIN, LUNGS or LIVER. Those in the brain can cause blindness and epilepsy.

echovirus a VIRUS that can cause symptoms of the common COLD, mild MENINGITIS and intestinal and respiratory INFECTSIONS.

eclampsia CONVULSIONS that occur during PREGNANCY, usually at the later stages or during delivery. Although the cause is not known, the start of convulsions may be associated with cerebral OEDEMA or a sudden rise in BLOOD PRESSURE. KIDNEY function is usually badly affected. It requires immediate treatment as it threatens both mother and baby. Treatment is by drugs and reduction of outside stimuli, and a CAESAREAN SECTION is needed.

E. coli *see* ESCHERICHIA.

ectopic a term used to refer to something or some event that is not in its usual place or at its usual time, e.g. an ectopic PREGNANCY is one in which the fertilized egg implants outside the UTERUS.

ectopic beat *see* EXTRASYSTOLE.

eczema an INFLAMMATION of the SKIN that causes itching, a red rash and often small blisters that weep and become encrusted. This may be followed by the skin thickening and then peeling off in scales. There are several types, atopic, the hereditary tendency to form allergic reactions because of an antibody in the skin, being one of the most common. A form of atopic eczema is infantile eczema, which starts at three or four months, and it is often the case that eczema, HAY FEVER and ASTHMA are found in the family history. Many children improve markedly as they approach the age of 10 or 11. Treatment usually involves the use of HYDROCORTISONE and other STEROID creams and ointments.

effector a motor or sensory NERVE ending that terminates in a muscle, gland or organ and stimulates contraction or secretion.

efferent a term meaning 'outwards from an organ, etc', especially the BRAIN or SPINAL CORD, e.g. an efferent NERVE.

elastin *see* FIBROUS TISSUE.

electrolyte strictly, a compound that dissolves in water to produce a solution, containing ions, that is able to conduct an electrical charge. In the body, electrolytes occur in the blood PLASMA, all fluid and interstitial fluid, and correct concentrations are essential for normal metabolic activity. Some diseases alter the electrolyte balance, either through vomiting or diarrhoea or because the kidney is malfunctioning. The correct balance can be restored through oral or intravenous dosage or by DIALYSIS.

elephantiasis a dramatic and debilitating enlargement of SKIN and underlying CONNECTIVE TISSUE because of inflammation of the skin, subcutaneous tissue and the blocking of lymph vessels, preventing drainage. Inflammation and blocking of vessels is caused by parasitic worms (filariae), which are carried to humans by mosquitoes. The parts of the body most commonly affected are the legs, scrotum and breasts, in some cases to enormous proportions. Associated muscles of a limb may degenerate as a result of the abnormal pressure on them, and eventually overall health suffers. Prevention is the key, by eradication of the mosquitoes, but some relief is gained by using certain drugs early in the disease.

embolism the state in which a small BLOOD VESSEL is blocked by an EMBOLUS. This plug may be fragments of a CLOT, a mass of BACTERIA, air bubbles that have entered the system during an operation or a particle of a TUMOUR. The blockage leads usually to the destruction of that part of the organ supplied by the vessel. The most common case is a pulmonary embolism. Treatment utilizes an ANTICOAGULANT drug such as warfarin or heparin, surgical removal or STREPTOKINASE, an ENZYME capable of dissolving blood clots.

embolus (*pl* **emboli**) material carried by the BLOOD which then lodges elsewhere in the body (*see* EMBOLISM). The material may be a blood clot, fat, air, a piece of tumour, etc.

embryo the first stage of development of a FOETUS after the fertilized OVUM is implanted in the UTERUS until the second month.

embryo transfer the FERTILIZATION of an OVUM by SPERM and its development into an early EMBRYO, outside the mother, and its subsequent implantation in the mother's UTERUS. *See also* IN VITRO FERTILIZATION.

emesis the medical term for VOMITING.

emetic a substance that causes VOMITING. Direct emetics, such as mustard in water, copper sulphate, alum or a lot of salty water, irritate the stomach while indirect emetics, such as apomorphine and ipecacuanha, act on the centre of the brain that controls the act of vomiting. Tickling the throat is also classed as an emetic (indirect). Great care must be exercised if their use is advocated.

emphysema an abnormal condition of the LUNGS in which the walls of the alveoli (*see* ALVEOLUS) are over-inflated and distended and changes in their structure occur. This destruction of parts of the walls produces large air-filled spaces that do not contribute to the respiratory process. Acute cases may be caused by whooping cough or bronchopneumonia, and chronic cases often accompany chronic bronchitis, which itself is caused in great part by smoking. Emphysema is also developed after TUBERCULOSIS, when the lungs are stretched until the fibres of the alveolar walls are destroyed. Similarly, in old age, the alveolar membrane may collapse, producing large air sacs, with decreased surface area.

enamel *see* TOOTH.

encephalin a PEPTIDE that acts as a NEUROTRANSMITTER. Two have been identified, both acting as ANALGESICS when their release controls pain. They are found in the brain and in nerve cells of the spinal cord.

encephalitis INFLAMMATION of the BRAIN. It is usually a viral infection and sometimes occurs as a complication of some common infectious diseases, e.g. MEASLES or CHICKENPOX. There are several forms of the disease, including encephalitis lethargica (SLEEPING SICKNESS or epidemic encephalitis), which attacks and causes swelling in the basal ganglia, cerebrum and brain stem that may result in tissue destruction. Other forms are Japanese encephalitis, which is caused by a virus carried by mosquitoes, and tick-borne encephalitis, which occurs in Europe and Siberia. In most cases there is no readily available treatment.

encephalomyelitis INFLAMMATION of the BRAIN and SPINAL CORD, typified by headaches, fever, stiff neck and back pain, with vomiting. Depending on the extent of inflammation and the patient's condition, it may cause paralysis, personality changes, coma or death.

encephalopathy any disease affecting the BRAIN or an abnormal condition of the brain's structure and function. It refers in particular to degenerative and chronic conditions.

endemic the term used to describe, for example, a disease that is indigenous to a certain area.

endocarditis inflammation of the ENDOCARDIUM, heart valves and muscle, caused by a bacterium, virus or rheumatic fever. At greatest risk are those with a damaged endocardium from a CONGENITAL deformity or alteration of the immune system by drugs.

endocardium a fine MEMBRANE lining the HEART, which forms a continuous membrane with the lining of veins and arteries. At the cavities of the heart it forms cusps on the valves, and its surface is very smooth to facilitate blood flow.

endocrine glands DUCTLESS GLANDs that produce HORMONES for secretion directly into the bloodstream (or lymph). Some organs, e.g. the PANCREAS, also release secretions via a DUCT. In addition to the pancreas, the major endocrine glands are the THYROID, PITUITARY, PARATHYROID, OVARY and TESTIS. Imbalances in the secretions of endocrine glands produce a variety of diseases.

endogenous a term used to refer to what is within the body, whether growing within, originating from within or the result of internal causes.

endolymph *see* EAR.

endometriosis the occurrence of ENDOMETRIUM in other parts of the body, e.g. within the muscle of the UTERUS, in the ovary, FALLOPIAN TUBES, PERITONEUM and possibly the bowel. Because of the nature of the tissue, it acts in a way similar to that of the uterus lining and causes pelvic pain, bleeding and painful menstruation. It occurs between puberty and the menopause and ceases during pregnancy. Treatment may include total hysterectomy, but occasionally the administration of a STEROID hormone will alleviate the symptoms.

endometritis inflammation of the ENDOMETRIUM caused commonly by bacteria but also by a virus, parasite or foreign body. It is associated with fever and abdominal pain and occurs mainly after abortion or childbirth or in women with an INTRAUTERINE CONTRACEPTIVE DEVICE.

endometrium the UTERUS'S MUCOUS MEMBRANE lining that changes in structure during the menstrual cycle, becoming thicker with an increased blood supply later in the cycle. This is in readiness for receiving an EMBRYO, but if this does not happen, the endometrium breaks down and most is lost in MENSTRUATION.

endorphin one of a group of PEPTIDES that occur in the BRAIN and have pain-relieving qualities similar to MORPHINE. They are derived from a substance in the PITUITARY and are involved in ENDOCRINE control. In addition to their opiate effects, they are involved in urine output, depression of respiration, sexual activity and learning (*see also* ENCEPHALIN).

endoscope an instrument used to inspect the interior of a body cavity. It is fitted with lenses and a light source and is usually inserted through a natural opening although an incision can be used.

endotoxin *see* TOXIN.

enema the procedure of putting fluid into the RECTUM for purposes of cleansing or therapy.

enteral a term meaning relating to the INTESTINE.

enteral feeding the procedure of feeding a patient who is very ill through a tube via the nose to the stomach.

enteritis INFLAMMATION of the INTESTINE, usually caused by a viral or bacterial infection, resulting in DIARRHOEA.

enterobacterium (*pl* **enterobacteria**) any of a class of Gram-negative (*see* GRAM'S STAIN) BACTERIA, including ESCHARICHIA and SALMONELLA, many of which are found in the human INTESTINE.

enteropeptidase *see* TRYPSIN.

enterovirus a VIRUS that enters the body via the gut, where it multiplies and from where it attacks the CENTRAL NERVOUS SYSTEM. Examples are POLIOMYELITIS and the Coxsackie viruses (the cause of severe throat infections, MENINGITIS and INFLAMMATION of heart tissue, some muscles and the brain).

enzyme any PROTEIN molecule that acts as a catalyst in the biochemical processes of the body. They are essential to life and are highly specific, acting on certain substrates at a set temperature and pH. Examples are the digestive enzymes amylase, lipase and TRYPSIN. Enzymes act by providing active sites (one or more for each enzyme) to which substrate molecules bind, forming a short-lived intermediate. The rate of reaction is increased, and after the product is formed, the active site is freed. Enzymes are easily rendered inactive by heat and some chemicals. They are vital for the normal functioning of the body, and their lack or inactivity can produce metabolic disorders.

epicardium *see* MYOCARDIUM.

epidemic a disease that affects a large proportion of the population at the same time, usually an infectious disease that occurs suddenly and spreads rapidly, e.g. influenza epidemics.

epidermis the outer layer of the SKIN, which comprises four layers and overlies the dermis. The top three layers are continually renewed as cells from the innermost germinative layer (called the Malpighian layer or stratum germinativum), which are pushed outwards. The topmost layer (stratum corneum) is made up of dead cells where the CYTOPLASM has been replaced by KERATIN. This layer is thickest on the palms and on the soles of the feet.

epididymis (*pl* **epididymides**) *see* TESTICLE.

epidural anaesthesia ANAESTHESIA in the region of the pelvis, abdomen or genitals produced by local anaesthetic injected into the epidural space of the SPINAL COLUMN (the epidural space being that space between the vertebral canal and the dura mater of the SPINAL CORD).

epiglottis situated at the base of the tongue, a thin piece of cartilage enclosed in MUCOUS MEMBRANE that covers the LARYNX. It prevents food from passing into the larynx and TRACHEA when swallowing. The epiglottis resembles a leaf in shape.

epiglottitis INFLAMMATION of the MUCOUS MEMBRANE of the EPIGLOTTIS. Swelling of the tissues may obstruct the airway and swift action may be necessary, i.e. a TRACHEOSTOMY, to avoid a fatality. The other symptoms of epiglottitis are sore throat, fever and a croup-like cough, and it occurs mainly in children, usually during winter.

epilepsy a neurological disorder involving convulsions, seizures and loss of consciousness. There are many possible causes, including cerebral trauma, brain tumour, cerebral haemorrhage and metabolic imbalances as in HYPO-GLYCAEMIA. Usually an epileptic attack occurs without warning, with complete unconsciousness and some muscle contractions and spasms. Some drugs are used in treatment although little can be done during the fit itself.

epineurium *see* NERVE.

epiphysis (*pl* **epiphyses**) the softer end of a long BONE that is separated from the shaft by a plate (the epiphyseal plate) of CARTILAGE. It develops separately from the shaft, but when the bone stops growing it disappears as the head and shaft fuse.

epinephrine *see* ADRENALINE.

epithelium (*pl* **epithelia**) tissue made up of cells packed closely together and bound by connective material. It covers the outer surface of the body and lines vessels and organs in the body. One surface is fixed to a basement membrane and the other is free, and it provides a barrier against injury, microorganisms and some fluid loss. There are various types of epithelium in single and multiple (or stratified) layers and differing shapes, namely, cuboidal, squamous (like flat pads) and columnar. The shape suits the function, so the SKIN is formed from stratified squamous (and KERATINIZED) epithelium while columnar epithelia, which can secrete solutions and absorb nutrients, line the INTESTINES and stomach.

Epstein-Barr virus a virus, similar to herpes, that causes infectious mononucleosis (GLANDULAR FEVER) and is implicated in HEPATITIS.

eruption an outbreak or RASH on the SKIN, usually in the form of a red and raised area, possibly with fluid-containing blisters or scales/crusts. It may be associated with a disease such as MEASLES or CHICKENPOX, a drug reaction or a physical or short-lived occurrence, e.g. nettle rash (URTICARIA).

erysipelas an infectious disease, caused by *Streptococcus pyogenes*. It produces an INFLAMMATION of the SKIN with associated redness. Large areas of the body may be affected, and other symptoms may include blisters, fever and pain with a feeling of heat and a tingling sensation. Patients are isolated and given PENICILLIN.

erythema an INFLAMMATION or redness of the SKIN in which the tissues are congested with BLOOD. The condition may be accompanied by pain or itching. There are numerous causes, some bacterial or viral and others physical, e.g. mild sunburn.

erythroblast a CELL occurring in the red BONE MARROW that develops into a red blood cell (ERYTHROCYTE). The cells are colourless at first but accumulate HAEMOGLOBIN and become red. In mammals, the NUCLEUS is lost.

erythrocyte the red blood cell that is made in the BONE MARROW and occurs as a red disc, concave on both sides, full of HAEMOGLOBIN. These cells are responsible for carrying oxygen to tissues and carbon dioxide away. The latter is removed in the form of the bicarbonate ion (HCO_3^-), in exchange for a chloride ion (Cl^-).

erythroderma *see* DERMATITIS.

erythromycin an ANTIBIOTIC used for bacterial and mycoplasmic infections. It is similar to PENICILLIN in its activity and can be taken for INFECTIONS that penicillin cannot treat.

eschar a SCAB or slough formed after living tissue has been destroyed by a BURN, CAUTERY or GANGRENE.

Escherichia *see page 24.*

essential amino acid of the 20 AMINO ACIDS required by the body, a number are termed essential because they must be included in the diet as they cannot be synthesized in the body. They are: isoleucine, leucine, lysine, methionine, phenylalanine, threonine, tryptophan and valine. In addition, infants require arginine and histidine. A lack leads to protein deficiency, but they are available in meat, cheese and eggs, and all eight would be obtained if the diet contained corn and beans.

essential fatty acid there are three polyunsaturated acids in this category, which cannot be produced in the body – arachidonic, linoleic and linolenic. These compounds are found in vegetable and fish oils and are vital for the proper functioning of the METABOLISM. A deficiency may cause such symptoms as allergic conditions, skin disorders, poor hair and nails, and so on.

Eustachian tube one of two tubes, one on each side, that connect the middle EAR to the PHARYNX. The short (about 35–40 mm) tube is fine at the centre and wider at both ends and is lined with mucous membrane. It is normally closed but opens to equalize air pressure on either side of the eardrum.

excision in general terms, a cutting out. More specifically, the removal of, for example, a gland or tumour from the body.

excoriation injury of the surface of the SKIN (or other part of the body) caused by the ABRASION or scratching of the area.

exhalation *see* RESPIRATION.

exocrine gland a GLAND that discharges its secretions through a DUCT, e.g. SALIVARY GLANDS and SWEAT GLANDS.

exogenous describing something originating outside the body.

expectorant one of a group of drugs that are taken to help in the removal of secretions from the LUNGS, BRONCHI and TRACHEA.

expiration *see* RESPIRATION.

extensor *or* **antagonist** a MUSCLE that extends or stretches to cause an arm, leg, etc, to move.

extrasystole *or* **ectopic beat** a heartbeat that is outside the normal rhythm of the HEART and is the result of an impulse generated outside the SINOATRIAL NODE. It may go unnoticed or it may seem that the heart has missed a beat. Extrasystoles are common in healthy people, but they may result from heart disease or nicotine from smoking, or caffeine from excessive intake of tea and coffee. Drugs can be taken to suppress these irregular beats.

eye the complicated organ of sight. Each eye is roughly spherical and contained within the bony ORBIT in the skull. The outer layer is fibrous and comprises the opaque SCLERA and transparent CORNEA. The middle layer is vascular and is made up of the choroid (the blood supply for the outer half of the retina), ciliary body (which secretes aqueous humour) and the IRIS. The inner layer is sensory, the RETINA. Between the cornea and the LENS is a chamber filled with liquid aqueous humour, and behind the lens is a much larger cavity with jelly-like vitreous humour. Light enters the eye through the cornea and thence via the aqueous humour to the lens, which focuses the light on to the retina. The latter contains CONE and ROD cells that are sensitive to light, and impulses are sent to the visual cortex of the brain via the optic nerve to be interpreted.

F

face the front-facing part of the head, which extends from the chin to the forehead. There are 14 bones in the skull, supporting the face, and numerous fine muscles are responsible for movements around the eyes, nose and mouth, producing expression. These are under the control of the seventh cranial nerve, which is a mixed sensory and motor nerve known as the FACIAL NERVE.

facial nerve a CRANIAL NERVE that has a number of branches and supplies the muscles that control facial expression. It also has branches to the middle EAR, TASTE BUDS, SALIVARY GLANDS and lacrimal glands. Some branches are MOTOR and others SENSORY in function.

facial paralysis PARALYSIS of the FACIAL NERVE, which leads to a loss of function in the muscles of the face, producing a lack of expression in the affected side. It occurs in BELL'S PALSY. The condition is often temporary, if caused by INFLAMMATION, and recovers in time. If the nerve itself is damaged by injury, however, or if the person has suffered a stroke, the condition is likely to be permanent.

factor VIII *or* **antihaemophilic factor** one of the COAGULATION FACTORs normally present in the BLOOD. If the factor is deficient in males, it results in HAEMOPHILIA.

factor IX *see* HAEMOPHILIA.

faeces *or* **stools** the end waste products of DIGESTION, which are formed in the COLON and discharged via the ANUS. They consist of undigested food, BACTERIA, MUCUS and other secretions, water and bile pigments, which are responsible for the colour. The condition and colour of the faeces are indicators of general health; e.g. pale stools are produced in JAUNDICE and COELIAC DISEASE and black stools often indicate the presence of bleeding in the digestive tract.

fainting *or* **syncope** a temporary and brief loss of consciousness caused by a sudden drop in the blood supply to the brain. It can occur in perfectly healthy people, brought about by prolonged standing or emotional shock. It may also result from an infection or severe pain or loss of blood through injury and may occur during pregnancy. It is often preceded by giddiness, blurred VISION, sweating and ringing in the ears. Recovery is usually complete, producing no lasting ill-effects, although this depends upon the underlying cause.

Fallopian tubes a pair of tubes, one of which leads from each OVARY to the UTERUS. At the ovary, the tube is expanded to form a funnel with finger-like projections (fimbriae) surrounding the opening. This funnel does not communicate directly with the ovary but is open to the abdominal cavity. However, when an egg is released from the ovary, the fimbriae move and waft it into the Fallopian tube. The tube is about 10 to 12 cm long and leads directly into the uterus at the lower end through a narrow opening.

false rib *see* RIB.

farmer's lung an allergic condition caused by sensitivity to inhaled dust and the fungal spores that are found in mouldy hay or straw. It is a form of allergic alveolitis (INFLAMMATION of the alveoli of the lungs, *see* ALVEOLI), characterized by increasing BREATHLESSNESS. The condition may be treated by CORTICOSTEROID drugs but can be cured only by avoidance of the ALLERGEN.

fascioliasis a disease of the LIVER and BILE ducts caused by the organism *Fasciola hepatica* or liver fluke. Human beings and animals are hosts to the adult flukes, and the eggs of the parasite are passed out in FAECES. These are taken up by a species of snail, which forms an intermediate host for the parasite and from which the larval stages are deposited on vegetation, especially wild watercress. Human beings are then infected, especially by eating wild watercress, which should always be avoided. Symptoms include fever, loss of appetite, indigestion, nausea and vomiting, diarrhoea, abdominal pain, severe sweating and coughing. In severe cases the liver may be damaged, and there may be jaundice and even death. CHEMOTHERAPY is required to kill the flukes.

fatty acid one of a group of organic compounds, each consisting of a long, straight hydrocarbon chain and a terminal carboxylic acid (COOH) group. The length of the chain varies from one to nearly 30 carbon atoms, and the chains may be saturated or unsaturated. Some fatty acids can be synthesized within the body, but others, the ESSENTIAL FATTY ACIDs, must be obtained from food. Fatty acids have three major roles within the body.

1. They are components of glycolipids (lipids containing carbohydrate) and phospholipids (lipids containing phosphate). These are of major importance in the structure of tissues and organs.

2. Fatty acids are important constituents of triglycerides (lipids that have three fatty acid molecules joined to a glycerol molecule). They are stored in the cytoplasm of many cells and are broken down when required to yield energy. They are the form in which the body stores fat.

3. Derivatives of fatty acids function as hormones and intracellular messengers.

favism an inherited disorder that takes the form of severe haemolytic ANAEMIA (destruction of red blood cells), brought on by eating broad beans. A person having this disorder is sensitive to a chemical present in the beans and also to certain drugs, particularly some antimalarial drugs. It is caused by the lack of a certain ENZYME, glucose 6-phosphate dehydrogenase, which plays an important role in glucose METABOLISM. The defective GENE responsible is passed on as a SEX-LINKED dominant characteristic and appears to persist in populations in which it occurs because it also confers increased resistance to malaria.

febrile having a FEVER.

femoral the term used to describe the FEMUR or that area of the thigh, e.g. femoral artery, vein, nerve and canal.

femur the thigh bone, which is the long BONE extending from the hip to the knee and is the strongest bone in the body. It is the weight-bearing bone of the body and fractures are common in old people who have lost bone mass.

fertilization the fusion of SPERM and OVUM to form a ZYGOTE, which then undergoes CELL division to become an EMBRYO. Fertilization in humans takes place high up in the FALLOPIAN TUBE near the OVARY, and the fertilized egg travels down and becomes implanted in the UTERUS.

fetus *see* FOETUS.

fever an elevation of body TEMPERATURE above the normal, which accompanies many diseases and infections. The cause is the production by the body of endogenous pyrogen, which acts on the thermoregulatory centre in the HYPO-THALAMUS of the brain. This responds by promoting mechanisms that increase heat generation and lessen heat loss. It is the main factor in many INFECTIONS caused by BACTERIA or VIRUSes and is the result of TOXINS produced by the growth of these organisms. In an intermittent fever body temperature fluctuates, sometimes returning to normal. In a remittent fever there is also a fluctuating body temperature but this does not return to normal. In a relapsing fever, caused by bacteria of the genus *Borella*, transmitted by ticks or lice, there is a recurrent fever every three to 10 days following the first attack, which lasts for about one week. Treatment depends on the underlying cause, but it may be necessary to reduce the temperature by direct methods such as sponging the body with tepid water or by giving drugs such as ASPIRIN. Symptoms also include headache, shivering, nausea, diarrhoea or constipation. Above 41°C (105°F) there may be DELIRIUM or CONVULSIONS, especially in young children.

FH *see* **growth hormone**.

fibrillation the rapid non-synchronized contraction or TREMOR of MUSCLES in which individual bundles of fibres contract independently. It applies especially to HEART muscle and disrupts the normal beating so that the affected part is unable to pump BLOOD. Two types of fibrillation may occur, depending on which muscle is affected. Atrial fibrillation, often resulting from ATHERO-SCLEROSIS or rheumatic heart disease, affects the muscles of the atria and is a common type of ARRHYTHMIA. The heartbeat and pulse are very irregular and cardiac output is maintained by the contraction of the ventricles alone. In ventricular fibrillation, the heart stops pumping blood, so this is, in effect, cardiac arrest. The patient requires emergency resuscitation or death ensues within minutes.

fibrin the end product of the process of blood COAGULATION, comprising threads of insoluble protein formed from a soluble precursor, FIBRINOGEN, by the activity of the ENZYME thrombin. Fibrin forms a network that is the basis of a BLOOD CLOT.

fibrinogen a COAGULATION FACTOR present in the blood, which is a soluble protein and the precursor of FIBRIN.

fibroid a type of BENIGN tumour found in the UTERUS, composed of fibrous and muscular tissue and varying in size from 1 or 2 mm to a mass weighing several kilograms. They more commonly occur in childless women and those over the age of 35. Fibroids may present no problems but, alternatively, can be the cause of pain, heavy and irregular menstrual bleeding, urine retention or frequency of MICTURITION and sterility. Fibroids can be removed surgically but often the complete removal of the UTERUS (HYSTERECTOMY) is carried out.

fibroma a BENIGN tumour composed of fibrous tissue.

fibrosarcoma a MALIGNANT tumour of CONNECTIVE TISSUE, particularly found in the limbs, especially the legs.

fibrosis the formation of thickened CONNECTIVE TISSUE or scar tissue, usually as a result of injury or inflammation. This may affect the lining of the alveoli (*see* ALVEOLUS) of the lungs (pulmonary interstitial fibrosis) and causes breathlessness. *See also* CYSTIC FIBROSIS.

fibrositis INFLAMMATION of fibrous CONNECTIVE TISSUE, muscles and muscle sheaths, particularly in the back, legs and arms, causing pain and stiffness.

fibrous tissue a tissue type that occurs abundantly throughout the body. White fibrous tissue consists of fibres of COLLAGEN, a PROTEIN with a high tensile strength and unyielding structure, and forms ligaments, sinews and scar tissue, and occurs in the skin. Yellow fibrous tissue is composed of the fibres of another protein, elastin. It is very elastic and occurs in ligaments that are subjected to frequent stretching, such as those in the back of the neck. It also occurs in arterial walls and in the walls of the alveoli (*see* ALVEOLUS), and in the dermis layer of the SKIN.

fibula (*pl* **fibulae**) the outer, thin, long BONE that articulates with the larger TIBIA in the lower leg.

filariasis a tropical and subtropical disease caused by nematode worms in the LYMPHATIC SYSTEM. These parasitic worms are carried to humans by mosquitoes, resulting in blockages in the lymph vessels, causing swelling (ELEPHANTIASIS).

filovirus a HAEMORRHAGIC FEVER virus. *See* page 126.

fimbria (*pl* **fimbriae**) *see* FALLOPIAN TUBES.

finger *see* HAND; PHALANGES.

fissure a natural cleft or groove or abnormal break in the SKIN or MUCOUS MEMBRANE, e.g. an anal fissure.

fistula an abnormal opening between two hollow organs or between such an organ or gland and the exterior.

fit any sudden convulsive attack; a term that is applied to an epileptic seizure, convulsion or bout of coughing. *See also* CONVULSIONS.

flexion bending of a joint or the term may also be applied to an abnormal shape in a body organ.

flexor *or* **agonist** any MUSCLE that contracts to cause a limb or other body part to bend (*see* VOLUNTARY MUSCLE).

flutter an abnormal disturbance of heartbeat rhythm that may affect the atria or ventricles but is less severe than FIBRILLATION.

foetus *or* **fetus** an unborn child after the eighth week of development.

folic acid a compound that forms part of the VITAMIN B complex. It is involved in the biosynthesis of some AMINO ACIDS and is used in the treatment of ANAEMIA.

follicle any small sac, cavity or secretory GLAND. Examples are HAIR follicles and the Graafian follicles of the ovaries, in and from which eggs mature and are released.

follicle-stimulating hormone (FSH) *see* GONADOTROPHINS.

fomentation *see* POULTICE.

fontanelle an opening in the SKULL of newborn and young infants in whom the BONE is not wholly formed and the SUTURES are incompletely fused.

food poisoning an illness of the digestive system caused by eating food contaminated by certain BACTERIA, VIRUSes or by chemical poisons (insecticides) and metallic elements such as mercury or lead. Symptoms include vomiting, diarrhoea, nausea and abdominal pain, and these may arise very quickly and usually within 24 hours. Bacteria are the usual cause of food poisoning and proliferate rapidly, producing TOXINS that cause the symptoms of the illness. Those involved include members of the genera *Salmonella, Staphylococcus, Campylobacter* and also *Clostridium botulinum*, the causal organism of BOTULISM. Food poisoning may be fatal, the old and the young being especially at risk.

foramen a hole or opening, usually referring to those that occur in some BONES. For example, the foramen magnum is a large hole at the base of the SKULL (in the OCCIPITAL BONE) through which the SPINAL CORD passes out from the brain.

forebrain the part of the BRAIN that consists of the THALAMUS and HYPOTHALAMUS.

foreskin the prepuce, which is a fold of skin growing over the end (glans) of the PENIS.

fossa (*pl* **fossae**) a natural hollow or depression on the surface or within the body. An example is the fossae within the SKULL, which house different parts of the BRAIN.

fovea (*pl* **foveae**) any small depression, often referring to the one that occurs in the RETINA of the EYE in which a large number of the light-sensitive cells called CONES are situated. It is the site of greatest visual acuity, being the region in which the image is focused when the eyes are fixed on an object.

fracture any break in a BONE, which may be complete or incomplete. In a simple or closed fracture, the skin remains more or less intact, but in a compound or open fracture there is an open wound connecting the bone with the surface. This type is more serious as it provides a greater risk of infection and more blood loss. If a bone that is already diseased suffers a fracture (as often occurs in OSTEOPOROSIS), this is known as a pathological fracture. A fatigue fracture occurs in a bone that suffers recurrent, persistent stress, e.g. the march fracture sometimes seen in the second toe of soldiers after long marches. A greenstick fracture occurs only in young children, whose bones are still soft and tend to bend. The fracture occurs on the opposite side from the causal force. A complicated fracture involves damage to surrounding soft tissue, including nerves and blood vessels. A depressed fracture refers only to the SKULL when a piece of bone is forced inwards and may damage the brain. *See also* COMMINUTED FRACTURE.

frenulum lingae *see* TONGUE.

Friedreich's ataxia an inherited disorder that is caused by degeneration of NERVE cells in the BRAIN and SPINAL CORD. It appears in children, usually in adolescence, and the symptoms include unsteadiness during walking and a loss of the knee-jerk REFLEX ACTION, leading progressively to tremors, speech impairment and curvature of the spine. *See also* ATAXIA.

frontal lobe the anterior part of each cerebral hemisphere of the CEREBRUM of the BRAIN, extending back to a region called the central sulcus, which is a deep cleft on the upper outer surface.

FSH *see* GONADOTROPHINS.

fulminant a term used to describe a pain that is sudden and sharp.

fundus (*pl* **fundi**) **1.** the enlarged base of an organ farthest from its opening. **2.** a point in the RETINA of the EYE opposite the pupil.

fungal diseases diseases or infections caused by fungi.

fungus (*pl* **fungi**) any of a large order of single-celled plants that lack chlorophyll and reproduce by spores. Some forms are infectious, in the same way as BACTERIA, e.g. RINGWORM, and others are used in the production of ANTIBIOTICS.

furuncle *see* BOIL.

G

gall another term for BILE.

gall bladder a SAC-like organ on the underside of the liver that stores and concentrates BILE. It is approximately 8 cm long and 2.5 cm at its widest, and its volume is a little over 30 cm^2. When fats are digested, the gall bladder contracts, sending bile into the DUODENUM through the common bile duct. GALLSTONES, the most common gall bladder disease, may form in certain circumstances.

gallstones stones of varying composition that form in the GALL BLADDER. Their formation seems to be caused by a change in BILE composition rendering CHOLESTEROL less soluble. Stones may also form around a foreign body. There are three types of stone: cholesterol, pigment and mixed, the last being the most common. Although gallstones may be present for years without symptoms, they can cause severe pain and may pass into the common bile duct, where the obstruction results in JAUNDICE.

gamete a mature germ or sexual cell, male or female, that can participate in FERTILIZATION, e.g. OVUM and SPERM.

gamma globulin *or* **immune gamma globulin** a concentrated form of the ANTIBODY part of human BLOOD. It is used for IMMUNIZATION against certain infectious diseases, e.g. measles, poliomyelitis, hepatitis A, etc. It is of no use when the disease is diagnosed but can prevent or modify it if given before. *See also* GLOBULIN.

ganglion (*pl* **ganglia**) **1.** a mass of nervous tissue containing nerve cells and SYNAPSES. Chains of ganglia are situated on each side of the SPINAL CORD while other ganglia are sited near to or in the appropriate organs. Within the CENTRAL NERVOUS SYSTEM, some well-defined masses of nerve cells are called ganglia, e.g. basal ganglia (*see* BASAL GANGLION). **2.** a BENIGN swelling that often forms in the sheath of a TENDON and is fluid-filled. It occurs particularly at the wrist and may disappear quite suddenly.

gangrene death of tissue because of loss of BLOOD supply or bacterial infection. There are two types of gangrene, dry and moist. Dry gangrene is caused purely by loss of blood supply and is a late-stage complication of DIABETES MELLITUS in which ATHEROSCLEROSIS is present. The affected part becomes cold and turns brown and black and there is an obvious line between living and dead tissue. In time the gangrenous part drops off. Moist gangrene is the more common type and is the result of bacterial infection which leads to putrefaction and issuing of fluids from the tissue, accompanied by an obnoxious smell. The patient may suffer from fever and ultimately die of blood poisoning. (*See also* GAS GANGRENE.)

gaseous exchange the exchange of respiratory gases (oxygen and carbon dioxide) by diffusion across the walls of the alveoli (*see* ALVEOLUS) in the LUNGS.

gas gangrene a form of GANGRENE that occurs when wounds are infected with soil BACTERIA of the genus *Clostridium*. It produces TOXINS that cause decay and putrefaction with the generation of gas. The gas spreads into muscles and CONNECTIVE TISSUE, causing swelling, pain, fever and possibly toxic DELIRIUM, and if untreated the condition quickly leads to death. Some of these bacteria are anaerobic (i.e. they exist without air or oxygen) hence surgery, oxidizing agents and PENICILLIN can all be used in treatment.

gastric a term used to describe anything relating to the STOMACH.

gastric juice the secretion from the gastric GLANDS in the STOMACH. The main constituents are hydrochloric acid, rennin, mucin and pepsinogen, the last forming pepsin in the acid conditions. The acidity (around pH 1–1.5) also destroys unwanted bacteria.

gastric glands GLANDS that are situated in the MUCOUS MEMBRANE of the STOMACH and secrete GASTRIC JUICE. The glands are the cardiac, pyloric and fundic.

gastric ulcer an erosion of the MUCOSA in the STOMACH caused by such agents as acid and BILE. It may penetrate the muscle and perforate the stomach wall (*see* PERFORATION). Typical symptoms include burning pain, belching and possibly nausea when the stomach is empty or soon after eating. Relief may be found with ANTACID compounds, but surgery may be necessary.

gastrin a HORMONE that stimulates excess production of acidic GASTRIC JUICE

gastritis INFLAMMATION of the STOMACH lining (MUCOSA). It may be caused by BACTERIA or excessive alcohol intake.

gastroenteritis INFLAMMATION of both the STOMACH and INTESTINES, leading to VOMITING and DIARRHOEA. It is most commonly caused by viral or bacterial infection and fluid loss can be serious in children.

gastroenterology the study of diseases that affect the gastrointestinal tract, including the PANCREAS, GALL BLADDER and BILE DUCT in addition to the STOMACH and INTESTINES.

gastrointestinal tract *see* ALIMENTARY CANAL.

gene the fundamental unit of genetic material found at a specific location on a CHROMOSOME. It is chemically complex and responsible for the transmission of information between older and younger generations. Each gene contributes to a particular trait or characteristic. There are more than 100,000 genes in humans, and gene size varies with the characteristic, e.g. the gene that codes for the hormone INSULIN is 1,700 base pairs long. There are several types of gene, depending on their function, and in addition genes are said to be dominant or recessive. A dominant characteristic is one that occurs whenever the gene is present while the effect of a recessive gene (e.g. a disease) requires that the gene be on both members of the chromosome pair, i.e. it must be homozygous. *See also* SEX-LINKED DISORDERS.

genetic code specific information, carried by DNA molecules, that controls the particular AMINO ACIDS and their positions in every PROTEIN and thus all the proteins synthesized within a cell.

genetic screening the procedure whereby individuals are tested to determine whether their GENE make-up suggests they carry a particular disease or condition. If it is shown that someone carries a genetically linked disease, then decisions can be taken regarding future children. *See also* SEX-LINKED DISORDERS.

genetics the study of heredity and variation in individuals and the means whereby characteristics are passed from parent to offspring.

genital the term used to describe anything relating to reproduction or the organs of the REPRODUCTIVE SYSTEM.

genitalia the male or female organs of the REPRODUCTIVE SYSTEM, often referring to the external parts only.

genito-urinary tract the GENITAL and URINARY ORGANS and associated structures: KIDNEYS, URETER, BLADDER, URETHRA and GENITALIA.

genome the total genetic information stored in the CHROMOSOMES of an organism, the number of chromosomes being characteristic of that particular species.

German measles *or* **rubella** a highly infectious viral disease, occurring mainly in childhood, which is mild in effect. Spread occurs through close contact with infected individuals, and there is an incubation period of two to three weeks. Symptoms include headache, shivering, and sore throat with a slight fever. There is some swelling of the neck, and soon after the onset a rash of pink spots appears, initially on the face and/or neck and subsequently spreading over the body. The rash disappears in roughly one week, but the condition remains infectious for three or four more days. IMMUNITY is usually conferred by the infection, and although it is a mild disease it is important because an attack during the early stages of PREGNANCY may cause foetal abnormalities. Girls are therefore immunized around the age of 12.

gestation the length of time from FERTILIZATION of the OVUM to birth (*see also* PREGNANCY).

giddiness *see* VERTIGO.

gigantism *or* **giantism** excessive growth of the body, usually as a result of over-production of GROWTH HORMONE from the PITUITARY GLAND during childhood or adolescence.

gingivitis INFLAMMATION of the gums.

gland an organ or group of CELLS that secretes a specific substance or substances. ENDOCRINE GLANDS secrete directly into the blood, while exocrine glands secrete on to an epithelial surface via a duct. Some glands produce fluids, e.g. milk from the mammary glands, saliva from the sublingual bland. The THYROID gland is an endocrine gland that releases hormones into the bloodstream. A further system of glands, the lymphatic glands, occur throughout the body in association with the lymphatic vessels (*see* LYMPH).

glandular fever *or* **infectious mononucleosis** an infectious viral disease caused by the EPSTEIN-BARR VIRUS. It produces a sore throat and swelling in neck LYMPH NODES (also those in the armpits and groin). Other symptoms include headache, fever and a loss of appetite. The LIVER may be affected, and the SPLEEN may become enlarged or even ruptured and then requires surgery.

glans the head of the PENIS, normally covered by the FORESKIN.

glaucoma a condition that results in loss of VISION because of high pressure in the EYE, although there is usually no associated disease of the eye. There are several types, which occur at differing rates but are all characterized by high intraocular pressure (because of the outflow of aqueous HUMOUR being restricted), which damages nerve fibres in the RETINA and optic nerve. Treatment involves reduction of the pressure with drops and tablets (to reduce production of aqueous humour), and if necessary surgery is undertaken to create another outlet for the aqueous humour.

glia *or* **neuroglia** *or* **glial cells** CONNECTIVE TISSUE in the CENTRAL NERVOUS SYSTEM composed of a variety of cells. The macroglia are divided into astrocytes, which surround brain capillaries, and oligodendrocytes, which form MYELIN sheaths. The microglia perform a mainly scavenging function. Glial cells are present at 10 to 50 times the number of NEURONS in the nervous system.

globin *see* HAEMOGLOBIN.

globulin one of a group of globular PROTEINS that occur widely in milk, blood, eggs and plants. There are four types in blood SERUM: a1, a2, b and g. The alpha and beta types are carrier proteins, like HAEMOGLOBIN, and GAMMA GLOB-ULINS include the IMMUNOGLOBULINS involved in the immune response.

glomerulus *see* KIDNEY; NEPHRITIS.

glottis 1. the opening between the VOCAL CHORDS. **2.** the part of the LARYNX involved with sound production.

glucagon a HORMONE important in maintaining the level of the body's BLOOD SUGAR. It works antagonistically with INSULIN, increasing the supply of blood sugar through the breakdown of GLYCOGEN to glucose in the liver. Glucagon is produced by the ISLETS OF LANGERHANS when blood-sugar level is low.

glucocorticosteroid *see* CORTICOSTEROID.

glue ear *or* **secretory otitis media** a form of OTITIS, common in children, which occurs as an INFLAMMATION of the middle EAR, with the production of a persistent sticky fluid. It can cause deafness and may be associated with enlarged ADENOIDS. In treatment of the condition, the adenoids may be removed and GROMMETS inserted.

gluteal the term used to describe the buttocks or the muscles forming them.

gluten enteropathy *see* COELIAC DISEASE.

gluteus *or* **glutaeus** (*pl* **glutei** *or* **glutaei**) one of the three muscles of each buttock. The gluteus maximus shapes the buttock and extends the thigh, the gluteus medius and gluteus minimus abduct the thigh (i.e. move the limb away from the body) while the former also rotates it.

glycerol a transparent colourless liquid with a very sweet taste, which is obtained from fats.

glycogen *or* **animal starch** a carbohydrate (polysaccharide) stored mainly in the LIVER. It acts as an energy store that is liberated upon hydrolysis (*see* GLUCAGON).

glycoprotein *see* INTERFERON.

glycosuria the presence of sugar (glucose) in the urine, which is usually because of DIABETES MELLITUS.

goitre swelling of the neck because of THYROID GLAND enlargement. The thyroid tries to counter the dietary lack of iodine necessary to produce thyroid hormone by increasing the output, thereby becoming larger. The endemic or simple goitre is the result. Other types are caused by HYPERPLASIA and autoimmune diseases, e.g. when antibodies are produced against antigens in the thyroid gland.

gonadotrophins *or* **gonadotrophic hormone** HORMONES secreted by the anterior PITUITARY GLAND. Follicle-stimulating hormone (FSH) is produced by males and females, as is luteinizing hormone, LH, (interstitial cell-stimulating hormone, ICSH, in males). FSH controls, directly or indirectly, growth of the ova and sperm, while LH/ICSH stimulates reproductive activity in the GONADS.

gonads the reproductive organs that produce the GAMETES and some hormones. In the male and female, the gonads are the TESTICLES and ovaries (*see* OVARY) respectively.

gonorrhoea the most common VENEREAL DISEASE, which is spread primarily by sexual intercourse but may be contracted through contact with infected discharge on clothing, towels, etc. The causative agent is the bacterium *Neisseria gonorrhoeae*, and it affects the MUCOUS MEMBRANE of the VAGINA or, in the male, the URETHRA. Symptoms develop approximately one week after infection and include pain on urinating with a discharge of pus.

Inflammation of nearby organs may occur (testicle, prostate in men; uterus, Fallopian tubes and ovaries in women), and prolonged inflammation of the urethra may lead to formation of FIBROUS TISSUE, causing STRICTURE. Joints may also be affected, and later complications include ENDOCARDITIS, arthritis and CONJUNCTIVITIS. Treatment is usually very effective through the administration of penicillin, sulphonamides or tetracycline.

gout a disorder caused by an excess of URIC ACID in the bloodstream, which is deposited in JOINTS as salts (urates) of the acid. This causes INFLAMMATION of the affected joints and painful gouty ARTHRITIS with destruction of the joints. The KIDNEYS may also be damaged, with formation of stones. Deposits of the salts (called tophi) may reach the stage where they prohibit further use of the joints, causing hands and feet to be set in a particular position. Treatment of gout is through drugs that increase the excretion of the urate salts or slow their formation.

Graafian follicle *see* FOLLICLE.

graft the removal of some tissue or an organ from one person for application to or IMPLANTATION into the same person or another individual. For example, a SKIN graft involves taking healthy skin from one area of the body to heal damaged skin, and a KIDNEY (or renal) graft (or transplant) is the removal of the organ from one person (usually a recently dead individual) to another. Numerous types of graft are now feasible, including skin, bone, cornea, cartilage, nerves and blood vessels, and whole organs such as kidney, heart and lung.

Gram's stain a technique described by H. C. J. Gram, the Danish bacteriologist, in 1884, which involves using a stain to differentiate between certain BACTERIA. Bacteria on a microscope slide are first stained with a violet dye and iodine, then rinsed in ethanol to decolorize and a second red stain added. Gram-positive bacteria keep the first stain and appear violet when examined under the microscope, while Gram-negative forms lose the first but take up the second stain, thus appearing red. The difference in staining is because of the structure of the bacteria cell walls.

grand mal a convulsive epileptic fit involving involuntary muscular contractions and lack of respiration. The latter produces bluish skin and lips (CYANOSIS). Convulsive movements follow, and often the tongue is bitten and bladder control is lost. On awakening, the patient has no recall of the event.

granulocyte *see* LEUCOCYTE.

Graves' disease a disorder typified by THYROID GLAND overactivity (*see* HYPERTHYROIDISM), an enlargement of the gland and protruding eyes. It is caused by antibody production and is probably an autoimmune response.

greenstick fracture *see* FRACTURE.

grey matter a part of the CENTRAL NERVOUS SYSTEM comprising the central part of the spinal cord and the CEREBRAL CORTEX and outer layer of the CEREBELLUM in the brain. It is brown-grey in colour and is the coordination point between the nerves of the central nervous system. It is composed of nerve cell bodies, DENDRITES, SYNAPSES, glial cells (supporting cells, *see* GLIA) and BLOOD VESSELS.

groin the area where the ABDOMEN joins the THIGHS.

grommet a small tube with a lip at either end that is inserted into the eardrum to permit fluid to drain from the middle EAR. It is used in the treatment of secretory otitis media (GLUE EAR).

growth hormone *or* **somatotrophin** *or* **FH** a HORMONE produced and stored by the anterior PITUITARY GLAND that controls protein synthesis in muscles and the growth of long BONES in legs and arms. Low levels result in DWARFISM in children and overproduction produces GIGANTISM.

guanine *see* NUCLEOTIDE.

gullet another term for the OESOPHAGUS.

Guthrie test *see* PHENYLKETONURIA.

H

haem a compound containing iron, composed of a PIGMENT, known as a porphyrin, that confers colour. It combines with a PROTEIN called globin in the blood to form HAEMOGLOBIN.

haem- a prefix that indicates anything relating to BLOOD.

haemangioma a benign TUMOUR of the BLOOD VESSELS. It may be visible on the skin as a type of naevus (BIRTHMARK), e.g. a strawberry haemangioma.

haemarthrosis bleeding into a JOINT, which causes swelling and pain and may be the result of injury or disease. It can be a symptom of HAEMOPHILIA.

haematemesis vomiting of blood, which may occur for a number of different reasons. Common causes are ulcers, either GASTRIC or DUODENAL, or GASTRITIS, especially when this is caused by irritants or poisons such as alcohol. Also, blood may be swallowed and subsequently vomited as a result of a nosebleed.

haematinic a substance that increases the amount of HAEMOGLOBIN in the BLOOD, e.g. ferrous sulphate. Haematinic drugs are often prescribed during PREGNANCY.

haematocoele leakage of BLOOD into a cavity, causing a swelling. It usually forms as a result of an injury caused by the rupture of blood vessels and the leaking of blood into a natural body cavity.

haematoma a collection of blood forming a firm swelling, a bruise. It may occur as a result of injury, a clotting disorder of the blood or if blood vessels are diseased.

haematuria the presence of BLOOD in the URINE, which may have come from the kidneys, ureters, bladder or urethra. It indicates the presence of inflammation or disease, such as a stone in the bladder or kidney.

haemodialysis the use of an artificial KIDNEY to remove waste products from a person's BLOOD using the principle of DIALYSIS. It involves passing blood from an ARTERY into the dialyser on one side of a semipermeable membrane. On the other side of the membrane, a solution of ELECTROLYTES of similar composition to the blood is circulated. Water and waste products pass through the membrane into this solution while cells and proteins are retained within the blood. The purified blood is then returned to the patient's body through a vein.

haemoglobin the respiratory substance contained within the red BLOOD cells, which contains a PIGMENT responsible for the red colour of blood. It consists of the pigment HAEM and the protein globin and is responsible for the transport of oxygen around the body. Oxygen is picked up in the lungs by arterial blood and transported to the tissues, where it is released. This (venous) blood is then returned to the lungs to repeat the process (*see* OXYHAEMOGLOBIN).

haemoglobinopathy any of a number of inherited diseases in which there is an abnormality in the formation of HAEMOGLOBIN. Examples are THALASSAEMIA and SICKLE CELL ANAEMIA.

haemoglobinuria the presence of HAEMOGLOBIN in the URINE caused by disintegration of red BLOOD cells, conferring a dark red or brown colour. It can sometimes result from strenuous exercise or after exposure to cold in some people. It is also caused by the ingestion of poisons, such as arsenic, and is a symptom of some infections, particularly BLACKWATER FEVER.

haemolysis the destruction (LYSIS) of red blood cells (ERYTHROCYTES), which may result from INFECTION, poisoning or as an antibody response (*see* ANTI-BODIES).

haemolytic disease of the newborn a serious disease affecting FOETUSes and newborn babies, which is characterized by HAEMOLYSIS, leading to ANAEMIA and severe JAUNDICE.

haemophilia an hereditary disorder of blood COAGULATION in which the blood clots very slowly. It is a SEX-LINKED DISORDER, a recessive condition carried on the X-CHROMOSOME, and hence it affects males, with females being the carriers. There are two types of haemophilia because of a deficiency of either one of two COAGULATION FACTORS in the blood. Haemophilia A is caused by deficiency of FACTOR VIII and haemophilia B by deficiency of factor IX (Christmas factor). The severity of the disease depends on how much less of the coagulation factor than normal is present. The symptoms are prolonged bleeding from wounds and also into joints, muscles and other tissues. Now the condition can be treated by injections or transfusions of plasma containing the missing coagulation factor and, with care, a sufferer can hope to lead a normal life.

haemopoiesis formation of BLOOD cells (particularly ERYTHROCYTES, the red blood cells) and platelets, which takes place in the BONE MARROW in adults but in a foetus occurs in the liver and spleen.

haemoptysis *see* HAEMORRHAGE.

haemorrhage bleeding – a flow of blood from a ruptured BLOOD VESSEL, which may occur externally or internally. A haemorrhage is classified according to the type of vessels involved: arterial H – bright red blood spurts in pulses from an ARTERY; venous H – a darker coloured steady flow from a VEIN; CAPILLARY L – blood oozes from torn capillaries at the surface of a wound. In addition, a haemorrhage may be primary, i.e. it occurs at the moment of injury. It is classed as reactionary when it occurs within 24 hours of an injury and results from a rise in BLOOD PRESSURE. A secondary haemorrhage occurs after a week or ten days as a result of infection (SEPSIS). Haemorrhage from a major artery is the most serious kind as large quantities of blood are quickly lost and death can occur within minutes. Haemorrhages at specific sites within the body are designated by special names, e.g. HAEMATURIA (from the KIDNEY or URINARY TRACT), haemoptysis (from the LUNGS) and HAEMATEMESIS (from the STOMACH).

haemorrhagic fever virus a viral disease with a high mortality rate. *See* page 126.

haemorrhoids *or* **piles** varicose and inflamed VEINS around the lower end of the bowel, situated in the wall of the ANUS. They are classified as internal, external and mixed, depending on whether they appear beyond the anus. They are commonly caused by constipation or diarrhoea, especially in middle and older age, and may be exacerbated by a sedentary lifestyle. They may also occur as a result of childbearing. Symptoms of haemorrhoids are bleeding and pain, and treatment is by means of creams, injections and suppositories (*see* SUPPOSITORY) and sometimes surgery.

haemostasis 1. the natural process to arrest bleeding (*see* HAEMORRHAGE), involving blood COAGULATION and contraction of a ruptured BLOOD VESSEL. 2. One of a number of surgical procedures designed to arrest bleeding, such as the use of LIGATURES.

haemothorax a leakage of BLOOD into the PLEURAL CAVITY of the chest, usually as a result of injury.

hair a threadlike outgrowth from the EPIDERMIS layer of the SKIN, which is a dead structure consisting of KERATINic cells. The part above the skin has three layers: an outer CUTICLE, a CORTEX containing PIGMENT that confers colour, and an inner core. The lower end of the hair (root) lies within the skin and is expanded to form the bulb, which contains dividing cells that are continuously pushed upwards. This is contained within a tubular structure known as the hair follicle. A small erector pili muscle, attached to the hair follicle in the dermis of the skin, operates to erect the hair.

hammer toe *see* CORN.

hamstring any of four TENDONs at the back of the knee, which are attached to the hamstring muscles and anchor these to the TIBIA and FIBULA. They are responsible for the bending of the knee joint.

hand the extremity of the upper limb below the wrist, which has a highly complex structure and an 'opposable' thumb, unique to humans. The human hand is highly developed in terms of structure, nervous supply and function, and communicates with a large area on the surface of the BRAIN. It is capable of performing numerous functions with a high degree of precision. When there is brain damage and PARALYSIS, the uses of the hand tend to be lost earlier and more permanently compared to movements in the leg and face. The hand consists of eight small carpal bones in the wrist (*see* CARPUS), five METACARPAL BONES in the region of the palm and three PHALANGES in each finger.

hantavirus a HAEMORRHAGIC FEVER VIRUS. *See* page 126.

hare lip a congenital developmental deformity that results in the presence of a cleft in the upper lip. It is brought about by a failure in the fusion of three blocks of embryonic tissue and is often associated with a CLEFT PALATE. It is routinely corrected by surgery.

hay fever an allergic reaction to pollen, e.g. that of grasses, trees and many other plants, which affects numerous individuals. The symptoms are a blocked and runny nose, sneezing and watering eyes because of the release of HISTAMINE. Treatment is by means of ANTIHISTAMINE drugs.

HCG *see* CHORIONIC GONADOTROPHIC HORMONE; HUMAN CHORIONIC GONADOTROPHIN.

heart the hollow, muscular organ that acts as a pump and is responsible for the CIRCULATION OF THE BLOOD. The heart is cone-shaped, with the point downwards, and is situated between the LUNGS, slightly to the left of the midline. The heart projects forwards and lies beneath the fifth rib. The wall consists mainly of CARDIAC MUSCLE, lined on the inside by the ENDOCARDIUM. An external membrane, the PERICARDIUM, surrounds the heart. A SEPTUM divides the heart into right and left halves, each of which is further divided into an upper chamber, the ATRIUM, and a lower one, the VENTRICLE. Four valves control the direction of blood flow at each outlet, the aortic, pulmonary, tricuspid and mitral. These prevent back flow once the blood has been forced from one chamber into the next.

heart attack *see* MYOCARDIAL INFARCTION.

heart block a condition describing a failure in the conduction of electrical impulses from the natural PACEMAKER (the SINOATRIAL NODE) through the HEART, which can lead to slowing of the pumping action. There are three types:
1. First degree (partial or incomplete) heart block – a delay in conduction between atria (*see* ATRIUM) and VENTRICLES, but this does not cause slowing.
2. Second degree heart block – an intermittent slowing because not all the impulses are conducted between atria and ventricles.

3. Third degree (or complete) heart block – there is no electrical conduction, the heartbeats are slow, and the ventricles beat at their own intrinsic slow rhythm. This causes blackouts and can lead to HEART FAILURE.

Heart block is more common in elderly people where degenerative changes have occurred. It may, however, also be CONGENITAL or result from other forms of heart disease, such as MYOCARDITIS, CORONARY THROMBOSIS, CARDIOMYOPATHY and VALVE DISEASE. For second and third degree heart block, treatment involves use of an artificial pacemaker.

heartburn a burning pain or discomfort felt in the region of the heart and often rising upwards to the throat. It is caused by regurgitation of the STOMACH contents, the burning being caused by the acid in GASTRIC JUICE or by oesophagitis (INFLAMMATION of the OESOPHAGUS). It is relieved by taking ANTACID tablets or alkaline substances such as sodium bicarbonate.

heart failure the inability of the HEART to sustain effective CIRCULATION OF THE BLOOD. It is usually the result of weakness of the MYOCARDIUM or inefficiency in the rhythmical action of the heart. Acute heart failure is caused most frequently by CORONARY THROMBOSIS. Chronic heart failure is a more gradual degenerative condition and is secondary to other diseases, such as ARTERIOSCLEROSIS or respiratory conditions such as EMPHYSEMA and BRONCHITIS.

heat exhaustion exhaustion and collapse as a result of overheating of the body and loss of fluid following unaccustomed or prolonged exposure to excessive heat. It is more common in hot climates and results from excessive sweating, leading to loss of fluids and salts and disturbance of the ELECTROLYTE balance in body fluids. In the mildest form, which is heat collapse, BLOOD PRESSURE and PULSE rate fall, accompanied by FATIGUE and light-headedness, and there may be muscular CRAMPS. Treatment involves taking a salt solution and avoidance by gradual acclimatization to the heat, especially if hard physical work is to be carried out.

heat rash *see* PRICKLY HEAT.

heat stroke *or* **heat hyperpyrexia** a severe condition following exposure of the body to excessive heat, characterized by a rise in TEMPERATURE and failure of sweating and temperature regulation. There is a loss of consciousness, followed by coma and death, which can occur rapidly. The body must be cooled by sponging and salt solutions given either by mouth or intravenously.

Heimlich's manoeuvre a procedure to dislodge a foreign body that is blocking the LARYNX and causing CHOKING.

hemiplegia *see* PARALYSIS.

Henle's loop *see* KIDNEY.

heparin an ANTICOAGULANT substance naturally present in the body and produced by liver and some white blood cells and in some other sites. It acts by inhibiting and neutralizing the action of the ENZYME thrombin (*see* BLOOD COAGULATION). It is used medically to prevent blood coagulation in patients with THROMBOSIS and also in blood collected for sampling.

hepatic the term used to describe the LIVER, e.g. the hepatic VEIN, which drains blood from the liver to the inferior VENA CAVA.

hepatitis *see* page 53.

hepatoma a malignant TUMOUR of the LIVER, which is rare in Western countries except among people with CIRRHOSIS. It is common in parts of the Far East and Africa, and a suspected cause is the aflatoxin, or poison, produced by a fungus that contaminates stored peanuts and cereals. The cancer often produces alpha fetoprotein, which is detectable in the blood and is an indicator of the presence of the malignancy.

heredity the principle applied to the passing on of all bodily characteristics from parents to offspring. *See* GENETICS.

hernia the protrusion of a part or whole of an organ from out of its normal position within the body cavity. Most commonly, a hernia involves part of the INTESTINE. A CONGENITAL hernia is present at birth. An acquired hernia occurs after birth, a common example being an inguinal hernia, in which part of the bowel bulges through a weak part of the abdominal wall. Another common type is a hiatus hernia, in which the stomach passes through the hiatus (a hole allowing passage of the OESOPHAGUS), from the abdomen into the chest cavity. A reducible hernia is freely movable and can be returned by manipulation into its rightful place. An irreducible hernia is the opposite, and an incarcerated hernia is one that has become swollen and fixed in its position. An obstructed hernia is one involving the bowel. The contents of the hernia are unable to pass farther down and are held up and obstructed. The most dangerous is a strangulated hernia, in which the blood supply has been cut off because of the protrusion itself. This becomes painful and eventually gangrenous and requires immediate surgery. Strenuous physical activity can lead to a hernia, which usually develops gradually. Although short-term measures are employed to control a hernia or reduce its size, the usual treatment is by means of surgery to return and retain the protrusion in its proper pace.

heroin a white crystalline powder that is derived from morphine. It is a very potent ANALGESIC but is highly addictive and dangerous.

herpes infectious inflammation of the SKIN and MUCOUS MEMBRANES, characterized by the development of small blisters and caused by a number of different *Herpes* viruses. The *Herpes simplex* virus, types I and II, are the cause of cold sores, which usually affect the lips, mouth and face. The virus is usually acquired in childhood and, once present, persists for life. It can be contracted without causing any symptoms but tends to flare up from time to time, producing the cold sores. *Herpes simplex* is also the cause of genital herpes, in which the blisters affect the genital region. Herpes zoster or shingles is produced by a virus that causes chickenpox in children. The virus affects the course of a nerve, producing severe pain and small yellowish blisters on the skin. Often the affected areas are the abdomen, back, face and chest, and although the disease subsides after about three weeks, the blisters form scabs that eventually drop off and the pain can persist for months. This is known as post-herpetic neuralgia, and pain-relieving drugs are needed to help relieve the condition. Other Herpes viruses are the cytomegalovirus and EPSTEIN-BARR virus.

hiatus hernia *see* HERNIA.

hindbrain the part of the BRAIN that consists of the MEDULLA OBLONGATA, PONS and CEREBELLUM.

hip the region on either side of the body where the FEMUR (thigh bone) articulates with the pelvis.

hip girdle *see* PELVIC GIRDLE.

hip joint a 'ball and socket' JOINT made up of the head of the FEMUR, which rests inside a deep, cup-shaped cavity (the acetabulum) in the hip bone. The hip bone (or innominate bone) is itself made up of three fused bones: the PUBIS, ISCHIUM and ILIUM, which form part of the PELVIS.

histamine a substance, derived from histidine that is an amino acid. It is widely found throughout all the body tissues and is responsible for the dilation of blood vessels (arterioles and capillaries) and the contraction of smooth MUSCLE, including that of the BRONCHI of the lungs. Histamine is released in great quantities in allergic conditions and ANAPHYLAXIS (*see also* ALLERGY).

histidine *see* ESSENTIAL AMINO ACID; HISTAMINE.

HIV the human immunodeficiency virus responsible for the condition known as AIDS. *See* page 39.

hives a common name for URTICARIA, or nettle rash.

Hodgkin's disease a malignant disease of unknown cause affecting the LYMPHATIC SYSTEM, in which there is a gradual and increasing enlargement of lymph glands and nodes throughout the body. The accompanying symptoms include loss of weight, sweating, ANAEMIA and a characteristic type of fever (Pel-Ebstein fever). The person becomes gradually weaker and the glands may attain a very large size. The outlook is good, especially if it is detected early.

hormone a chemical substance that is naturally produced by the body and acts as a messenger. A hormone is produced by CELLS or GLANDS in one part of the body and passes into the bloodstream. When it reaches another specific site, its 'target organ', it causes a reaction there, modifying the structure or function of cells, perhaps by causing the release of another hormone. They are secreted by the ENDOCRINE GLANDS, and examples are the sex hormones, e.g. TESTOSTERONE, secreted by the testes (*see* TESTICLE), and oestradiol and PROGESTERONE, secreted by the ovaries (*see* OVARY).

hormone replacement therapy (HRT) *see* MENOPAUSE.

housemaid's knee *or* **bursitis** a painful condition resulting from a swelling of the BURSA (fluid-filled fibrous sac) in front of the kneecap.

HRT *see* MENOPAUSE.

human chorionic gonadotrophin (HCG) a HORMONE secreted by the PLACENTA during early PREGNANCY, under the influence of which the OVARY produces OESTROGEN, PROGESTERONE and relaxin, which are essential for the maintenance of pregnancy. Pregnancy can be detected early on by a laboratory procedure that tests for the presence of HCG in the URINE. *See* CHORIONIC GONADOTROPHIC HORMONE.

human T-cell lymphocytotrophic virus (HTLV) one of a group of viruses, including the HIV virus that causes AIDS (HTLV III), which are responsible for LYMPHOMAS.

humerus (*pl* **humeri**)the bone of the upper arm that articulates with the shoulder blade (SCAPULA) of the PECTORAL GIRDLE and the ULNA and RADIUS at the elbow.

humour a natural fluid in the body, the best-known examples being the aqueous and vitreous humours of the EYE.

Huntington's chorea *see* **chorea**.

hydrocephalus *or* **water on the brain** an abnormal collection of CEREBROSPINAL FLUID within the SKULL that causes, in babies and children, a great increase in the size of the head. It results either from an excessive production of fluid or from a defect in the mechanism for its reabsorption or from a blockage in its circulation. The cause may be CONGENITAL, and it often accompanies SPINA BIFIDA or infection (MENINGITIS) or the presence of a TUMOUR. Hydrocephalus causes pressure on the BRAIN, with drowsiness, irritability and mental subnormality in children. Treatment involves surgery to redirect the fluid but is not always successful. About 50 per cent of children survive if the progress of the condition is halted, and one-third of these go on to enjoy a normal life.

hydrocortisone a STEROID glucocorticoid HORMONE produced and released by the CORTEX of the ADRENAL GLANDS (a CORTICOSTEROID). It is closely related to CORTISONE, being released in response to stress and playing a significant part in carbohydrate METABOLISM. Medically it has a number of uses, especially in the treatment of ADDISON'S DISEASE, inflammatory, allergic and rheumatic conditions, e.g. eczema and rheumatoid arthritis. Prolonged use may cause SIDE EFFECTS, including PEPTIC ULCERS, stunting of growth in children, CUSHING'S SYNDROME and damage to bone and muscle tissue.

hydrophobia *see* RABIES.

hymen a thin MEMBRANE that covers the lower end of the VAGINA at birth and usually tears before a girl reaches PUBERTY.

hyperadrenalism a condition in which the ADRENAL GLANDS are overactive, producing the symptoms of CUSHING'S SYNDROME.

hyperalgesia an extreme sensitivity to pain.

hyperemesis VOMITING to excess. Hyperemesis gravidarum is excessive vomiting during PREGNANCY, which often begins as an exaggerated form of MORNING SICKNESS. Medical intervention is imperative in this condition.

hyperglycaemia the presence of excess sugar (glucose) in the blood, as in DIABETES MELLITUS, caused by insufficient INSULIN to cope with carbohydrate intake. The condition can lead to a diabetic coma.

hyperlipidaemia *or* **hyperlipaemia** the presence of an excess concentration of fat in the blood. An excess of CHOLESTEROL in the blood may lead to CORONARY ARTERY DISEASE and ATHEROMA. An excess of TRIGLYCERIDES may lead to PANCREATITIS.

hyperplasia increased growth in size and number of the normal CELLs of a tissue so that the affected part enlarges, e.g. the BREASTS during PREGNANCY. *Compare* HYPERTROPHY and NEOPLASM.

hypersensitivity abnormal allergic response to an ANTIGEN to which the person has previously been exposed. Hypersensitive responses vary from quite mild, such as HAY FEVER, to very severe and life-threatening, e.g. ANAPHYLAXIS. (*See also* ALLERGY.)

hypertension high BLOOD PRESSURE (in the arteries). Essential hypertension may be the result of an unknown cause or KIDNEY or ENDOCRINE diseases. MALIGNANT hypertension will prove fatal if not treated. It may be a condition in itself or an end stage of essential hypertension. It tends to occur in a younger age group, and there is high diastolic blood pressure (*see* DIASTOLE) and kidney failure. ARTERIOSCLEROSIS is a complication of, and often associated with, hypertension. Other complications include cerebral HAEMORRHAGE, HEART FAILURE and kidney failure. Previously a fatal condition, antihypertensive drugs have revolutionized treatment and given sufferers a near-normal life. *See also* PULMONARY HYPERTENSION.

hyperthermia 1. extremely high and abnormal body TEMPERATURE, i.e. a FEVER. **2.** a method of treatment of certain diseases by inducing a state of fever, achieved by a variety of techniques.

hyperthyroidism excessive activity of the THYROID GLAND – an overactive thyroid. It may be caused by increased growth of the gland, by the presence of a tumour or by GRAVES' DISEASE.

hypertonicity *see* SPASTICITY.

hypertrophy an increase in the size of an organ because of enlargement of its CELLs (rather than in their number), often in response to a greater demand for work, e.g. the increase in size of the remaining kidney if the other is removed. *Compare* HYPERPLASIA.

hyperventilation breathing at an abnormally rapid rate when at rest, which may be a response to stress and, if not checked, results in unconsciousness because the concentration of carbon dioxide in the BLOOD falls. If the carbon dioxide level in the blood is abnormally high, because of impaired gas exchange in the LUNGS, e.g. in pulmonary OEDEMA and PNEUMONIA, hyperventilation may occur. (*See also* HYPOVENTILATION.)

hypochondria an abnormal preoccupation by an individual with the state of his or her health. In its severest form, the person wrongly believes that he or she is suffering from a number of illnesses and is anxious and depressed. Treatment is by means of psychotherapy and antidepressant drugs, but it tends to be difficult to cure.

hypodermic literally 'beneath the skin', the term usually used in reference to INJECTIONS given by means of a hypodermic syringe.

hypoglycaemia a lack of sugar in the blood, which occurs in starvation and also with DIABETES MELLITUS when too much INSULIN has been given and insufficient carbohydrates have been eaten. Symptoms include weakness, sweating, light-headedness and tremors, and can lead to coma. They are alleviated by taking in glucose, either by mouth or by injection in the case of hypoglycaemic coma.

hypoparathyroidism *or* **tetany** *see* PARATHYROID GLAND.

hypophysis *see* PITUITARY GLAND.

hypoplasia underdevelopment of a tissue or organ, such as can occur in the teeth as a result of illness or starvation (dental hypoplasia). It is marked by lines across the teeth of brown enamel.

hypothalamus an area of the BRAIN in the floor of the third VENTRICLE, with the THALAMUS above and PITUITARY GLAND below. It contains centres controlling vital processes, e.g. fat and carbohydrate METABOLISM, thirst and water regulation, hunger and eating, thermal regulation and sexual function. It also plays a part in the emotions and regulation of sleep. It controls the SYMPATHETIC and PARASYMPATHETIC NERVOUS SYSTEMS and secretions from the pituitary.

hypothermia 1. the bodily state when the core TEMPERATURE falls below 35°C (95°F) as a result of prolonged exposure to cold. At first, shivering occurs and the heart works harder to increase the flow of blood around the body. Eventually shivering ceases and, with increasing chilling, the function of the body organs becomes disturbed and cardiac output falls. The tissues require less oxygen as their functions start to fail, but eventually the heart is unable to supply even this reduced demand. The symptoms are fatigue and confusion followed by unconsciousness and death. **2.** A state of artificial hypothermia is occasionally induced during surgery to reduce the oxygen requirements of the tissues and enable the circulation to be briefly halted.

hypoventilation an abnormally slow rate of shallow breathing that may result from injury or the effects of drugs on the respiratory centre in the brain. The effect is to increase the amount of carbon dioxide in the blood and lessen that of oxygen. Eventually this leads to death from a lack of oxygen supply to cells and tissues.

hysterectomy the surgical removal of the UTERUS, either by means of an abdominal incision or through the VAGINA. It is commonly carried out if FIBROIDS are present or if the uterus is cancerous, and also if there is excessive bleeding.

I

ichthyosis a generally hereditary SKIN condition in which the skin is very dry and looks cracked, producing a resemblance to fish scales. There is no particular medication to take but vitamin A may help. The treatment is thus external and involves special baths and the application of ointments.

ICSH *see* GONADOTROPHINS.

idiopathic a term given to a disease to indicate that its cause is not known.

ileitis INFLAMMATION of the ILEUM, with pain, bowel irregularity and loss of weight. The intestinal wall may become thickened, and if the tract becomes blocked, surgery is required immediately. The specific cause is not known, but it may occur in association with TUBERCULOSIS, bacterial infection (by *Yersinia enterocolitica*), CROHN'S DISEASE and TYPHOID.

ileostomy a surgical procedure in which an opening is made in the abdominal wall to which the ILEUM is joined. This creates an artificial ANUS through which the waste contents of the INTESTINES are collected in a special bag. This procedure is undertaken to allow the COLON to heal after surgery or COLITIS, or in association with other surgery in treating cancer of the RECTUM.

ileum the lower part of the small INTESTINE between the JEJUNUM and the CAECUM.

ileus an obstruction of the INTESTINE (often the ILEUM), which may be mechanical, as a result of worms or a gallstone from the GALL BLADDER, or because of loss of PERISTALSIS. This latter condition may be caused by surgery, injury to the spine or PERITONITIS.

ilium (*pl* **ilia**) the largest of the BONES that form each half of the PELVIC GIRDLE. It has a flattened wing-like part fastening it to the SACRUM by means of LIGAMENTS.

immune the term used to mean being protected against an INFECTION by the presence of ANTIBODIES specific to the organism concerned.

immune gamma globulin *see* **gamma globulin**.

immunity the way in which the body resists infection because of the presence of ANTIBODIES and white blood cells (LEUCOCYTES). Antibodies are generated in response to the presence of ANTIGENS of a disease. There are several types of immunity: active immunity is when the body produces antibodies and continues to be able to do so during the course of a disease, whether occurring naturally (also called ACQUIRED immunity) or by deliberate stimulation. Passive immunity is short-lived and is provided by the injection of ready-made antibodies from someone who is already immune.

immunization the production of IMMUNITY to disease by artificial means. Injection of an ANTISERUM will produce temporary passive immunity, while active immunity is produced by making the body generate its own ANTIBODIES. This is done by the use of treated ANTIGENS (VACCINATION or INOCULATION). VACCINE is used for immunization, and it may be derived from live BACTERIA or VIRUSES or dead organisms or their products.

immunoglobulin any of a group of high molecular weight PROTEINS that act as ANTIBODIES and are present in SERUM and secretions. Designated Ig, there are five groups, each with different functions identified by a particular letter. Immunoglobulin A (Ig A) is the most common and occurs in all secretions of the body. It is the main antibody in the MUCOUS MEMBRANE of the INTESTINES, BRONCHI, saliva and tears. Ig D is found in the SERUM in small amounts but increases during allergic reaction. Ig E is found primarily in the LUNGS, SKIN and mucous membrane cells and is an anaphylactic antibody (*see* ANAPHYLAXIS). Ig G is synthesized to combat BACTERIA and VIRUSES in the body. Ig M, or macroglobulin, has a very high molecular weight (about five or six times that of the others) and is the first produced by the body when ANTIGENS occur. It is also the main antibody in BLOOD GROUP incompatibilities.

immunosuppression the use of drugs (immunosuppressives) that affect the body's IMMUNE system and lower its resistance to disease. These drugs are used to maintain the survival of transplanted organs in transplant surgery and to treat AUTOIMMUNE DISEASES. The condition may also be produced as a side effect, e.g. after chemotherapy treatment for cancer. In all instances, there is an increased risk of infection.

impacted a descriptive term for things being locked or wedged together or stuck in position, e.g. a wisdom tooth when it cannot erupt normally because of other tissues blocking it.

impetigo a staphylococcal and infectious SKIN disease found primarily in children. It spreads quickly over the body, starting as a red patch that forms pustules that join to create crusted yellowish sores. It is easily spread by contact or through towels, etc, and must be treated quickly otherwise it may continue on an individual for months. Treatment with ANTIBIOTICS is usually effective.

implant a drug, tissue or artificial object inserted or grafted into the skin or other organ. Drugs are often inserted into the skin for controlled release, and in RADIOTHERAPY treatment of prostate tumours or head/neck cancers can include embedding a capsule of radioactive material in tissue. A surgical implant includes a tissue graft (e.g. a BLOOD VESSEL), insertion of a PACEMAKER or a hip PROSTHESIS.

impotence the condition when a man is unable to have sexual intercourse because of lack of penile ERECTION or, less commonly, to ejaculate having gained an erection. It may be the result of a condition or disease (DIABETES, ENDOCRINE GLAND disorder) or, more commonly, a psychological or emotional problem.

incision a surgical cut into tissue or an organ and the act of making this cut.

incisor a TOOTH with a chisel edge, used for biting. The four front teeth in the jaw are incisors.

incontinence an inability to control bowel movements or the passage of URINE. Urinary incontinence may be caused by a lesion in the brain or spinal cord, injury to the sphincter or damage to the nerves of the bladder. Stress incontinence occurs during coughing or straining and is common in women because of the weakening of muscles in childbirth.

incubation 1. the time between a person being exposed to an infection and the appearance of symptoms. Incubation periods for diseases tend to be quite constant, some commoner ones being: measles 10 to 15 days; German measles 14 to 21; chicken pox 14 to 21; mumps 18 to 21; and whooping cough 7 to 10 days. **2.** the time taken to start and grow microorganisms in culture media. **3.** the process of caring for a premature baby in an INCUBATOR.

incubator 1. the transparent box-like container in which a premature baby is kept in controlled, infection-free conditions. **2.** a heated container for growth of bacterial cultures in a laboratory.

incus (*pl* **incudes**) *see* EAR.

indigestion *see* DYSPEPSIA.

induction 1. the commencement of LABOUR by artificial means, either by administering drugs to produce uterine contractions or by AMNIOTOMY. **2.** in ANAESTHESIA, the process prior to the required state of anaesthesia, including premedication with a sedative.

infant a child from birth to 12 months.

infantile paralysis *see* POLIOMYELITIS.

infarction the formation of an infarct, or dead area of tissue, in an organ or vessel because of the obstruction of the ARTERY supplying blood. The obstruction may be caused by a blood clot or an EMBOLUS.

infection the invasion of the body by PATHOGENs and the resulting condition. BACTERIA, VIRUSES, fungi (*see* FUNGUS), etc, are all included, and they enter the body, multiply and, after the INCUBATION period, symptoms may appear. The organisms reach the body in many ways: by airborne droplets, direct contact, sexual intercourse, or by VECTORS, from contaminated food or drink, etc.

infectious mononucleosis *see* GLANDULAR FEVER.

infertility the condition in which a person is unable to produce offspring naturally. Female infertility may be because of irregular or absence of ovulation, blocked FALLOPIAN TUBES, ENDOMETRIOSIS; while a low sperm count or other deficiency in the SPERMATOZOA can lead to male infertility. Treatment can include drug therapy, surgery or, more recently, the technique of IN VITRO FERTILIZATION.

inflammation the response of the body's tissues to injury or infection, which involves pain, redness, heat and swelling (acute inflammation). The first sign, when the tissues are infected or injured physically or chemically, is a dilation of BLOOD VESSELS in the affected area, increasing blood flow and resulting in heat and redness. The circulation then slows a little, and white blood cells migrate into the tissues producing the swelling. The white blood cells engulf invading BACTERIA, dead tissue and foreign particles. After this, either the white blood cells migrate back to the circulation or there is the production and discharge of PUS as healing commences. Chronic inflammation is when repair is not complete and there is formation of SCAR tissue.

influenza a highly infectious disease caused by a VIRUS that affects the RESPIRATORY TRACT. Symptoms include headache, weakness and fever, appetite loss and general aches and pains. Sometimes there is the complication of a lung infection, which requires immediate treatment. There are three main strains of influenza virus, designated A, B and C. The viruses quickly produce new strains, which is why an attack of one is unlikely to provide protection against a later bout of the disease. Epidemics occur periodically.

ingestion 1. the process of chewing and swallowing food and fluid that then go into the STOMACH. **2.** the means whereby a PHAGOCYTE takes in cell debris, foreign particales, microorganisms, etc.

inhalant a substance taken into the body by INHALATION. The substances can be in several forms: the steam of a hot solution; a pressurized aerosol of droplets of particles; or a powdered medication that is drawn into the body by breathing in deeply from a nonpressurized passive inhaler. Sufferers of ASTHMA use inhalers to deliver drugs to the BRONCHI (BRONCHODILATORS) for relief from attacks.

inhalation 1. *or* **inspiration** the act of drawing air into the lungs (*see* RESPIRATION). **2.** the medication breathed in, whether in gas, vapour of particulate form, to ensure contact with and/or treatment of conditions of the throat, BRONCHI or LUNGS.

injection the means whereby a liquid (often a drug) is introduced into the body by using a syringe in cases where it would otherwise be destroyed by digestive processes. The location depends on the speed with which the drug is to be absorbed and the target site. Thus, injections may go into the skin (intradermal) or beneath the skin (subcutaneous, as with INSULIN). For slow absorption an intramuscular injection is used, and INTRAVENOUS for fast delivery.

inner ear *see* EAR.

innervation the NERVE system serving a particular organ, tissue or area of the body that carries MOTOR impulses to the target and SENSORY impulses away from it towards the BRAIN.

innominate artery *or* **brachiocephalic trunk** a branch of the AORTA. *See also* CAROTID ARTERY.

innominate bone *see* HIP JOINT.

innoculation the process whereby a small quantity of solution is injected into the body to produce or increase IMMUNITY to the disease related to the solution (*see* IMMUNIZATION; VACCINATION).

insemination the introduction of SEMEN into the VAGINA, whether by sexual intercourse or artificial means.

insomnia the condition of being unable to remain asleep or to fall asleep, resulting in debilitating tiredness. It may be caused by a painful condition but is more likely to be the result of anxiety.

inspiration *see* INHALATION; RESPIRATION.

insulin a pancreatic HORMONE, produced in the ISLETS OF LANGERHANS, that initiates uptake of glucose by body CELLS and thereby controls the level of glucose in the blood. It works by stimulating proteins on cell surfaces within muscles and other tissues to take up glucose for their activity. A lack of hormone results in the sugar derived from food being excreted in the urine (DIABETES MELLITUS), In such cases, insulin can be administered by injection.

intercalated disc *see* MUSCLE.

intercostal the term used to describe nerves, muscles, etc, that are situated between the RIBS.

interferon PROTEINS released from CELLS infected with a VIRUS that restrict, or interfere with, the growth of that virus. They limit the growth of cells, hence their use in cancer treatment (which is as yet of indeterminate value).

interleukin one of several cytokines (molecules secreted by a cell to regulate other cells nearby, e.g. INTERFERON) that act between LEUCOCYTES. There are eight currently recognized, and some are involved in functions such as the recognition of ANTIGENS, enhancing the action of MACROPHAGES and the production of other cytokines.

interstitial cell-stimulating hormone *see* GONADOTROPHIN.

intervertebral disc fibrous cartilaginous discs that connect adjacent VERTEBRAe and permit rotational and bending movements. The discs make up approximately 25 per cent of the backbone length, and they act as shock absorbers, providing cushioning for the BRAIN and SPINAL CORD. With age, the discs lose their effectiveness and may be displaced (*see* PROLAPSED INTERVERTEBRAL DISC).

intestinal flora the BACTERIA usually found in the INTESTINE, some of which synthesize VITAMIN K. Acidic surroundings are produced by the bacteria, and this helps lessen infection by PATHOGENS unable to withstand the conditions.

intestine the part of the ALIMENTARY CANAL or tract between STOMACH and ANUS where final digestion and absorption of food matter occur, in addition to the removal of water and production of FAECES. The intestine is divided into the small intestine, comprising the DUODENUM, ILEUM and JEJUNUM, and the large intestine, which is made up of the CAECUM, vermiform APPENDIX, COLON and RECTUM. The length of the intestine in humans is about 9 metres (30 feet).

intracranial a term meaning 'within the SKULL', applied to diseases, structures, etc.

intracranial pressure the pressure within the CRANIUM; more specifically, the pressure is maintained by all tissues: BRAIN, BLOOD, CEREBROSPINAL FLUID, etc. An increase in the pressure can occur as a result of injury, haemorrhage or tumour, and treatment is necessary to restore it to normal.

intramuscular a term meaning 'within a muscle', e.g. an intramuscular INJECTION.

intrauterine device (IUD) a plastic or metal contraceptive device, often in the shape of a coil about 25 mm long, that is placed in the UTERUS. It probably prevents CONCEPTION by preventing potential implantation of the EMBRYO.

There are sometimes SIDE EFFECTS, e.g. back pain, but it is reasonably effective.

intravenous a term meaning 'relating to the inside of a VEIN', hence intravenous INJECTIONS are made into a vein, as are BLOOD TRANSFUSIONS.

intubation the insertion of a tube into the body through a natural opening. It is commonly used to keep an airway open by insertion into the mouth or nose and through the LARYNX. It may also be adopted to enable an ANAESTHETIC gas or oxygen to be delivered.

intussusception an eventual obstruction of the bowel caused by one part of the bowel slipping inside another part beneath it. The commonest sufferers are young children, and symptoms include pain, vomiting and the passage of a jelly-like bloodstained MUCUS. If the condition does not right itself, corrective treatment is essential.

invasion 1. the state when BACTERIA enter the body. **2.** the process whereby malignant CANCER cells move into nearby normal and deeper tissues and gain access to the BLOOD VESSELS.

in vitro a term used to refer to a biological or biochemical reaction or process that occurs literally 'in glassware', i.e. in a test-tube.

in vitro fertilization (IVF) the process of fertilizing an OVUM outside the body. The technique is used when a woman has blocked FALLOPIAN TUBES or when there is some other reason for SPERM and ovum not uniting. The woman produces several ova (because of hormone therapy treatment), which are removed by a LAPAROSCOPE and mixed with sperm and incubated in CULTURE medium until they are fertilized. Some are later implanted in the mother's UTERUS. The first successful live birth using this technique was in 1978.

in vivo a term used to refer to biological processes that occur in a living organism.

involuntary muscle one of two types of MUSCLE not under voluntary or conscious control, such as those in the BLOOD VESSELS, STOMACH and INTESTINES. The CARDIAC MUSCLE is slightly different.

iris the part of the EYE that controls the amount of light that enters. It is, in effect, a muscular disc, and to reduce the amount of light entering, circular MUSCLEs contract, and to increase the aperture in dim light, radiating muscles contract. The varying-sized hole is the PUPIL. The iris can be seen through the CORNEA and is the coloured part of the eye. This latter feature is accounted for by PIGMENT cells containing melanin (blue is little; brown is more).

irradiation the use in treatment of any form of radiating energy, i.e. electromagnetic radiation in the form of X-RAYS, alpha, beta or gamma radiation and also heat and light. Some radiations are used in diagnosis or cancer treatments, others for relief of pain.

irritable bowel syndrome a condition caused by abnormal muscular contractions (or increased motility) in the COLON, producing effects in the large and small INTESTINES. The specific cause is unknown and no disease is present, so treatment is limited to relief of anxiety or stress (which may be contributory factors) and also some drug therapy to reduce muscle activity and careful choice of diet to include a high fibre content.

irritant a general term encompassing any agent that causes irritation of a tissue, e.g. nettle stings, chemicals and gases, etc.

ischaemic relating to a decrease in BLOOD supply to a part of the body or an organ, caused by a blockage or narrowing of the BLOOD VESSELS. It is often associated with pain.

ischium (*pl* **ischia**) one of the three BONES that comprise each half of the PELVIS. It is the most posterior of the three and supports the weight of the body when sitting.

islets of Langerhans clusters of cells within the PANCREAS, which are the ENDOCRINE part of the gland. There are three types of cells, termed alpha, beta and delta, the first two producing GLUCAGON and INSULIN respectively, both vital hormones in the regulation of BLOOD-SUGAR levels. The third hormone produced is somatostatin (also released by the HYPOTHALAMUS), which works antagonistically against GROWTH HORMONE by blocking its release by the PITUITARY GLAND.

isoleucine *see* ESSENTIAL AMINO ACID.

isometric a term meaning 'of equal measurement' – isometric exercises are undertaken to build up MUSCLE strength by increasing tension in the muscles without contract, e.g. by pushing against something that cannot move.

isotopes atoms that differ from other atoms of the same element because of a different number of neutrons in the nucleus. Isotopes have the same number of protons and therefore the same atomic number but a different mass number (total number of protons and neutrons). Radioactive isotopes decay into other elements or isotopes through the emission of alpha, beta or gamma radiation, and some radioactive isotopes can be produced in the laboratory. RADIOTHERAPY uses such isotopes in the treatment of cancer.

itching *or* **pruritis** a SKIN condition or sensation prompting scratching to obtain relief. The causes are numerous and include mechanical irritation, e.g. by clothing or lice, skin diseases or conditions such as ECZEMA, allergies, etc.

IUD *see* INTRAUTERINE CONTRACEPTIVE DEVICE.

IVF *see* IN VITRO FERTILIZATION.

J

Japanese encephalitis *see* ENCEPHALITIS and page 122.

jaundice a condition characterized by the unusual presence of BILE pigment (BILIRUBIN) in the blood. The bile produced in the LIVER passes into the blood instead of the INTESTINES, and because of this there is a yellowing of the skin and the whites of the eyes. There are several types of jaundice: obstructive jaundice, which is caused by bile not reaching the intestine as a result of an obstruction, e.g. a GALLSTONE; haemolytic jaundice, in which red blood cells are destroyed by HAEMOLYSIS; hepatocellular jaundice, which is caused by a liver disease such as HEPATITIS, which results in the liver being unable to use the bilirubin; neonatal jaundice, which is quite common in newborn infants when the liver is physiologically immature but usually lasts only a few days. The infant can be exposed to blue light, which converts bilirubin to biliverdin, another (harmless) bile pigment.

jaw the term for the BONES that carry the teeth and associated soft tissues. More specifically, they are the upper jaw (maxilla) and the lower jaw (mandible). The maxillae are fixed, while the mandible (which is one bone after the age of about 12 months) hinges on part of the temporal bone in front of the ear.

jejunum the part of the small INTESTINE lying before the ILEUM and after the DUODENUM. Its main function is the absorption of digested food, and its lining has numerous finger-like projections (villi) that increase the surface area for absorption. The villi are longer in the jejunum than elsewhere in the small intestine.

joint a connection between BONES (and CARTILAGES). Joints can be categorized by their structure and the degree to which they permit movement: fibrous joints are fixed by FIBROUS TISSUE binding bones together, e.g the bones of the skull; cartilaginous joints are slightly movable. These have discs of cartilage between bones so that only limited movement is permitted over one joint but over several adjacent joints considerable flexure is achieved, as with the spine; synovial joints can move freely. Each synovial joint comprises the bones, cartilage over the ends, then a capsule (sheath of fibrous tissue) from which the ligaments form, and a SYNOVIAL MEMBRANE containing synovia for lubrication. This type of joint then occurs in two forms: hinge joints allowing planar movement (e.g. the knee), and ball and socket joints permitting all-round movement (e.g. the hip). Joints are subject to various conditions and diseases, including SYNOVITIS, epiphysitis (inflammation of the EPIPHYSIS), GOUT, RHEUMATISM and dislocations.

jugular a general term used to describe structures in the neck.

jugular vein any of the VEINS in the neck, particularly the anterior, internal and external. The anterior jugular vein is an offshoot of the external jugular vein and runs down the front of the neck. The external jugular itself drains the scalp, face and neck, while the larger internal jugular vein drains the face, neck and brain and is sited vertically down the side of the neck.

K

kala-azar *see* LEISHMANIASIS.

Kaposi's sarcoma a condition involving malignant SKIN tumours that form from the blood vessels. Purple lumps, as a result of the tumours, form on the feet and ankles, spreading to arms and hands. The disease is common in Africa but less so in Western countries, although it is associated with AIDS. RADIOTHERAPY is the primary treatment but CHEMOTHERAPY may also be required.

keloid *or* **cheloid** SCAR tissue that forms because of the growth of FIBROUS TISSUE over a BURN or injury, creating a hard, often raised, patch with ragged edges.

keratin a fibrous, sulphur-rich PROTEIN made up of coiled polyPEPTIDE chains. It occurs in hair, fingernails and the surface layer of the skin.

keratoplasty *see* CORNEAL GRAFT.

keratosis a condition of the SKIN whereby there is a thickening and overgrowth of the horny layer (or stratum corneum). It is usually induced by excessive sunlight and can occur as scales and patchy skin pigmentation (actinic keratosis) or as yellow/brown warts (seborrhoeic keratosis). It is essential to avoid overexposing the skin to sunlight if the condition is to be prevented or treated.

Kernig's sign the inability of someone with MENINGITIS to straighten his or her legs at the knee when the thighs are at right angles to the body. It is symptomatic of the disease.

ketoaciduria *see* **ketonuria**.

ketogenesis the normal production of KETONES in the body because of METABOLISM of fats. Excess production leads to KETOSIS.

ketone an organic compound that contains a carbonyl group (C=O) within the compound. Ketones can be detected in the body when fat is metabolized for energy when food intake is insufficient.

ketone body one of several compounds (e.g. acetoacetic acid) produced by the LIVER as a result of METABOLISM of fat deposits. They normally provide energy, via KETOGENESIS, for the body's peripheral tissues. In abnormal conditions, when carbohydrate supply is reduced, ketogenesis produces excess ketone bodies in the blood (KETOSIS) which may then appear in the URINE (KETONURIA).

ketonuria *or* **acetonuria** *or* **ketoaciduria** the presence of ketone bodies in the URINE as a result of starvation or DIABETES MELLITUS, causing excessive KETOGENESIS and KETOSIS.

ketosis the build-up of KETONES in the body and bloodstream because of a lack of carbohydrates for METABOLISM or failure fully to use the available carbohydrates, resulting in fat breakdown (*see* KETOGENESIS and KETONURIA).

kidney one of two GLANDS/organs that remove nitrogenous wastes, mainly UREA, from the BLOOD and also adjust the concentrations of various salts. It is positioned at the back of the abdomen, below the diaphragm. Blood is supplied to the kidney by the renal ARTERY and leaves via the renal VEIN. Each kidney is held in place by fat and CONNECTIVE TISSUE, and comprises an inner MEDULLA and outer CORTEX. The kidneys produce and eliminate URINE by a complex process of filtration and reabsorption. The 'active' parts are the nephrons, which filter blood under pressure, reabsorbing water and other substances. A nephron comprises a renal TUBULE and BLOOD VESSELS. The tubule expands into a cup shape that contains a knot of capillaries, called the glomerulus, and this brings the water, UREA, salts, etc. Filtrate passes from the glomerulus through three areas of the tubule, which together form a shape resembling a hairpin, leaving as urine. The kidneys contain roughly two million nephrons and receive between one and two thousands litres of blood each day, processing 150 to 200 litres of filtrate, resulting in roughly 1.5 litres of urine.

kinin one of a group of polyPEPTIDES that lower BLOOD PRESSURE through dilation of the BLOOD VESSELS and cause smooth MUSCLE to contract. They are associated with INFLAMMATION, causing local increases in the permeability of tissue capillaries. In addition they play some part in the allergic response and ANAPHYLAXIS. Kinins do not normally occur in the blood but form under these conditions or when the tissue is damaged.

Klinefelter's syndrome a genetic imbalance in males in which there are 47 rather than 46 CHROMOSOMES, the extra one being an X-CHROMOSOME, producing a genetic make-up of XXY instead of the usual XY. The physical manifestations are small testes which atrophy, resulting in a lack of sperm production, enlargement of the breasts, long thin legs and little or no facial or body hair. There may be associated mental retardation and pulmonary disease.

knee the JOINT connecting the thigh to the lower leg and formed by the FEMUR, TIBIA and kneecap (PATELLA). It is a hinge type of synovial joint with very strong LIGAMENTS binding the bones together. Although it is a strong joint, it is complex and injuries can be serious.

kneejerk *see* REFLEX ACTION.

knock-knee *or* **genu valgum** an abnormal curvature of the legs so that when the knees are touching, the ankles are spaced apart. When walking, the knees knock, and severe cases can lead to stress on the JOINTs in the legs, with ARTHRITIS. Surgery may be performed to correct the condition, which in the past was commonly a result of RICKETS but is now mainly the result of poor MUSCLES.

knuckle *see* METACARPAL BONE.

Koplik spots *see* MEASLES.

kuru *see* SPONGIFORM ENCEPHALOPATHY.

kwashiorkor a type of MALNUTRITION seen especially among children in Africa. It is the result of a deficiency in dietary PROTEIN and foods normally eaten for energy. It occurs when a child is weaned from the breast onto an adult diet that is inadequate, so the child cannot eat enough to obtain sufficient protein. The result is appetite loss, diarrhoea, oedema, anaemia and other conditions caused by, for example, VITAMIN deficiencies. Initially the condition responds well to first-class protein, but it is less straightforward with more prolonged cases.

L

labia (*sing* **labium**) lips or something resembling lips, as in the folds of skin enclosing the VULVA (the labia majora and minora).

labial 1. pertaining to the lips. **2.** the TOOTH surface next to the lips.

labour the process of giving birth, from dilatation of the CERVIX to expulsion of the AFTERBIRTH. It usually commences naturally, although some labours are induced. The cervix expands, and at the same time the muscles of the UTERUS wall contract, pushing part of the AMNION down into the opening. The amnion ruptures, releasing the 'waters', but these two events do not necessarily occur at the same time. The second stage is the actual delivery of the child, who passes through the bony girdle of the PELVIS via the VAGINA to the outside. Initially the head appears at the cervix, and the uterine contractions strengthen. These contractions are augmented by abdominal muscular contractions when the baby is in the vagina. When the baby's head is clear, the whole body is helped out and the UMBILICAL CORD severed. The final stage, accomplished by some contractions, is expulsion of the PLACENTA and membranes.

labyrinth part of the inner EAR, consisting of canals, ducts and cavities, forming the organs of hearing and balance. There are two parts: the membranous labyrinth, comprising the semicircular canals and associated structures and the central cavity of the cochlea; and the bony labyrinth, a system of canals filled with PERILYMPH (a third) and surrounding the other parts.

laceration a WOUND with jagged edges.

lacrimal relating to, or about, tears.

lacrimal gland one of a pair of GLANDs, situated above and to the side of each EYE, that secrete saline and slightly alkaline tears that moisten the conjunctiva (the MUCOUS MEMBRANE lining the inside of the eyelid). The glands comprise part of the lacrimal apparatus, the remainder being the lacrimal ducts (or canaliculi) through which the tears drain to the lacrimal sacs and the nasal cavity.

lactase the ENZYME that acts on milk sugar (LACTOSE) to produce the simple sugars glucose and galactose.

lactation the process of milk secretion by the MAMMARY GLANDs in the breast, which begins at the end of PREGNANCY.

lacteal vessels part of the LYMPHATIC SYSTEM. They occur as projections with a closed end extending into villi in the small INTESTINE and take up digested fats as a milky fluid called chyle.

lactose milk sugar found only in mammalian milk and produced by the MAMMARY GLANDs. It is made up of one molecule of glucose and one molecule of galactose. People with a low level of activity of the enzyme LACTASE, or none at all, cannot absorb lactose, a condition called lactose intolerance.

lacuna (*pl* **lacunae**) an anatomical term meaning a small depression, cavity or pit, especially in compact BONE.

lamella (*pl* **lamellae**) a thin plate, especially of BONE.

lamina (*pl* **laminae**) a thin plate, e.g. of BONE or MUSCLE, such as the laminae propria of MUCOUS MEMBRANE.

laparoscope a type of ENDOSCOPE that is inserted into the abdominal cavity through a small incision. This allows a surgeon to view the organs in the cavity (laparoscopy) and a laparoscope is also used to enable some minor operations to be performed using instruments inserted through a second incision.

large intestine *see* INTESTINE.

laryngitis INFLAMMATION of the MUCOUS MEMBRANE that lines the LARYNX and VOCAL CORDS. It is mainly caused by viral infection but also by BACTERIA, chemical irritants, heavy smoking or excessive use of the voice. Acute laryngitis accompanies infections of the upper respiratory tract, and symptoms include pain, a cough and difficulty in swallowing. Chronic laryngitis may be a recurrence of the acute form but is often attributable to excessive smoking worsened by alcohol. Changes occurring in the vocal cords are more permanent, and the symptoms are as for the acute form, but longer lasting.

laryngotracheobronchitis an acute INFLAMMATION of the major parts of the respiratory tract, causing shortness of breath, a CROUP-like cough and hoarseness. It occurs usually because of viral infection and particularly in young children where there may be some obstruction of the LARYNX. The main airways, the BRONCHI, become coated with fluid generated by the inflamed tissues, resulting in the shortness of breath. Treatment is through INHALATIONS, ANTIBIOTICS, if appropriate, and, if the obstruction is serious, hospitalization may be necessary for INTUBATION, TRACHEOSTOMY, etc.

larynx part of the air passage connecting the PHARYNX with the TRACHEA and also the organ producing vocal sounds. It is situated high up in the front of the neck and is constructed of CARTILAGES with LIGAMENTS and MUSCLES. The ligaments bind together the cartilages, and one pair of these form the VOCAL CORDS. The larynx is lined with MUCOUS MEMBRANE and in all is about 5 cm long.

Lassa fever a highly contagious viral infection first reported from Lassa in Nigeria. It takes from three to 21 days to incubate and results in FEVER and headache, acute muscular pains, sore throat and some difficulty in swallowing. Death often occurs because of HEART or KIDNEY failure, and pregnant women show a high mortality rate. Little can be done as it is a viral infection, but treatment with PLASMA from patients who have recovered may help.

laxative a substance that is taken to evacuate the bowel or to soften stools (*see* FAECES). Typical laxatives include castor oil, senna and its derivatives (*see also* PURGATIVE).

l-dopa *or* **levadopa** *see* DOPA.

legionnaires' disease *see* page 64.

leishmaniasis a common tropical and subtropical disease (in Africa, Asia, South America and the Mediterranean) caused by the parasitic protozoa *Leishmania*, which are transmitted by the bites of sandflies. Depending on the region, it affects people of differing ages, and there are two forms, visceral and cutaneous. In the former, internal organs are affected while in the latter it affects the SKIN but also the MUCOUS MEMBRANES. Visceral leishmaniasis results in FEVER, enlargement of the GLANDS, LIVER and SPLEEN, and roughly three-quarters of untreated cases result in fatalities. Cutaneous leishmaniasis produces skin ulcers that go by various names and may include the nose and throat. The drug commonly used to treat it is a salt of sodium that contains antimony.

lens the part of the EYE that focuses incoming light onto the RETINA. It is composed of a fibrous PROTEIN, crystallin, and is enclosed in a thin CAPSULE.

leprosy a serious disease caused by the bacterium *Mycobacterium leprae* that attacks the SKIN, NERVES and MUCOUS MEMBRANES and has an INCUBATION period of several years. There are two forms: tuberculoid leprosy, which occurs in those with a higher degree of IMMUNITY and produces discoloured patches of skin with some numbness but is generally BENIGN and often heals untreated; and lepromatous leprosy, which is a much more serious and progressively destructive form, creating lumps, thickening of skin and nerves, inflammation of the IRIS, numbness with MUSCLE weakness and PARALYSIS. The more serious cases show deformity and considerable disfigurement and sometimes blindness. There is also an intermediate form with symptoms of both types (indeterminate leprosy). Drugs therapy is quite effective, providing a combination of ANTIBIOTICS is used (because the bacterium develops resistance to one of the SULPHONAMIDES commonly used).

leptomeninges *see* MENINGES.

leptomeningitis INFLAMMATION of two of the three MENINGES surrounding the BRAIN and SPINAL CORD. Specifically, the inner two (pia mater and arachnoid) are affected.

leptospirosis an acute infectious disease caused by BACTERIA of the genus *Leptospira*. The disease varies from the mild form of an influenza type of illness to the more serious cases involving FEVER, LIVER disease and therefore JAUNDICE, and possibly KIDNEY disease or MENINGITIS. *See* page 100.

lesion 1. a WOUND or injury to body tissues. **2.** an area of tissue that, because of damage caused by disease or wounding, does not function fully. Thus, primary lesions include TUMOURS and ULCERS, and from primary lesions secondary lesions may form.

leucine *see* ESSENTIAL AMINO ACID.

leucocyte *or* **leukocyte** a white BLOOD cell, so called because it contains no HAEMOGLOBIN. It also differs from red blood cells (ERYTHROCYTES) in having a nucleus. Leucocytes are formed in the BONE MARROW, SPLEEN, THYMUS and LYMPH NODES, and there are three types: granulocytes, comprising 70 per cent of all white blood cells, LYMPHOCYTES (25 per cent) and MONOCYTES (5 per cent). Granulocytes help combat bacterial and viral infection and may be involved in allergies. Lymphocytes destroy foreign bodies, either directly or through production of ANTIBODIES, and monocytes ingest BACTERIA and foreign bodies by the process called PHAGOCYTOSIS. In disease, immature forms of leucocytes may appear in the blood (ultimately forming both red and white blood cells).

leucocytosis except for during PREGNANCY, MENSTRUATION and exercise, an abnormal and temporary increase in the number of white blood cells (*see* LEUCOCYTE) in the blood. It usually accompanies bacterial but not viral infections, because the body's defence mechanism is fighting the bacteria by producing leucocytes. A blood sample may thus form a useful diagnostic tool for a condition that has not yet manifested any physical symptoms.

leucorrhoea a discharge of white or yellow-coloured MUCUS from the VAGINA. It may be a normal condition, increasing before and after MENSTRUATION, but a large discharge probably indicates an infection somewhere in the genital tract.

leukaemia a cancerous disease in which there is an uncontrolled proliferation of LEUCOCYTES in the BONE MARROW. The cells fail to mature to adult cells and thus cannot function as part of the defence mechanism against infections. This leads to ANAEMIA, bleeding and easy bruising, with enlargement of the SPLEEN, LIVER and LYMPH NODES. Acute leukaemia has a sudden onset and development, while the chronic form may take years to develop the same symptoms. The cause is unknown although it has been attributed to viruses, exposure to toxic chemicals or ionizing radiations. In addition to the acute and chronic forms, it is further classified by the predominant white blood cells: acute lymphoblastic leukaemia, acute myeloblastic leukaemia (myeloblast is an early form of granulocytes, *see* LEUCOCYTE) and chronic lymphatic leukaemia. Treatment involves RADIOTHERAPY, CHEMOTHERAPY and bone marrow transplants. The survival or REMISSION rate varies with the type of leukaemia, and a cure is achievable in some cases.

levodopa *or* **l-dopa** *see* DOPA.

LH *see* GONADOTROPHINS.

ligament 1. bands of fibrous CONNECTIVE TISSUE, composed chiefly of COLLAGEN, that join BONES together, restricting movement and preventing dislocation. Ligaments strengthen JOINTS, and most joints are surrounded by a capsular ligament. **2.** a layer of SEROUS MEMBRANE, e.g. the PERITONEUM, which supports or links organs.

ligation 1. the procedure of tying off a DUCT or BLOOD VESSEL to prevent flow during surgery, etc. **2.** the application of a LIGATURE.

ligature material for tying firmly around a BLOOD VESSEL or DUCT to stop bleeding or prevent flow. The material may be wire, silk, catgut, etc.

light reflex the mechanism whereby the PUPIL of the EYE opens in response to direct light or the stimulation of one pupil with light results in a response in the other.

lingual a term meaning 'relating to the TONGUE', or something close to it (e.g. lingual NERVE or the lingual surface of a TOOTH).

linoleic, linolenic *see* ESSENTIAL FATTY ACID.

lipase *see* ENZYME; LIPOLYSIS; PANCREAS.

lipid an organic compound in fats that is soluble in organic solvents (e.g. alcohol) but insoluble in water.

lipolysis the breakdown of LIPIDS into FATTY ACIDS via the action of the ENZYME lipase.

lipoma a benign TUMOUR, made up of fat cells, that can occur in the fibrous tissues of the body, often beneath the SKIN. The only problem associated with such structures may be their size and position.

liposarcoma a malignant TUMOUR of fat cells that is very rare, particularly under the age of 30. It occurs in the buttocks or thighs.

lipoprotein a PROTEIN that has a FATTY ACID molecule attached to it. They are important in certain processes, e.g. transporting CHOLESTEROL.

liposome a spherical droplet of microscopic size comprising fatty membranes around an aqueous vesicle. Liposomes are created in the laboratory by adding an aqueous solution to a phospholipid gel (phospholipids are compounds containing FATTY ACIDS and a phosphate group). Liposomes bear some resemblance to living cell components and are studied on this basis. Additionally, they can be introduced into living cells and are used to transport toxic drugs to a specific treatment site. The liposomes retain the drug while in the blood and on passing through the chosen organ the membrane is melted by selectively heating the organ and the drug is released. This technique is used for certain forms of cancer.

listeriosis *see* page 83.

Little's disease CEREBRAL PALSY on both sides of the body that affects the legs more than the arms.

liver a very important organ of the body, with many functions critical in regulating metabolic processes. The largest GLAND in the body, it occupies the top right-hand part of the abdominal cavity and is made up of four LOBES. It is fastened to the abdominal wall by LIGAMENTS and sits beneath the DIAPHRAGM and on the right KIDNEY, large INTESTINE, DUODENUM and STOMACH.

There are two BLOOD VESSELS supplying the liver: the hepatic ARTERY delivers oxygenated blood, while the hepatic PORTAL VEIN conveys digested food from the stomach. Among its functions, the liver converts excess glucose to glycogen for storage as a food reserve; excess amounts of AMINO ACIDS are converted to UREA for excretion by the kidneys; BILE is produced for storage in the GALL BLADDER and LIPOLYSIS occurs; some poisons are broken down (detoxified), hence the beneficial effect of the hepatic portal vein carrying blood to the liver rather than it going around the body first.

The liver also synthesizes blood-clotting substances such as FIBRINOGEN and prothrombin and the anticoagulant HEPARIN; it breaks down red blood cells (ERYTHROCYTES) at the end of their life and processes the HAEMOGLOBIN for iron, which is stored; VITAMIN A is synthesized and stored, and it also stores VITAMINS B12, D, E and K. In the EMBRYO it forms red blood cells. Such is the chemical and biochemical activity of the liver that significant energy is generated, and this organ is a major contributor of heat to the body.

lobe certain organs are divided by FISSURES into large divisions that are called lobes, e.g. the BRAIN, LIVER and LUNGS.

lobectomy the removal of a LOBE of an organ, e.g. lung or brain. A lobe of a lung may be removed in CANCER or other disease.

lobule a small LOBE or a subdivision of lobe in an organ, e.g. the lobules of the LIVER.

lockjaw the nonmedical name for TETANUS.

loin that area of the back between the lower RIBS and the PELVIS.

lumbago pain of any sort in the lower back. It can be muscular, skeletal or neurological in origin. A severe and sudden case may be caused by a strained MUSCLE or slipped disc (*see* PROLAPSED INTERVERTEBRAL DISC), and the latter is usually the cause of lumbago with SCIATICA.

lumbar a general term for anything relating to the LOINS, e.g. LUMBAR VERTEBRAE.

lumbar puncture the procedure wherein a hollow needle is inserted into the spinal canal in the lumbar region (usually between the third and fourth LUMBAR VERTEBRAE) to obtain a sample of CEREBROSPINAL FLUID for diagnosis of diseases or to introduce drugs, etc.

lumbar vertebrae the five vertebrae between the SACRUM and the thoracic VERTE-BRAE at the lowest part of the back. The lumbar vertebrae are not fused and have strong attachments points (PROCESSES) for the MUSCLES of the lower back.

lumpectomy the surgical removal of a TUMOUR with the tissue immediately around it but leaving intact the bulk of the tissue and the LYMPH NODES. The procedure is used in BREAST CANCER, when it is often followed by RADIO-THERAPY and is undertaken for patients with a small tumour and no metastases (*see* METASTASIS) to nearby lymph nodes or organs elsewhere in the body.

lungs the SAC-like, paired organs of RESPIRATION, situated with their base on the DIAPHRAGM and the top projecting into the neck. Each lung consists of fibrous, elastic sacs that are convoluted to provide a large surface area for GASEOUS EXCHANGE. Air enters the body through the windpipe, or TRACHEA, which branches into two BRONCHI, one to each lung. Further branching then occurs into numerous BRONCHIOLES. The bronchioles divide further and then end in alveoli (*see* ALVEOLUS), where the gaseous exchange occurs. The exchange of oxygen and carbon dioxide occurs between the many blood capillaries (*see* CAPILLARY) on one side of the MEMBRANE and the air on the other. The lungs are served by the pulmonary arteries (*see* ARTERY) and pulmonary veins.

lunula (*pl* **lunulae**) *see* NAIL.

lupus any of a number of skin diseases, of which lupus vulgaris and lupus erythematosus are the two main types. Lupus vulgaris is characterized by small yellow transparent nodules that, if left unreated, will ulcerate and thicken, causing scars. Lupus erythematosus is thought to be an AUTOIMMUNE disease and is characterized by red raised patches on the skin which may merge at the edges ('butterfly lesions'). *See also* SYSTEMIC LUPUS ERYTHEMATOSUS.

lutenizing hormone *see* GONADOTROPHINS; PROGESTERONE.

Lyme disease an arthritic disease with rashes, fever and possibly carditis (inflammation of the heart) and ENCEPHALITIS. It is caused by a spirochaete (a type of BACTERIUM) that is transmitted by a tick bite. Symptoms may not appear until some time after the bite but ANTIBIOTICS can be used in treatment.

lymph a colourless, watery fluid that surrounds the body tissues and circulates in the LYMPHATIC SYSTEM. It is derived from blood and is similar to PLASMA, comprising 95 per cent water with PROTEIN, sugar, salts and LYMPHOCYTES. The lymph is circulated by muscular action, and passes through LYMPH NODES, which act as filters, and is eventually returned to the BLOOD via the thoracic ~ct (one of the two main vessels of the lymphatic system).

lymphadenitis INFLAMMATION of the LYMPH NODES, which become enlarged, hard and tender. The neck lymph nodes are commonly affected in association with another inflammatory condition.

lymphadenoma *see* HODGKIN'S DISEASE.

lymphatic gland *see* GLAND.

lymphatic system *or* **lymphatics** the network of vessels, valves, nodes, etc, that carry LYMPH from the tissues to the bloodstream and help maintain the internal fluid environment of the body. Lymph drains into capillaries and larger vessels, passing through nodes and eventually into two large vessels (the thoracic duct and right lymphatic duct), which return it to the bloodstream by means of the innominate veins.

lymph node any of numerous small oval structures that occur at various points in the LYMPHATIC SYSTEM. They are found grouped in several parts of the body, including the neck, groin and armpit, and their main functions are to remove foreign particles and produce LYMPHOCYTES, important in the IMMUNE response.

lymphocyte a type of white blood cell (LEUCOCYTE) produced in the BONE MARROW and also present in the SPLEEN, THYMUS GLAND and LYMPH NODES, which forms a vital component of the IMMUNE system. There are two types: B-cells or B-lymphocyte and T-cells or T-lymphocyte. B-cells produce ANTIBODIES and search out and bind with particular ANTIGENS. T-cells circulate through the thymus gland, where they differentiate. When they contact an antigen, large numbers of T-cells are generated, which secrete chemical compounds to assist the B-cells in destroying foreign bodies, e.g. BACTERIA.

lymphoedema the build-up of LYMPH in soft tissues, causing swelling. It may be the result of obstruction of the vessels by PARASITES, TUMOUR or INFLAMMATION. A secondary form of lymphoedema may occur after removal of lymph vessels in surgery or by blocking. The condition occurs most often in the legs, and treatment comprises use of elastic bandages and DIURETIC drugs.

lymphoid tissue tissues that are involved in the formation of LYMPH, LYMPHOCYTES and ANTIBODIES, such as the spleen, thymus and lymph nodes.

lymphoma a TUMOUR, usually MALIGNANT, of the LYMPH NODES. Often several lymph nodes become enlarged and subsequent symptoms include fever, anaemia, weakness and weight loss. If much of the lymphoid tissue is involved, there may be enlargement of the LIVER and SPLEEN. Life expectancy is often very low although treatment with drugs usually produces a marked response.

RADIOTHERAPY may be used for localized varieties (*see also* HODGKIN'S DISEASE).

lymphosarcoma a TUMOUR of the LYMPHATIC SYSTEM resulting in enlargement of the GLANDS, SPLEEN and LIVER. In general an older term applied to LYMPHOMAS other than HODGKIN'S DISEASE.

lysin *see* LYSIS.

lysine *see* ESSENTIAL AMINO ACID.

lysis 1. the destruction of CELLS by ANTIBODIES called lysins. **2.** more generally, the destruction of cells or tissues because of breakdown of the cell MEMBRANES.

lysozyme an ENZYME, present in tears, nasal secretions and on the skin, that has an antibacterial action (by breaking the cell wall of the bacterium). Lysozyme also occurs in ALBUMIN.

M

macrocephaly an abnormal enlargement of the head when compared with the rest of the body, *see* MICROCEPHALY, HYDROCEPHALUS.

macrocyte a red blood cell (ERYTHROCYTE) that is abnormally large. Macrocytes are characteristic of PERNICIOUS ANAEMIA.

macrocytosis the condition in which abnormally large red blood cells (ERYTHRO-CYTES) are present in the blood. It is characteristic of macrocytic anaemias such as those caused by the deficiency of VITAMIN B12 (cyanocobalamin, *see also* PERNICIOUS ANAEMIA) and FOLIC ACID. Macrocytes are also produced in those anaemias in which there is an increased rate of production of erythrocytes.

macroglia *see* GLIA.

macroglobulin *see* IMMUNOGLOBULIN.

macrophage a large scavenger CELL (phagocyte), numbers of which are found in various tissues and organs including the LIVER, SPLEEN, BONE MARROW, LYMPH NODES, CONNECTIVE TISSUE and the microglia of the CENTRAL NERVOUS SYSTEM. They remove foreign bodies such as BACTERIA from blood and tissues. Fixed macrophages remain in one place in the connective tissue; free microphages are able to migrate between cells and gather at sites of infection to remove bacteria and other foreign material.

macula (*pl* **maculae**) *or* **macule 1.** a small area or spot of tissue that is distinct from the surrounding region, e.g. the yellow spot in the retina of the EYE. **2.** a spot of small pigmented area in the SKIN, which may be thickened. They appear as a result of PREGNANCY, sunburn, ECZEMA or PSORIASIS and may be symptomatic of other diseases such as SYPHILIS and those affecting internal organs.

mad cow disease an informal name for BOVINE SPONGIFORM ENCEPHALOPATHY.

malabsorption syndrome a group of diseases in which there is a reduction in the normal absorption of digested food materials in the small INTESTINE. The food materials involved are commonly fats, vitamins, minerals, amino acids and iron. The diseases include COELIAC DISEASE, PANCREATITIS, CYSTIC FIBROSIS, SPRUE and STAGNANT LOOP SYNDROME and also surgical removal of a part of the small intestine.

malaria *see* page 116.

malignant 1. a term used to describe a TUMOUR that proliferates rapidly and destroys surrounding healthy tissue and can spread via the LYMPHATIC SYSTEM and bloodstream to other parts of the body. **2.** a term used to describe a form of a disease that is more serious than the usual one and is life-threatening, e.g. malignant HYPERTENSION.

malignant pustule *see* ANTHRAX.

malleus *see* EAR; TYMPANIC MEMBRANE.

malnutrition a condition caused either by an unbalanced diet, i.e. too much of one type of food at the expense of others, or by an inadequate food intake (subnutrition), which can lead to starvation. The condition may also arise because of internal dysfunction, e.g. MALABSORPTION SYNDROME or other metabolic disturbance within the body.

Malpighian layer *see* EPIDERMIS; SKIN.

mammary gland a GLAND present in the female BREAST that produces milk after childbirth.

mandible *see* JAW.

mandibular nerve *see* TRIGEMINAL NERVE.

Mantoux test a test for the presence of a measure of IMMUNITY to TUBERCULOSIS. A PROTEIN called tuberculin, extracted from the TUBERCLE bacilli (BACTERIA), is injected in a small quantity beneath the skin of the forearm. If an inflamed patch appears within 18 to 24 hours, it indicates that a measure of immunity is present and that the person has been exposed to tuberculosis. The size of the reaction indicates the severity of the original tuberculosis infection, although it does not mean that the person is actively suffering from the disease at that time.

Marfan's syndrome an inherited disease of CONNECTIVE TISSUE. The person affected is abnormally tall and thin, has spindly, elongated fingers and toes (arachnodactyly), spine and chest deformities and weak LIGAMENTS. Heart defects include a hole in the septum separating the right and left atria and narrowing of the aorta. The lenses of the eyes are partially dislocated.

mastalgia pain in the BREAST.

mast cell a large CELL, many of which are found in loose CONNECTIVE TISSUE. The CYTOPLASM contains numerous granules with chemicals important in the body, including HISTAMINE, SEROTONIN, HEPARIN and the antibody IMMUNOGLOBULIN E. All are important in allergic and inflammatory responses.

mastectomy surgical removal of the BREAST, usually performed because of the presence of a TUMOUR. Mastectomy may be simple, leaving the skin (and possibly the nipple) so that an artificial breast (PROSTHESIS) can be inserted. Or it may be radical, in which case the whole breast, the pectoral MUSCLES and the LYMPH NODES beneath the armpit are all removed, generally performed because a CANCER has spread.

mastitis INFLAMMATION of the BREAST, usually caused by bacterial infection during breast-feeding, the organisms responsible gaining access through cracked nipples. Cystic mastitis does not involve INFLAMMATION, but the presence of CYSTS (thought to be caused by hormonal factors) causes the breast(s) to be lumpy.

mastoid *see* MASTOID PROCESS.

mastoiditis INFLAMMATION of the mastoid cells and mastoid ANTRUM, usually caused by bacterial infection that spreads from the middle EAR. Treatment is by means of ANTIBIOTIC drugs and sometimes surgery. *See* MASTOID PROCESS.

mastoid process *or* **mastoid** a projection of the TEMPORAL bone of the SKULL, which contains numerous air spaces (mastoid cells) and is situated behind the ear. It provides a point of attachment for some of the neck muscles and communicates with the middle EAR through an air-filled channel called the mastoid ANTRUM. *See* MASTOIDITIS.

maxilla (*pl* **maxillae**) *see* JAW.

maxillary nerve *see* TRIGEMINAL NERVE.

ME *see* MYALGIC ENCEPHALOMYELITIS.

measles an extremely infectious disease of children caused by a VIRUS and characterized by the presence of a RASH. It occurs in epidemics every two or three years. After an INCUBATION period of 10–15 days, the initial symptoms are those of a COLD, with coughing, sneezing and high fever. It is at this stage that the disease is most infectious and spreads in airborne droplets before measles has been diagnosed, the main factor responsible for the epidemic nature of the disease. Small red spots with a white centre (Koplik spots) may appear in the mouth on the inside of the cheeks. Then a characteristic rash develops on the skin, spreading from behind the ears and across the face and also affecting other areas. The small red spots may be grouped together in patches, and the child's fever is usually at its height while these are developing. The spots and fever gradually decline and no marks are left on the skin, most children making a good recovery. However, complications can occur, particularly pneumonia and middle EAR infections, which can result in deafness. A VACCINE now available has reduced the incidence and severity of measles in the UK.

meatus a passage or opening, e.g. the external auditory meatus linking the pinna of the outer EAR to the eardrum.

media (*pl* **mediae**) the middle layer of a tissue or organ. Usually it is applied to the middle layer of the wall of a VEIN or ARTERY, comprising alternating sheaths of smooth MUSCLE and elastic fibres.

mediastinum the space in the CHEST cavity between the two LUNGS, which contains the HEART, AORTA, OESOPHAGUS, TRACHEA, THYMUS GLAND and PHRENIC NERVES.

medication any substance introduced into or on the body for the purposes of medical treatment, e.g. drugs.

medulla the inner portion of a tissue or organ when there are two distinct parts. Examples include the ADRENAL medulla and the medulla of the KIDNEYS. *Compare* CORTEX.

medulla oblongata the lowest part of the BRAIN stem, which extends through the FORAMEN magnum to become the upper part of the SPINAL CORD. It contains important centres that govern RESPIRATION, CIRCULATION, swallowing and salivation.

megaloblast an abnormally large form of any of the CELLS that go on to produce ERYTHROCYTES (red blood cells). In certain forms of ANAEMIA (megaloblastic anaemias), they are found in the BONE MARROW, and their presence is the result of a deficiency of VITAMIN B12 or of FOLIC ACID. They indicate a failure in the maturation process of erythrocytes, which results in anaemia.

meiosis a type of CELL division that occurs in the maturation process of the GAMETES (sperm and ova) so that the sex cells eventually contain only half the number of CHROMOSOMES of the parent cells from which they are derived.

melanin a dark brown PIGMENT found in the SKIN and HAIR and also in the choroid layer of the EYE. Melanin is contained and produced within cells, known as melanocytes, in the dermis layer of the skin. When the skin is exposed to hot sunshine, more melanin is produced, giving a 'suntan'. In dark-skinned races, more melanin is produced by greater activity of the melanocytes, and it helps to protect the skin from harmful ultraviolet radiation.

melanocyte *see* MELANIN; MELANOMA.

melanoma an extremely malignant TUMOUR of the melanocytes, the cells in the SKIN that produce MELANIN. Melanomas are also found, although less commonly, in the MUCOUS MEMBRANES and in the EYE. There is a link between the occurrence of melanoma of the skin and exposure to harmful ultraviolet light during sunbathing. A highly malignant form can also arise from the pigmented cells of MOLES. It can be successfully treated by surgery if it is superficial and caught at an early stage. It commonly spreads, however, especially to the LIVER and LYMPH NODES, when the outlook is poor. The incidence of MALIGNANT melanoma is increasing and has attracted much attention in connection with the formation of holes in the ozone layer, which screens the earth from harmful UV radiation. It is recommended that people should cover exposed skin, use sunscreen creams and avoid the sun at the hottest part of the day.

membrane 1. a thin composite layer of LIPOPROTEIN surrounding an individual CELL. **2.** a thin layer of tissue surrounding an organ, lining a cavity or tube or separating tissues and organs within the body.

Ménière's disease a disease that affects the inner EAR, causing deafness and TINNITUS (ringing in the ears), VERTIGO, VOMITING and sweating. It is most common in middle-aged men, with severe attacks of VERTIGO followed by VOMITING. The time interval between attacks varies from one week to several months, but the DEAFNESS gradually becomes more pronounced. The symptoms are caused by an over-accumulation of fluid in the LABYRINTHS of the inner ears, but the reason for this is not known. Treatment is by a variety of drugs and surgery, neither of which is completely successful.

meningeal sarcoma *see* MENINGIOMA.

meninges (*sing* **meninx**) the three CONNECTIVE TISSUE membranes that surround the SPINAL CORD and BRAIN. The outermost layer, or meninx, is called the dura mater, which is fibrous, tough and inelastic, and also called the pachymeninx, closely lining the inside of the SKULL and helping to protect the brain. It is thicker than the middle layer, the arachnoid mater, which surrounds the brain. The innermost layer, the pia mater, is thin and delicate and lines the brain. CEREBROSPINAL FLUID circulates between it and the arachnoid mater, and both these inner layers are richly supplied with BLOOD VESSELS that supply the surface of the brain and skull. These two inner membranes are sometimes collectively called the pia-arachnoid or leptomeninges.

meningioma a slow-growing TUMOUR affecting the MENINGES of the BRAIN or SPINAL CORD that exerts pressure on the underlying nervous tissue. It may cause PARAPLEGIA or other losses of sensation if present in the spinal cord. In the brain it causes increasing neurological disability. A meningioma can be present for many years without being detected. The usual treatment is surgical removal if the tumour is accessible. MALIGNANT meningiomas, known as meningeal sarcomas, can invade surrounding tissues. These are treated by means of surgery and also RADIOTHERAPY.

meningitis INFLAMMATION of the MENINGES of the BRAIN (cerebral meningitis) or SPINAL CORD (spinal meningitis), or the disease may affect both regions. *See* page 43.

menopause *or* **climacteric** the time in a woman's life when the ovaries (*see* OVARY) no longer release an egg cell every month and MENSTRUATION ceases. The woman is normally no longer able to bear a child and the age at which the menopause occurs is usually between 45 and 55. There may be a gradual decline in menstruation or in its frequency, or it may cease abruptly. There is a disturbance in the balance of SEX HORMONES, causing a number of physical symptoms, including palpitations, hot flushes, sweats, vaginal dryness, loss of libido and DEPRESSION. In the long term, there is a gradual loss of BONE (OSTEO-POROSIS) in postmenopausal women, which leads to greater risk of FRACTURES, especially of the FEMUR. These symptoms are relieved by hormone replacement therapy (HRT), involving OESTROGEN and PROGESTERONE, which is now generally recognized to be of great benefit.

menstrual cycle *and* **menstruation** the cyclical nature of the reproductive life of a sexually mature female. One OVUM develops and matures within a Graafian FOLLICLE in one of the ovaries (*see* OVARY). When the egg is mature, the follicle ruptures to release it, and it passes down the FALLOPIAN TUBE to the UTERUS. The ruptured follicle becomes a temporary ENDOCRINE GLAND, which secretes the hormone PROGESTERONE, under the influence of which the uterus wall (ENDOMETRIUM) thickens and its blood supply increases in readiness for the implantation of a fertilized egg. If the egg is not fertilized and there is no PREGNANCY, the thickened endometrium is shed along with a flow of blood through the VAGINA (menstruation). The usual age at which menstruation starts is 12 to 15. The duration varies and can be anything from 2 to 8 days, the whole cycle usually occupying about 29 to 30 days.

metronidazole *see* TRICHOMONIASIS.

mesencephalon *or* **mid-brain** the part of the BRAIN that connects the PONS and CEREBELLUM with the CEREBRUM.

mesentery a double layer of the peritoneal MEMBRANE (PERITONEUM), which is attached to the back wall of the ABDOMEN. It supports a number of abdominal organs, including the STOMACH, small INTESTINE, SPLEEN and PANCREAS, and contains associated NERVES, LYMPH and BLOOD VESSELS.

mesothelioma a malignant TUMOUR of the PLEURA of the chest cavity and also of the PERICARDIUM or PERITONEUM. It is usually associated with exposure to asbestos dust but may arise independently with no known cause. Most mesotheliomas are in sites that render them inoperable, and CHEMOTHERAPY and RADIOTHERAPY are used but often with limited success.

metabolism the sum of all the physical and chemical changes within CELLS and tissues that maintain life and growth. The breakdown processes that occur are known as catabolic (CATABOLISM), and those that build materials up are called anabolic (anabolism). The term may also be applied to describe one particular set of changes, e.g. PROTEIN metabolism. Basal metabolism is the minimum amount of energy required to maintain the body's vital processes, e.g. heartbeat and respiration, and is usually assessed by means of various measurements taken while a person is at rest.

metabolite *see* ANTIMETABOLITE; DRUG METABOLISM.

metacarpal bone one of the five BONES of the middle of the HAND, between the PHALANGES of the fingers and the carpal bones of the wrist (*see* CARPUS) forming the metacarpus. The heads of the metacarpal bones form the knuckles.

metaplasia an abnormal change that has taken place within a tissue e.g. myeloid metaplasia, where elements of BONE MARROW develop within the SPLEEN and LIVER. Also squamous metaplasia, which involves a change in the EPITHELIUM lining the BRONCHI of the LUNGS.

metastasis the process by which a malignant TUMOUR spreads to a distant part of the body and also the secondary growth that results from this. The spread is accomplished three routes: the blood CIRCULATION, LYMPHATIC SYSTEM and across body cavities.

metatarsal bone one of the five BONES in the FOOT, lying between the toes and the TARSAL bones of the ankle, together forming the metatarsus. The metatarsal bones are equivalent to the METACARPAL BONES in the HAND.

methicillin an ANTIBIOTIC drug used in staphylococcal infecions.

methicillin-resistant Staphylococcus aureus (MRSA) *see* page 3.

methionine *see* ESSENTIAL AMINO ACID.

metritis inflammation of the UTERUS.

microcephaly the condition in which there is abnormal smallness of the head compared to the rest of the body. *See also* MACROCEPHALY.

microglia *see* MACROPHAGE.

microorganism an organism that is too small to be studied with the naked eye and must be studied under a microscope. Microorganisms include BACTERIA and VIRUSes..

microsurgery surgery performed with the aid of an operating microscope using high precision miniaturized instruments. It is routine for some operations on the EYE, LARYNX and EAR and increasingly in areas inaccessible to normal surgery, e.g. parts of the BRAIN and SPINAL CORD.

micturition the act of URINATION.

mid-brain *see* MESENCEPHALON.

middle ear *see* EAR.

migraine a very severe throbbing HEADACHE, usually on one side of the head, which is often accompanied by disturbances in vision, NAUSEA and VOMITING. It is a common condition and seems to be triggered by any one or several of a number of factors. These include anxiety, FATIGUE, watching television or video screens, loud noises, flickering lights (e.g. strobe lights) and certain foods such as cheese and chocolate or alcoholic drinks. The cause is unknown but thought to involve constriction followed by dilation of BLOOD VESSELS in the BRAIN and an outpouring of fluid into surrounding tissues. Attacks can last up to 24 hours and treatment is by means of bed rest in a darkened, quiet room and pain-relieving drugs.

miliaria *see* PRICKLY HEAT.

miliary a term meaning 'resembling tiny seeds', used to describe a disease or condition of the skin that is characterized by small LESIONS that look like seeds, e.g. miliary TUBERCULOSIS.

mineralocorticosteroid *see* CORTICOSTEROID.

miscarriage *see* ABORTION.

mitochondrion (*pl* **mitochondria**) a tiny rodlike structure, numbers of which are present in the CYTOPLASM of every CELL. Mitochondria contain ENZYMES and ATP involved in cell METABOLISM.

mitosis *see* CELL.

mitral incompetence a condition in which the MITRAL VALVE of the HEART is defective and allows BLOOD to leak back from the left VENTRICLE into the left ATRIUM. It is often caused by RHEUMATIC FEVER or can be a CONGENITAL defect or the result of MYOCARDIAL INFARCTION. The left ventricle is forced to work harder and enlarges but eventually may be unable to cope, and this can result in left-sided HEART FAILURE. Other symptoms include atrial FIBRILLATION, BREATHLESSNESS and EMBOLISM. Drug treatment and/or surgery to replace the valve may be required (mitral prosthesis, *see* MITRAL STENOSIS).

mitral stenosis a condition in which the opening between the left ATRIUM and left VENTRICLE is narrowed because of scarring and adhesion of the MITRAL VALVE. This scarring is often caused by RHEUMATIC FEVER, and the symptoms are similar to those of MITRAL INCOMPETENCE, accompanied also by a diastolic MURMUR. It is treated surgically by widening the STENOSIS (mitral VALVOTOMY) or by valve replacement – mitral PROSTHESIS.

mitral valve a VALVE located between the ATRIUM and VENTRICLE of the left side of the HEART, attached to the walls at the opening between the two. It has two cusps or flaps and normally allows BLOOD to pass into the ventricle from the atrium but prevents any back flow.

MMR vaccine a VACCINE, introduced in 1988, that protects against MEASLES, MUMPS and RUBELLA (German measles). It is normally given to children during their second year.

molar *see* TOOTH.

mole a dark-coloured PIGMENTed spot in the SKIN, which is usually brown. It may be flat or raised and may have hair protruding from it. Some types can become MALIGNANT (*see* MELANOMA).

monocyte the largest type of white blood cell (LEUCOCYTE) with a kidney-shaped nucleus and found in the blood and LYMPH. It ingests foreign bodies such as BACTERIA and tissue particles.

mononucleosis *see* GLANDULAR FEVER.

morbidity the state of being diseased, the morbidity rate being expressed as the number of cases of a disease occurring within a particular number of the population.

moribund a term meaning dying.

morning sickness VOMITING and NAUSEA, most common during the first three months of PREGNANCY. *See also* HYPEREMESIS.

morphine a NARCOTIC and very strong ANALGESIC drug that is an alkaloid derived from OPIUM. It is used for the relief of severe pain but tolerance and dependence may occur, leading to ADDICTION.

motility the ability to move without outside aid.

motor nerve a nerve, containing MOTOR-NEURON fibres, that carries electrical impulses outwards from the CENTRAL NERVOUS SYSTEM to a MUSCLE or GLAND to bring about a response there.

motor neuron one of the units or fibres of a MOTOR NERVE. An upper motor neuron is contained entirely within the CENTRAL NERVOUS SYSTEM, having its CELL body in the BRAIN and its AXON (a long process) extending into the SPINAL CORD where it SYNAPSES with other neurons. A lower motor neuron has its cell body in the spinal cord or brain stem and an axon that runs outwards via a spinal or cranial motor nerve to an effector muscle or gland.

motor-neuron disease a disease of unknown cause that most commonly occurs in middle age and is a degenerative condition of elements of the CENTRAL NERVOUS SYSTEM (i.e. the fibres of the CEREBRAL CORTEX and SPINAL CORD, motor nuclei in the BRAIN stem and the cells of the anterior horn of the spinal cord). It causes increasing PARALYSIS involving nerves and MUSCLES and is ultimately fatal.

mouth the opening that forms the beginning of the ALIMENTARY CANAL, through which food enters the digestive process. The entrance is guarded by the lips, behind which lie the upper and lower sets of teeth (*see* TOOTH) embedded in the JAW. The roof of the mouth is the PALATE, the front part being hard and immobile while behind lies the mobile soft palate. The TONGUE is situated behind the lower teeth, and SALIVARY GLANDS which are present secrete saliva into the mouth through small ducts. Saliva contains the ENZYME ptyalin, which begins the breakdown of starch while the chewing action of the teeth and manipulation of the tongue reduce the food to a more manageable size so that it can be swallowed.

MRSA *see* METHICILLIN-RESISTANT STAPHYLOCOCCUS AUREUS.

mucosa another term for MUCOUS MEMBRANE.

mucous membrane a moist MEMBRANE that lines many tubes and cavities within the body and is lubricated with MUCUS. The structure of a mucous membrane varies according to its site, and they are found, for example, lining the mouth, respiratory, urinary and digestive tracts. Each has a surface EPITHELIUM, a layer containing various cells and glands that secrete mucus. Beneath this lie CONNECTIVE TISSUE and MUSCLE layers, the laminae propria and muscularis mucosa respectively, the whole forming a pliable layer.

mucus a slimy substance secreted by MUCOUS MEMBRANES as a lubricant. It is a clear viscous fluid that may contain ENZYMES and has a protective function. It is normally present in small amounts but the quantity increases if INFLAMMATION or INFECTION is present.

multiple sclerosis a disease of the BRAIN and SPINAL CORD that affects the MYELIN sheaths of NERVES and disrupts their function. It usually affects people below the age of 40 and its cause is unknown. It is characterized by the presence of patches of hardened (sclerotic) CONNECTIVE TISSUE irregularly scattered through the brain and spinal cord. At first the fatty part of the nerve sheaths breaks down and is absorbed, leaving bare nerve fibres, and then connective tissue is laid down. Symptoms depend on the site of the patches in the CENTRAL NERVOUS SYSTEM, and the disease is characterized by periods of progression and REMISSION. However, they include unsteady gait and apparent clumsiness, tremor of the limbs, involuntary eye movements, speech disorders, bladder dysfunction and paralysis. The disease can progress very slowly, but generally there is a tendency for the paralysis to become more marked.

mumps an infectious disease of childhood, usually occurring in those between the ages of five to 15 and caused by a virus that produces INFLAMMATION of the PAROTID GLANDS. The INCUBATION period is two to three weeks, followed by symptoms including feverishness, headache, sore throat and vomiting, before or along with a swelling of the parotid gland on one side of the face. The swelling may be confined to one side or spread to the other side of the face and also may go on to include the submaxillary and sublingual SALIVARY GLANDS beneath the jaw. Generally, after a few days the swelling subsides and the child recovers but remains infectious until the glands have returned to normal. The infection may spread to the pancreas and, in 15–30 per cent of males, to the TESTICLES. In adult men this can cause sterility. More rarely, inflammation in females can affect the ovaries and breasts, and MENINGITIS is another occasional complication, especially in adults. A protective vaccine is now available (*see* MMR VACCINE).

murmur a characteristic sound caused by uneven blood flow through the HEART or BLOOD VESSELS when these are diseased or damaged. Heart murmurs can also be present in normal individuals, especially children, without indicating disease.

muscle the contractile tissue of the body, which produces movements of various structures both internally and externally. There are three types of muscle:

1. striated or VOLUNTARY MUSCLE, which has a striped appearance when viewed under a microscope and is attached to the SKELETON. It is called 'voluntary' because it is under the control of the will and produces movements, e.g. in the limbs.

2. smooth or INVOLUNTARY MUSCLE, which has a plain appearance when viewed microscopically and is not under conscious control but is supplied by the AUTONOMIC NERVOUS SYSTEM. Examples are the muscles that supply the digestive and respiratory tracts.

3. CARDIAC MUSCLE, the specialized muscle of the walls of the HEART, which is composed of a network of branching, elongated fibres that rejoin and interlock, each having a nucleus. It has a somewhat striated appearance, and

where there are junctions between fibres, irregular transverse bands occur, known as intercalated discs. This muscle is involuntary, and contracts and expands rhythmically throughout a person's life. However, rate of heartbeat is affected by activity within the VAGUS NERVE.

muscle cramp *see* CRAMP.

muscular dystrophy *or* **myopathy** any of a group of diseases that involve wasting of MUSCLES and in which an hereditary factor is involved. The disease is classified according to the groups of muscles that it affects and the age of the person involved. It usually appears in childhood and causes muscle fibres to degenerate and to be replaced by fatty and FIBROUS TISSUE. The affected muscles eventually lose all power of contraction, causing great disability, and affected children are prone to chest and other infections, which may prove fatal. The cause is not entirely understood but the commonest form, Duchenne muscular dystrophy, is a SEX-LINKED DISORDER and recessive, so it nearly always affects boys, with the mother as a carrier, and appears in very early childhood.

muscularis mucosa *see* MUCOUS MEMBRANE.

mutagen any substance or agent that increases the rate of MUTATION in body CELLS, examples being various chemicals, viruses and radiation. Mutagens increase the number, rather than the range, of mutations beyond what might be expected.

mutation a change that takes place in the DNA (the genetic material) of the CHROMOSOMES of a cell, which is normally a rare event. It may involve the structure or number of whole chromosomes or take place at one GENE site. Mutations are caused by faulty replication of the cell's genetic material at cell division. If normal body (somatic) cells are involved, there may be a growth of altered cells or a TUMOUR, or these may be attacked and destroyed by the IMMUNE system, but this type cannot be passed on. If the sex cells (ova or sperm) are involved in the mutation, the alteration may be passed on to the offspring, producing a changed characteristic.

myalgia pain in a MUSCLE.

myalgic encephalomyelitis (ME) *or* **post-viral fatigue syndrome** a disorder characterized by muscular pain, FATIGUE, general DEPRESSION and loss of memory and concentration. The cause is not understood but seems to follow on from viral infections such as INFLUENZA, hence its alternative name. Recovery may be prolonged and there is no specific treatment.

myasthenia gravis a serious and chronic condition of uncertain cause, which may be an AUTOIMMUNE DISEASE. It is more common among young people, especially women (men tend to be affected over 40). Rest and avoidance of unnecessary exertion is essential to conserve MUSCLE strength as there is a reduction in the ability of the neurotransmitter, ACETYLCHOLINE, to effect MUSCLE contraction. There is a weakening that affects skeletal muscles and those for breathing and swallowing, etc, but little wasting of the muscles themselves. It seems the body produces ANTIBODIES that interfere with the acetylcholine receptors in the muscle and that the THYMUS GLAND may be the original source of these receptors. Surgical removal of the THYMUS GLAND is one treatment. Other treatment is by means of drugs that inhibit the activity of the ENZYME cholinesterase, which destroys excess acetylcholine. Other IMMUNOSUPPRESSIVE drugs are used to suppress production of the antibodies that interfere with the receptors.

mycoplasma a microorganism of the *Mycoplasma* genus, several species of which cause disease.

mycosis any disease caused by a FUNGUS, e.g. THRUSH and RINGWORM.

myelin a sheath of phospholipid (*see* LIPOSOME) and PROTEIN that surrounds the axons of some NEURONS. It is formed by specialized CELLS known as Schwann cells, each of which encloses the axon in concentric folds of its cell MEMBRANE. These folds then condense to form myelin, the neuron then being described as myelinated. Schwann cells produce myelin at regular intervals along the length of the axon, and electrical impulses pass more rapidly along myelinated nerve fibres than along non-myelinated ones.

myelitis 1. any inflammatory condition of the SPINAL CORD such as often occurs in MULTIPLE SCLEROSIS. **2.** inflammation of BONE MARROW, *see* OSTEOMYELITIS.

myeloblast *see* LEUKAEMIA.

myelocyte a CELL that is an immature type of granulocyte (*see* LEUCOCYTE) responsible for the production of white blood cells.

myelofibrosis a disease, the cause of which is unknown, in which FIBROSIS takes place within the BONE MARROW, and many immature red and white blood cells (*see* ERYTHROCYTE, LEUCOCYTE) appear in the circulation because of the resultant ANAEMIA. There is an enlargement of the SPLEEN, and blood-producing (MYELOID) tissue is abnormally found both here and in the LIVER.

myeloid like or relating to BONE MARROW or like a MYELOCYTE.

myeloma a MALIGNANT disease of the BONE MARROW in which TUMOURS are present in more than one bone at the same time. The bones may show 'holes' when X-rayed because of typical deposits, and certain abnormal PROTEINS may be present in the blood and urine. Treatment is by chemotherapy and radiotherapy. Myelomatosis is the production of myeloma, which is usually fatal.

myocardial infarction NECROSIS of part of the MYOCARDIUM, usually as a result of a CORONARY THROMBOSIS.

myocarditis INFLAMMATION of the MUSCLE in the wall of the HEART.

myocardium the middle of the three layers of the HEART wall, which is the thick, muscular area. The outer layer is the epicardium (forming part of the PERICARDIUM) and the inner the ENDOCARDIUM.

myoglobin an iron-containing PIGMENT that is similar to HAEMOGLOBIN and occurs in MUSCLE cells. It binds oxygen from haemoglobin and releases it in the muscle cells.

myometrium the muscular tissue of the UTERUS, composed of smooth MUSCLE and surrounding the ENDOMETRIUM. Its contractions are influenced by the presence of certain HORMONES and are especially strong during LABOUR.

myopathy *see* MUSCULAR DYSTROPHY.

myofibril *see* VOLUNTARY MUSCLE.

myopia short-sightedness, which is corrected by wearing spectacles with concave lenses.

myxoedema a disease caused by underactivity of the THYROID gland (HYPOTHYROIDISM). There is a characteristic development of a dry, coarse skin and swelling of subcutaneous tissue. There is intellectual impairment, with slow speech and mental dullness, lethargy, muscle pain, weight gain and constipation. The hair thins and there may be increased sensitivity to cold. As the symptoms are caused by the deficiency of thyroid HORMONES, treatment consists of giving THYROXINE in suitable amounts.

N

naevus *see* BIRTHMARK.

nail the horny structure at the end of a finger or toe. It is formed of KERATIN.

The body is the part of the nail showing, while the root is beneath the skin. The pale crescent is called the lunula.

narcosis a state induced by NARCOTIC drugs in which a person is unconscious or nearly so but can respond a little to stimuli. It is the result of the depressant action of the drugs on the body.

narcotic a drug that leads to a stupor and loss of awareness. In particular, OPIATES derived from MORPHINE or produced synthetically induce various conditions: deep sleep, euphoria, mood changes and mental confusion. In addition, respiration and the cough reflex are depressed and muscle spasms may be produced. Because of the dependence resulting from the use of morphine-like compounds, they have largely been replaced as sleeping drugs.

nasal cavity one of two cavities in the NOSE, divided by a SEPTUM, which lie between the roof of the MOUTH and the floor of the CRANIUM.

nasogastric tube a tube of small diameter that is passed through the NOSE into the STOMACH for purposes of introducing food or drugs or removing fluid (ASPIRATION).

nausea a feeling of being about to vomit. It may be caused by MIGRAINE, MOTION SICKNESS, early PREGNANCY, pain, FOOD POISONING or a VIRUS.

navel *see* UMBILICAL CORD.

nebulizer a device for producing a fine spray. Many inhaled drugs are administered in this way, and it is an effective method of delivering a concentrated form of medication, e.g. BRONCHODILATORS.

neck 1. the part of the body between the head and the trunk. **2.** the narrow part of a BONE or organ.

necrosis death of tissue in a localized area or organ, caused by disease, injury or loss or interruption of BLOOD supply.

necrotizing fasciitis *see* page 35.

neonatal a term meaning 'relating to the first 28 days of life'.

neoplasm a new and abnormal growth of CELLS, i.e. a TUMOUR, which may be BENIGN or MALIGNANT.

nephritis INFLAMMATION of the KIDNEY, which may be the result of one of several causes. Types of nephritis include glomerulonephritis (when the glomerulus is affected), hereditary nephritis, etc.

nephroblastoma *see* WILM'S TUMOUR.

nephron *see* KIDNEY.

nerve a bundle of fibres comprising NEURONs and glial (supporting) cells (*see* GLIA), all contained in a fibrous sheath, the epineurium. MOTOR NERVES carry (efferent) impulses in motor neurons from the BRAIN (or SPINAL CORD) to MUSCLES or GLANDS, and a SENSORY nerve carries (afferent) impulses in sensory neurons from sensory organs to the brain or spinal cord. Most large nerves are mixed nerves containing both motor and sensory nerves.

nerve block *or* **conduction anaesthesia** the blocking of SENSORY nerves sending pain impulses to the brain, thus creating ANAESTHESIA in that part of the body. It is achieved by injecting the tissue around a nerve with local ANAESTHETIC to permit minor operations.

nerve impulse the transmission of information along a NERVE fibre by electrical activity, which has its basis in the formation of chemical substances and the generation of the action potential. This is a change in electrical potential across the cell membrane (between inside and outside) of an AXON (nerve cell) as an impulse moves along. It is a temporary and localized occurrence caused by a stimulus that travels down the axon. When the stimulus has passed, the membrane is restored to its resting potential. When a stimulus

is continually received, several hundred pulses travel along the nerve per
second.

nervous system the complete system of tissues and CELLS, including NERVES,
NEURONS, SYNAPSES and RECEPTORS (a special cell sensitive to a particular stimulus which then sends an impulse through the nervous system). The nervous
system operates through the transmission of NERVE IMPULSES that are conducted
rapidly to and from muscles, organs, etc. It consists of the CENTRAL NERVOUS
SYSTEM (brain and spinal cord) and the PERIPHERAL NERVOUS SYSTEM, which
includes the CRANIAL NERVES and spinal nerves (*see* AUTONOMIC NERVOUS SYSTEM).

nettle rash *see* URTICARIA.

neuralgia strictly, pain in some part or the whole of a NERVE (without any physical change) but used more widely to encompass pain following the course of
a nerve or its branches, whatever the cause. Neuralgia often occurs at the same
time each day and is frequently an agonizing pain. It occurs in several forms
and is named accordingly, e.g. SCIATICA, trigeminal neuralgia (affecting the
face, *see* TRIGEMINAL NERVE) and intercostal neuralgia (affecting the RIBS).
Treatment often involves the application of ointments and the taking of
painkilling drugs. If such treatments do not bring relief, it is possible to freeze
the nerve or destroy part of it by surgery.

neuritis INFLAMMATION of a NERVE or nerves, which may be the result of inflammation from nearby tissues or a more general condition in which the nerve
fibres degenerate. This latter condition (polyneuritis) is caused by a systemic
poison such as alcohol or long-term exposure to solvents such as naphtha.

neuroendocrine system one of a number of dual control systems regulating
bodily functions through the action of NERVES and HORMONES.

neurofibromatosis *see* VON RECKLINGHAUSEN'S DISEASE.

neuroglia the fine web of tissues that support nerve fibres (*see* GLIA).

neurohormone a HORMONE that is secreted by the NERVE endings of specialized
nerve CELLS (i.e. neurosecretory cells) and not by an ENDOCRINE GLAND. They
are secreted into the bloodstream or directly into the target tissue. Included
are NORADRENALINE and VASOPRESSIN.

neurohypophysis *see* PITUITARY GLAND.

neuroleptic any drug that induces neurolepsis, i.e. reduced activity, some indif-
ference to the surroundings and possibly sleep. They are used to quieten
disturbed patients suffering from DELIRIUM, BRAIN damage or behavioural
disturbances.

neuromuscular junction the area of MEMBRANE between a MUSCLE cell and a
MOTOR NEURON, forming a SYNAPSE between the two. NERVE IMPULSES travel
down the neuron, and each releases ACETYLCHOLINE, which slightly depolar-
izes the enlarged end of the neuron (the motor end plate). These small
depolarizations are totalled until a threshold of -50mV is reached, and this
results in the production of an 'action potential' that crosses the synapse into
the muscle fibre, thereby producing a muscle contraction.

neuron a NERVE cell, vital in the transmission of NERVE IMPULSES. Each CELL has
an enlarged portion (the cell body) from which extends the long, thin AXON
for carrying impulses away. Shorter, more numerous DENDRITES receive
impulses. The transmission of impulses is faster in axons that are covered in
a sheath of MYELIN.

neuropathy any disease that affects the peripheral NERVES, whether singly
(mononeuropathy) or more generally (polyneuropathy).

neurosecretory cell *see* NEUROHORMONE.

neurotransmitter one of several chemical substances released in minute quantities by axon tips into the SYNAPSE to enable a NERVE IMPULSE to cross. It diffuses across the space and may depolarize the opposite MEMBRANE, allowing the production of an action potential. Outside the central nervous system, ACETYL-CHOLINE is a major neurotransmitter, and NORADRENALINE is released in the SYMPATHETIC NERVOUS SYSTEM. Acetylcholine and noradrenaline also operate within the CENTRAL NERVOUS SYSTEM, as does DOPAMINE, amongst others.

nicotinic acid *see* PELLAGRA.

night blindness *or* **nyctalopia** poor VISION in dim light or at night because of a deficiency within the cells responsible for such vision (*see* ROD). The cause may be a lack of VITAMIN A in the diet or a CONGENITAL defect.

non-steroidal anti-inflammatory drugs (NSAID) a large group of drugs used to relieve pain and also inhibit INFLAMMATION. They are used for conditions such as rheumatoid arthritis, sprains, etc, and include ASPIRIN. The main SIDE EFFECT is gastric ulcer or haemorrhage, but the synthesis of new compounds has led to some with milder side effects.

noradrenaline *or* **norepinephrine** (US) a NEUROTRANSMITTER of the SYMPATHETIC NERVOUS SYSTEM secreted by nerve endings and also the ADRENAL GLANDS. It is similar to ADRENALINE in structure and function. It increases BLOOD PRESSURE by constricting the vessel, slowing heartbeat and increasing breathing both in rate and depth.

nose the olfactory organ and also a pathway for air entering the body, by which route it is warmed, filtered and moistened before passing into the LUNGS. The 'external' nose leads to the NASAL CAVITY, which has a MUCOUS MEMBRANE with olfactory (smell) cells.

notifiable diseases diseases that must be reported to the health authorities to enable rapid control and monitoring to be undertaken. The list varies between countries but in the UK includes acute POLIOMYELITIS, AIDS, CHOLERA, DYSENTERY, FOOD POISONING, MEASLES, MENINGITIS, RABIES, German MEASLES (rubella), SCARLET FEVER, SMALLPOX, TETANUS, TYPHOID, viral HEPATITIS and WHOOPING COUGH.

NSAID *see* NON-STEROIDAL ANTI-INFLAMMATORY DRUGS.

nucleic acid a linear molecule that occurs in two forms: DNA (deoxyribonucleic acid) and RNA (ribonucleic acid), composed of four NUCLEOTIDES. DNA is the major part of CHROMOSOMES in the cell nucleus while RNA is also found outside the nucleus and is involved in PROTEIN synthesis.

nucleotide the basic molecular building block of the nucleic acids RNA and DNA. A nucleotide comprises a five-carbon sugar molecule with a phosphate group and an organic base. The organic base can be a purine, e.g. adenine and guanine, or a pyrimidine, e.g. cytosine and thymine as in DNA. In RNA uracil replaces thymine.

nucleus the large ORGANELLE in a MEMBRANE-bounded CELL that contains the DNA. Unless it is dividing, a nucleolus with RNA is present. During cell division, the DNA, which is normally dispersed with PROTEIN (as chromatin), forms visible CHROMOSOMES.

nyctalopia *see* NIGHT BLINDNESS.

O

occipital bone a BONE of the SKULL, which is shaped like a saucer and forms the back of the CRANIUM and part of its base. Arising from the base of this bone are two occipital CONDYLES, which articulate with the first cervical VERTEBRA (the atlas) of the SPINAL COLUMN.

oculomotor nerve either of a pair of CRANIAL NERVES that are involved in EYE movements, including movement of the eyeball and alterations in the size of the PUPIL and LENS.

odontoblast *see* DENTINE.

oedema an accumulation of fluid in the body, possibly beneath the skin or in cavities or organs. With an injury the swelling may be localized, or it can be more general, as in cases of KIDNEY or HEART failure. Fluid can collect in the chest cavity, abdomen or lung (PULMONARY OEDEMA). The causes are numerous, e.g. CIRRHOSIS of the liver, heart or kidney failure, starvation, acute NEPHRITIS, allergies or drugs. To alleviate the symptom, the root cause has to be removed. Subcutaneous oedema commonly occurs in women before MENSTRUATION, as swollen legs or ankles, but subsides if the legs are rested in a raised position.

oesophagitis INFLAMMATION of the OESOPHAGUS. *See also* HEARTBURN.

oesophagus the first part of the ALIMENTARY CANAL, lying between the PHARYNX and STOMACH. The MUCOUS MEMBRANE lining produces secretions to lubricate food as it passes, and the movement of the food to the stomach is achieved by waves of muscular contractions called peristalsis.

oestradiol the major female SEX HORMONE. It is produced by the OVARY and is responsible for development of the BREASTs, sexual characteristics and premenstrual uterine changes.

oestrogen one of a group of STEROID hormones secreted mainly by the ovaries and, to a lesser extent, by the ADRENAL CORTEX and PLACENTA. (The TESTICLES also produce small amounts.) Oestrogens control the female SECONDARY SEXUAL CHARACTERISTICS, i.e. enlargement of the breasts, change in the profile of the PELVIC GIRDLE, pubic hair growth and deposition of body fat. High levels are produced at ovulation and, with PROGESTERONE, they regulate the female reproductive cycle. Naturally occurring oestrogens include OESTRADIOL, oestriol and oestrone. Synthetic varieties are used in the contraceptive pill and to treat gynaecological disorders.

olfaction the sense of smell, *see* NOSE.

olfactory nerve one of a pair of SENSORY nerves for smell. It is the first CRANIAL NERVE and comprises many fine threads connecting RECEPTORS in the MUCOUS MEMBRANE of the olfactory area of the NOSE, which pass through holes in the SKULL, fuse to form one fibre and then pass back to the BRAIN.

oncogene any GENE directly involved in CANCER, whether in viruses or in the individual.

oncogenic any factor that gives rise to TUMOURS. This may be an organism, a chemical or some environmental condition. Some VIRUSES are oncogenic and make a normal CELL cancerous.

oocyte a cell in the OVARY that undergoes MEIOSIS to produce an OVUM, the female reproductive CELL. A newborn female already has numerous primary oocytes, of which only a small number survive to puberty and only a fraction are ovulated (*see* OVULATION).

ophthalmic nerve *see* TRIGEMINAL NERVE.

ophthalmoplegia PARALYSIS of the muscles serving the EYE, which may be internal (affecting the IRIS and ciliary muscle) or external (those muscles moving the eye itself).

opiate one of several drugs derived from OPIUM and including MORPHINE. They act by depressing the CENTRAL NERVOUS SYSTEM, thus relieving pain and suppressing coughing. Morphine and HEROIN, synthetic derivatives of opium, are NARCOTICS.

opium a milky liquid extracted from the unripe seed capsules of the poppy *Papaver somniferum*, which has almost 10 per cent of anhydrous (i.e. containing no water) MORPHINE. Opium is a NARCOTIC and ANALGESIC.

opportunistic a term used to describe an INFECTION that is contracted by someone with a lowered RESISTANCE. This may be because of drugs or disease, such as DIABETES MELLITUS, CANCER or AIDS. In normal circumstances, in a healthy person, the infecting organism would not cause the disease.

optic atrophy a deterioration and wasting of the OPTIC DISC as a result of degeneration of fibres in the OPTIC NERVE. It may accompany numerous conditions, including DIABETES, ARTERIOSCLEROSIS or GLAUCOMA, or may be because of a congenital defect, inflammation or injury, or toxic poisoning from alcohol, lead, etc.

optic chiasma *or* **optic commissure** the cross-shaped structure formed from a crossing over of the OPTIC NERVE running back from the eyeballs to meet beneath the brain in the midline.

optic disc an oval area on the RETINA of the EYE where the OPTIC NERVE enters the eyeball.

optic nerve the second CRANIAL NERVE. It is a SENSORY nerve, sending messages from the RETINA to the BRAIN. *See also* OPTIC CHIASMA.

organ any distinct and recognizable unit within the body that is composed of two or more types of tissue and is responsible for a particular function or functions, e.g. LIVER, KIDNEY, HEART, BRAIN.

organelle a functional entity that is bound by a MEMBRANE to separate it from other CELL constituents, e.g. a MITOCHONDRION.

orthopnoea a severe difficulty in breathing that is so bad that a patient cannot lie down and has to sleep in a sitting position. It usually occurs only with serious conditions of the heart and lungs.

osmosis the process whereby solvent molecules (usually water) move through a semipermeable MEMBRANE to a more concentrated solution. CELL membranes function as semipermeable membranes, and osmosis is important in regulating water content in living systems.

ossicle a small BONE, particularly in the middle EAR, e.g. the auditory ossicles that transmit sound to the inner ear from the eardrum.

ossification *or* **osteogenesis** BONE formation, which occurs in several stages via special cells called OSTEOBLASTS. COLLAGEN fibres form a network in CONNECTIVE TISSUE and then a cement of polysaccharide is laid down. Finally, calcium salts are distributed among the cement as tiny crystals. The osteoblasts are enclosed as bone cells (OSTEOCYTES).

osteitis INFLAMMATION of BONE, caused by damage, INFECTION or bodily disorder. Symptoms include swelling, tenderness, a dull aching SKIN pain and redness of the affected area.

osteitis deformans *see* PAGET'S DISEASE OF BONE.

osteoarthritis a form of ARTHRITIS involving joint CARTILAGE with accompanying changes in the associated BONE. It usually involves the loss of cartilage and the development of OSTEOPHYTES at the bone margins. The function of the JOINT (most often the thumb, knee and hip) is affected and it becomes painful. The condition may be caused by overuse and affects those past middle age. It also may complicate other joint diseases. Treatment usually involves administering ANALGESICS, possibly anti-inflammatory drugs and the use of corrective or replacement surgery.

osteoblast a specialized CELL responsible for the formation of BONE.

osteochondritis INFLAMMATION of BONE and CARTILAGE.

osteochondrosis a disease affecting the OSSIFICATION centres of BONE in children. It begins with degeneration and NECROSIS, but the bone regenerates and calcifies again.

osteclast *see* OSTEOSCLEROSIS.

osteocyte a bone CELL formed from an OSTEOBLAST that is no longer active and has become embedded in the matrix of the BONE.

osteogenesis *see* OSSIFICATION.

osteogenesis imperfecta *or* **brittle bone disease** an hereditary disease that results in the BONES being unusually fragile and brittle. It may have associated symptoms, e.g. transparent teeth, unusually mobile JOINTS, DWARFISM, etc. It may be caused by a disorder involving COLLAGEN, but there is little that can be done in treatment.

osteomalacia a softening of the BONES and the adult equivalent of RICKETS, which is caused by a lack of VITAMIN D. This vitamin is obtained from the diet and is produced on exposure to sunlight, and it is necessary for the uptake of calcium from food.

osteomyelitis INFLAMMATION of BONE MARROW caused by INFECTION. This may happen after a compound FRACTURE or during bone surgery. It produces pain, swelling and fever, and high doses of ANTIBIOTICS are necessary.

osteophyte a bony projection that occurs near a joint or intervertebral disc where CARTILAGE has degenerated or been destroyed (*see* OSTEOARTHRITIS). Osteophytes may, in any case, occur with increasing age, with or without loss of cartilage.

osteoporosis a loss of BONE tissue because of its being resorbed, resulting in bones that become brittle and likely to fracture. It is common in menopausal women and can also be a result of long-term steroid therapy. Hormone replacement therapy is a treatment available to women (*see* MENOPAUSE).

osteosarcoma the commonest and most malignant TUMOUR of the BONE found most commonly in older children. The FEMUR is usually affected but metastases (*see* METASTASIS) are common. It produces pain and swelling. Amputation used to be the standard treatment, but surgery is now possible, with replacement of the diseased bone and associated CHEMOTHERAPY and/or RADIOTHERAPY.

osteosclerosis a condition in which the density of BONE tissue increases abnormally. It is caused by TUMOUR, INFECTION or poor BLOOD supply and may be the result of an abnormality involving osteoclasts, cells that resorb calcified bone.

otitis INFLAMMATION of the EAR. This may take several forms, depending on the exact location, which produces diverse symptoms. For example, inflammation of the inner ear (otitis interna) affects balance, causing VERTIGO and VOMITING, while otitis media is usually a bacterial infection of the middle ear, resulting in severe pain and a fever requiring immediate antibiotic treatment. Secretory otitis media is otherwise known as GLUE EAR.

otosclerosis an hereditary condition in which there is overgrowth of BONE in the inner EAR, which restricts and then stops sound being conducted to the inner ear from the middle ear. The person affected becomes progressively more deaf, often beginning with TINNITUS, but surgery is effective.

ovarian cyst a sac filled with fluid that develops in the OVARY. Most are benign but their size may cause swelling and pressure on other organs. For those CYSTS that do become MALIGNANT, it is possible that discovery comes too late to allow successful treatment.

ovary the reproductive organ of females, which produces eggs (ova) and hormones (mainly OESTROGEN and PROGESTERONE). There are two ovaries, each the size of an almond, on either side of the UTERUS, and each contains numerous Graafian FOLLICLES in which the eggs develop. At OVULATION an egg is released from a follicle. The follicles secrete oestrogen and progesterone, which regulate the MENSTRUAL CYCLE and the UTERUS during PREGNANCY.

ovulation the release of an egg from an OVARY, which then moves down the FALLOPIAN TUBE to the UTERUS. It is brought about by secretion of luteinizing hormone by the anterior PITUITARY GLAND.

ovum (*pl* **ova**) the mature, unfertilized female reproductive CELL, which is roughly spherical with an outer MEMBRANE and a single nucleus.

oxytocin a HORMONE from the PITUITARY GLAND that causes the UTERUS to contract during LABOUR and prompts LACTATION because of contraction of muscle fibres in the milk ducts of the BREASTS.

P

pacemaker 1. the part of the HEART that regulates the beat, the SINOATRIAL NODE. **2.** in patients with a HEART BLOCK, a device inserted into the body to maintain a normal heart rate. There are different types of pacemaker, some being permanent, others temporary; some stimulate the beat while others are activated only when the natural rate of the heart falls below a certain level.

pachymeningitis *see* MENINGITIS.

pachymeninx *see* MENINGES.

Paget's disease of bone *or* **osteitis deformans** a chronic BONE disease, particularly of the long bones (e.g. the FEMUR), SKULL and SPINE, that results in them becoming thickened, disorganized and soft, causing them to bend. The cause is unknown, and although there is no cure, good results are being obtained with calcitonin, which is a HORMONE produced by the THYROID GLAND that regulates levels of calcium in the BLOOD. The main symptom is pain.

palate the roof of the MOUTH, which separates the cavity of the mouth below from that of the nose above. It consists of the hard and soft palate. The hard palate is located at the front of the mouth and is a bony plate covered by MUCOUS MEMBRANE. The soft palate is a muscular layer also covered by mucous membrane. The movable soft palate is important in the production of sounds and speech.

palliative a medicine or treatment that is given to effect some relief from symptoms, if only temporarily, but does not cure the ailment. This is often the case in the treatment of CANCER.

pallor abnormal paleness of the SKIN because of reduced BLOOD flow or a lack of the normal PIGMENTS. It may be a direct result of ANAEMIA or SHOCK or spending an excessive amount of time indoors.

palpation examination of the surface of the body by carefully feeling with hands and fingertips. By doing this, it is often possible to distinguish between solid lumps or swelling and cystic structures.

palpitation when the HEART beats noticeably or irregularly and the person becomes aware of it. The heartbeat is not normally noticed but, with fear, emotion or exercise, it may be felt, unpleasantly so. Palpitations may also be caused by neuroses (*see* NEUROSIS), ARRHYTHMIA or heart disease, and a common cause is too much tea, coffee, alcohol or smoking. Where an excess is the cause (tea, coffee, etc) this can be eliminated. For disease-associated palpitations, drugs can be used for control.

palsy the term used formerly for PARALYSIS and retained for the names of some conditions, e.g. BELL'S PALSY.

pancreas a GLAND with both ENDOCRINE and EXOCRINE functions. It is located between the DUODENUM and SPLEEN, behind the STOMACH, and is about 15 cm long. There are two types of cells producing secretions. The acini produce pancreatic juice that goes to the intestine via a system of DUCTS. This contains an alkaline mixture of salt and ENZYMES – TRYPSIN and chymotrypsin to digest proteins, amylase to break down starch and lipase to aid digestion of fats. The second cell types are in the ISLETS OF LANGERHANS, and these produce two hormones, INSULIN and GLUCAGON, secreted directly into the blood for control of sugar levels (*see also* DIABETES MELLITUS, HYPOGLYCAEMIA and HYPERGLY-CAEMIA).

pancreatitis INFLAMMATION of the PANCREAS, occurring in several forms but often associated with GALLSTONES or alcoholism. Any bout of the condition that interferes with the function of the pancreas may lead to DIABETES and MALAB-SORPTION.

pandemic an EPIDEMIC that is so widely spread that it affects large numbers of people in a country or countries or even globally.

pantothenic acid *see* VITAMIN B3.

Papanicolaou test *or* **Pap test** another name for a CERVICAL SMEAR.

papilla (*pl* **papillae**) any small protuberance, such as the papillae on the TONGUE.

papilloma (*pl* **papillomata**) a usually BENIGN growth on the SKIN surface or MUCOUS MEMBRANE, e.g. WARTS.

Pap test *see* PAPANICOLAOU TEST.

papule *see* PIMPLE.

paracentesis the procedure of tapping or taking off (excess) fluid from the body by means of a hollow needle or CANNULA.

parainfluenza viruses a group of VIRUSES that cause respiratory tract infections with usually mild INFLUENZA-like symptoms. Infants and young children seem to be affected most. There are four types of the virus, virulent at different times of the year.

paralysis MUSCLE weakness or total loss of muscle movement, depending on the causal disease and its effect on the BRAIN. Various descriptive terms are used to qualify the parts of the body affected. Thus, hemiplegia affects one side of the body (*see also* DIPLEGIA, PARAPLEGIA, QUADRIPLEGIA). Paralysis is really a symptom of another condition or disease, e.g. BRAIN disease such as a cerebral haemorrhage or THROMBOSIS causing hemiplegia; disease or injury of the SPINAL CORD leading to paraplegia; and POLIOMYELITIS (infantile paralysis). In addition, there is the paralysis associated with MOTOR-NEURON DISEASE.

paraphimosis constriction of the PENIS because of retraction of an abnormally tight FORESKIN, which contracts on the penis behind the GLANS and cannot be easily moved. Swelling and pain may be caused and usually CIRCUMCISION is necessary.

paraplegia PARALYSIS of the legs. It may be caused by injury or disease of the SPINAL CORD, and often the BLADDER and RECTUM are also affected.

parasite any organism that obtains its nutrients by living in or on the body of another organism (the host). The extent to which the host is damaged by the parasite ranges from virtually no effect to, in extreme cases, death. Parasites in humans include worms, VIRUSES, fungi (*see* FUNGUS), etc.

parasympathetic nervous system one of the two parts of the AUTONOMIC

NERVOUS SYSTEM, which acts antagonistically with the SYMPATHETIC NERVOUS SYSTEM. The parasympathetic nerves originate from the BRAIN and lower portion of the SPINAL CORD (sacral region). The AXONS of this system tend to be longer than sympathetic nerves, and SYNAPSES with other neurons are close to the target organ. The parasympathetic system contracts the BLADDER, decreases HEART rate, stimulates the sex organs, promotes DIGESTION, etc.

parathyroid gland one of four small glands, located behind or within the THYROID GLAND, that control the METABOLISM of calcium and phosphorus (as phosphate) in the body. The HORMONE responsible, parathormone or parathyroid hormone, is produced and released by the glands. A deficiency of the hormone leads to lower levels of calcium in the BLOOD, with a relative increase in phosphorus. This produces tetany or hypoparathyroidism, a condition involving muscular spasms that can be treated by injection and is often caused by the removal or injury of the glands. If the hormone is at high levels, calcium is transferred from bones to the blood, causing weakness and susceptibility to breaks.

paratyphoid fever *see* page 92.

parietal 1. pertaining to the walls of a CAVITY of the body. **2.** pertaining to the BONES that form the sides and upper part of the SKULL.

Parkinsonism a progressive condition, occurring in mid to late life, that results in a rigidity of MUSCLES affecting the voice and FACE rather than those in the limbs. A TREMOR also develops, possibly in one hand initially and then spreading to other limbs, and it appears most pronounced when sitting. The disease is usually caused by a deficiency in the DOPAMINE (a NUEROTRANS-MITTER) because of degeneration of the basal ganglia of the brain (*see* BASAL GANGLION). There is no cure, but a number of drugs are able, in varying degrees, to control the condition (*see* DOPA).

parotid gland one of a pair of SALIVARY GLANDS situated in front of each ear and opening inside on the cheek near the second-last molar of the upper JAW.

parotitis INFLAMMATION of the PAROTID GLAND, which, as EPIDEMIC or infectious parotitis, is called MUMPS.

paroxysm 'a sudden attack', a term used about CONVULSIONS.

parturition *see* LABOUR.

pasteurization the STERILIZATION of food by heating it to a certain TEMPERATURE to destroy potentially harmful BACTERIA. Milk, for example, is heated to 62–65°C for 30 minutes, followed by rapid cooling. INFECTIONS avoided by this process include TUBERCULOSIS and TYPHOID, SCARLET FEVER, DIPHTHERIA and FOOD POISONING.

patch test a test undertaken to identify the substances causing a person's ALLERGY. Different ALLERGENs are placed in very small amounts on the skin. A red flare with swelling will develop if the person is allergic. This commonly happens within 15 minutes but may take up to 72 hours.

patella (*pl* **patellae**) the kneecap, an almost flat bone shaped somewhat like an oyster shell, that lies in front of the knee in the TENDON of the thigh muscle.

patellar reflex *see* REFLEX ACTION.

pathogen an organism that causes disease. Most pathogens affecting humans are BACTERIA and VIRUSES.

pectoral the descriptive term for anything relating to the CHEST.

pectoral girdle *or* **shoulder girdle** the skeletal structure to which the BONES of the upper limbs are attached. It is composed of two shoulder blades (SCAPULAe) and two collar bones (CLAVICLES) attached to the vertebral column and STERNUM respectively.

pediculosis parasitic infestation with LICE. Head lice are a common problem in school-age children. Pubic lice infest the pubic hair and are generally less common, except in conditions of poor hygiene. Both can be cleared with insecticide preparations.

Pel-Epstein fever *see* HODGKIN'S DISEASE.

pellagra a DEFICIENCY DISEASE caused by a lack of nicotinic acid, part of the VITAMIN B complex. It occurs when the diet is based on maize (rather than wheat) with an associated lack of first-class PROTEIN (meat and milk). The reason is that although maize contains nicotinic acid it is in an unusable form and also it does not contain the AMINO ACID tryptophan, which the body can use to produce nicotinic acid. The symptoms are DERMATITIS, DIARRHOEA and DEPRESSION.

pelvic girdle *or* **hip girdle** the skeletal structure to which the bones of the lower limbs are attached. It is made up of the two HIP bones, each comprising the ILIUM, PUBIS and ISCHIUM, fused together.

pelvic inflammatory disease (PID) an acute or chronic INFECTION of the UTERUS, ovaries (*see* OVARY) or FALLOPIAN TUBES. It is the result of infection elsewhere, e.g. in the APPENDIX, which spreads, or one that is carried by the BLOOD. It produces severe abdominal pain, which usually responds to ANTIBIOTICS but surgery may sometimes be necessary to remove diseased tissue.

pelvis 1. the skeletal structure that is formed by the HIP bones, SACRUM and COCCYX and connects with the SPINAL COLUMN and legs. The female pelvis is shallower and the ilia (*see* ILIUM) are wider apart and there are certain angular differences from the male pelvis, all of which relate to childbearing. The pelvis is a point of contact for the MUSCLES of the legs, and it partially envelops the BLADDER and RECTUM. In males it also houses the PROSTATE GLAND and seminal vesicles while in females it contains the UTERUS and ovaries (*see* OVARY). **2.** a basin-shaped cavity in the body, e.g. the renal pelvis, the hollow interior of the KIDNEY that opens out into the URETER, into which URINE is drained.

penicillin the ANTIBIOTIC, derived from the mould *Penicillium notatum*, that grows naturally on decaying fruit, bread or cheese. The genus used for production of the drug is *P. chrysogenum*. It is active against a large range of BACTERIA and is nontoxic. Usually given by INJECTION, it can be taken orally. There are many semisynthetic penicillins acting in different ways. Some patients are allergic to penicillin but there tend to be very few serious SIDE EFFECTS.

penis the male organ through which the URETHRA passes, carrying URINE or SEMEN. It is made up of tissue that is filled with blood during sexual arousal, producing an erection that enables penetration of the VAGINA and ejaculation of semen. The GLANS is the end part, normally covered by the FORESKIN (prepuce).

pepsin a digestive ENZYME that is active in the breakdown of PROTEINS contained in GASTRIC JUICE.

peptic ulcer an ULCER in the STOMACH (GASTRIC ULCER), OESOPHAGUS, DUODENUM (DUODENAL ULCER) or JEJUNUM. It is caused by a break in the mucosal lining as a result of the action of acid and pepsin, either because of their high concentrations or other factors affecting the mucosal protective mechanisms.

peptide an organic compound made up of two or more AMINO ACIDS and collectively named by the number of amino acids. A dipeptide therefore contains two, and a polypeptide many.

percussion the tapping of parts of the body (particularly on the back or chest) with the fingers to produce a vibration and a note-like sound. The sound produced gives an indication of abnormal enlargement of organs and the presence of fluid in the LUNGS.

perforation a hole that forms in a hollow organ, tissue or tube, e.g. the stomach, eardrum, etc. In particular, it is a serious development of an ULCER in the STOMACH or bowels because, on perforation, the INTESTINE contents, with BACTERIA, enter the peritoneal cavity (*see* PERITONEUM), causing PERITONITIS, accompanied by severe pain and SHOCK. Usually corrective surgery is required.

pericarditis INFLAMMATION of the PERICARDIUM. It may be a result of URAEMIA, CANCER or viral infection and produces fever, chest pain and possible accumulation of fluid.

pericardium the smooth MEMBRANE surrounding the HEART. The outer fibrous part covers the heart and is connected to the large vessels coming out of it. The inner serous part is a closed SEROUS MEMBRANE attached both to the fibrous part and the heart wall. Some fluid in the resulting SAC enables smooth movement as the heart beats.

pericranium *see* SCALP.

perilymph the fluid that separates the bony LABYRINTH and the membranous labyrinth of the EAR.

perineum the area of the body between the ANUS and the opening of the URETHRA.

periodontal a descriptive term relating to the tissues surrounding the teeth (*see* TOOTH).

periosteum *see* BONE.

peripheral nervous system those parts of the NERVOUS SYSTEM excluding the CENTRAL NERVOUS SYSTEM (BRAIN and SPINAL CORD). It comprises the afferent (SENSORY) and EFFERENT (motor) nerves, which include 12 pairs of CRANIAL NERVES and 31 pairs of spinal nerves. The motor nervous system then comprises the SOMATIC NERVOUS SYSTEM, carrying impulses to the skeletal muscles, and the AUTONOMIC NERVOUS SYSTEM, which is further divided into the SYMPATHETIC and the PARASYMPATHETIC NERVOUS SYSTEMS.

peristalsis the wave-like contraction and relaxation of MUSCLES in the OESOPHAGUS and INTESTINES that move ingested food gradually along the ALIMENTARY CANAL.

peritonsillar abscess *see* QUINSY.

peritoneum the SEROUS MEMBRANE that lines the abdominal cavity. That lining the abdominal walls is the parietal peritoneum, while the visceral peritoneum covers the organs. The folds of peritoneum from one organ to another are given special names, e.g. MESENTERY. Both are continuous and form a closed sac at the back of the abdomen in the male, while in the female there is an opening for the FALLOPIAN TUBE on either side.

peritonitis INFLAMMATION of the PERITONEUM. It may be caused by a primary INFECTION caused by BACTERIA in the bloodstream (e.g. tuberculous peritonitis), resulting in pain and swelling, fever and weight loss. Secondary infection results from entry into the abdominal cavity of bacteria (e.g. from APPENDICITIS) and irritants (e.g. digestive juices) from a perforated or ruptured organ, e.g. duodenum or stomach. This produces severe pain and SHOCK, and surgery is often necessary.

pernicious anaemia a type of ANAEMIA caused by VITAMIN B12 deficiency, which results from dietary lack or the failure to produce the substance that enables B12 to be absorbed from the bowel. This in turn results in a lack of red blood cell (ERYTHROCYTE) production and MEGALOBLASTS in the BONE MARROW. The condition is easily treated by regular injections of the vitamin.

perspiration *or* **sweat** the excretion from millions of tiny SWEAT GLANDS in the skin. Sweat that evaporates from the skin immediately is insensible perspiration, while that forming drops is sensible perspiration. Sweat is produced in two types of sweat glands. The EXOCRINE GLANDS are found mainly on the soles of the feet and palms of the hands. The APOCRINE glands are in the armpits and around the anus and genitalia. Sweat is produced in response to stimuli such as fear and sexual arousal, but the major function of sweating is the regulation of body TEMPERATURE.

pertussis *see* WHOOPING COUGH.

pessary 1. an instrument that fits into the VAGINA to treat a PROLAPSE. **2.** a soft solid substance that is shaped for insertion into the vagina and contains drugs for some gynaecological disorder (also used for inducing LABOUR).

petit mal the lesser type of epileptic seizure, which is IDIOPATHIC. It consists of brief periods (seconds) of unconsciousness, when the eyes stare blankly but posture is maintained. Children suffering from it frequently may have learning difficulties but the condition may disappear in adult life.

PG *see* PROSTAGLANDIN.

phage a short form of BACTERIOPHAGE.

phagocyte any of various CELLS able to absorb and digest BACTERIA and dead or harmful matter, such phagocytic cells including white blood cells (LEUCO-CYTES). *See also* INGESTION; MACROPHAGE.

phagocytosis the process by which a phagocytes, e.g. LEUCOCYTES, engulf microorganisms and cell debris to remove them from the body.

phalanges (*sing* **phalanx**) the BONES of the digits (fingers and toes) which number 14 in each hand and foot. The thumb and big toe comprise two while all the other digits have three phalanges.

phallus 1. the PENIS or a penis-like object. **2.** the term used for the embryonic penis before the final development of the URETHRA.

pharyngitis INFLAMMATION of the PHARYNX and therefore the throat, commonly caused by a virus and resulting in a sore throat. It is often associated with TONSILLITIS.

pharynx the region extending from the beginning of the OESOPHAGUS up to the base of the SKULL at the cavity into which the NOSE and MOUTH open. It is muscular, with a MUCOUS MEMBRANE, and acts as the route for both food (to the oesophagus) and air (to the LARYNX). The EUSTACHIAN TUBES open from the upper part of the pharynx.

phenotype the detectable, observable chatracteristics of an individual, which are determined by the interaction of his or her GENES and the environment in which he or she develops. The expression of the dominant gene masks the presence of a recessive one, as only the expressed gene affects the phenotype.

phenylalanine *see* ESSENTIAL AMINO ACID.

phenylketonuria a genetic disorder that results in the deficiency of an ENZYME that converts phenylalanine, an ESSENTIAL AMINO ACID, to tyrosine. Children can be severely mentally retarded by an excess of phenylalanine in the blood, damaging the nervous system. The responsible GENE is recessive, so the condition occurs only if both parents are carriers. However, there is a test for newborn infants (the Guthrie test) that ensures the condition can be detected and the diet can be modified to avoid phenylalanine and thus any brain damage.

phimosis a condition in which the edge of the FORESKIN is narrowed and cannot be drawn back over the GLANS of the PENIS. To avoid INFLAMMATION and an exacerbation of the problem, CIRCUMCISION may be necessary. *See also* PARA-PHIMOSIS.

phlebitis inflammation of a VEIN. This commonly occurs as a complication of VARICOSE VEINS, producing pain and a hot feeling around the vein, with possible THROMBOSIS development. Drugs and elastic support are used in treatment.

phlebothrombosis the obstruction of a VEIN by a BLOOD CLOT, common in the deep veins of the leg (in particular the calf) and resulting from HEART failure,

PREGNANCY, injury and surgery, which may change the clotting factors in the blood. The affected leg may swell, and there is the danger that the clot may move, creating a PULMONARY EMBOLISM. Large clots may be removed surgically, otherwise the treatment involves ANTICOAGULANT drugs and exercise.

phlegm a general term (non-medical) for SPUTUM, MUCUS.

phobia an anxiety disorder and irrational fear of certain objects, animals, situations, events, etc. Avoiding the situation can lead to significant disruption, restriction of normal life or even suffering.

phospholipid *see* LIPOSOME.

photophobia an atypical sensitivity to light. Exposure produces discomfort and actions to evade the light source. The condition may be associated with medication or MIGRAINE, MENINGITIS, etc.

photoreceptor *see* CONE.

phrenic nerve the NERVE to the muscles of the DIAPHRAGM, arising from the 3rd, 4th and 5th cervical spinal nerves.

phthisis *see* TUBERCULOSIS.

physiotherapy the use of physical methods to help healing. It may involve exercise, massage and manipulation, heat treatment and the use of light and ultraviolet radiation, etc.

pia-arachnoid *see* MENINGES.

pia mater *see* BRAIN; MENINGES.

pigment an organic colouring agent, e.g. the blood pigment HAEMOGLOBIN, BILE pigments, rhodopsin (found in the RODS of the RETINA) and MELANIN.

piles *see* HAEMORRHOIDS.

pilus (*pl* **pili**) a HAIR or a structure like a hair.

pimple *or* **papule** a small swelling on the SKIN that is inflamed and may contain PUS. The cause is often INFECTION of a PORE that is blocked with fatty secretions from the SEBACEOUS GLANDS.

pinna *see* EAR.

pituitary gland *or* **hypophysis** a small, but very important ENDOCRINE GLAND at the base of the HYPOTHALAMUS. It has two LOBES, the anterior adenohypophysis and the posterior neurohypophysis. It secretes HORMONES that control many functions and is itself controlled by hormonal secretions from the hypothalamus. The neurohypophysis stores and releases PEPTIDE hormones produced in the hypothalamus, OXYTOCIN and VASOPRESSIN. The adenohypophysis secretes GROWTH HORMONE, GONADOTROPHIN, prolactin (involved in stimulating LACTATION), ACTH and THYROID-stimulating hormones.

placebo an inactive substance, taken as medication, that nevertheless may help to relieve a condition. The change occurs because the patient expects some treatment (even if nothing need, in reality, be done) and an improvement reflects the expectations of the patient. New drugs are tested in trials against placebos, when the effect of the drug is measured against the placebo response, which happens even when there is no active ingredient.

placenta the organ attaching the EMBRYO to the UTERUS. It is a temporary and comprises maternal and embryonic tissues. It allows oxygen and nutrients to pass from the mother's BLOOD to that of the embryo, but there is no direct contact of blood supplies. The embryo also receives salt, glucose, AMINO ACIDS, some PEPTIDES and ANTIBODIES, fats and VITAMINS. Waste molecules from the embryo are diffused into the maternal circulation. It also stores GLYCOGEN for conversion to glucose, if required, and secretes HORMONES to regulate the PREGNANCY. It is expelled after birth.

plague any EPIDEMIC disease that results in a high death rate and specifically the bubonic plague, which is transmitted to humans from infected rats by the rat flea. After an INCUBATION period of two to six days, the symptoms occur as headache, weakness, fever, aches in the limbs and delirium. The LYMPH NODES (especially in the groin) swell and become painful (buboes –po hence 'bubonic') and may burst, releasing PUS. In other cases, the infective fluid may not be released and there may be SUBCUTANEOUS bleeding with creation of black patches (gangrenous) on the skin, leading to ULCERS (hence the old term, black death). If the BACTERIA enter the BLOOD (septicaemic plague), death follows rapidly, but the most serious is pneumonic plague, when the LUNGS are affected. Preventive actions are very important in such cases, particularly to eliminate the carriers. However, the disease can be treated effectively with ANTIBIOTICS and SULPHONAMIDES.

plantar a descriptive term meaning 'relating to the sole of the foot'.

plaque a surface layer on teeth formed from BACTERIA and food debris and, later, calcium salts.

plasma a light-coloured fluid component of BLOOD in which the various CELLS are suspended. It contains inorganic salts with PROTEIN and some trace substances. One protein present is FIBRINOGEN.

plastic surgery a branch of surgery that deals with the repair or rebuilding of damaged, deformed or missing parts of the body. Cosmetic plastic surgery is merely for the improvement of appearance but most is to repair burns, accident damage or congenital defects.

platelet *or* **thrombocyte** a disc-like structure in the BLOOD involved in the halting of bleeding.

plegmasia alba dolens *see* THROMBOPHLEBITIS.

pleura (*pl* **pleurae**) the SEROUS MEMBRANE that covers the LUNGS (visceral) and the inside of the CHEST wall (parietal). The membranes have a smooth surface that is moistened to allow them to slide over each other.

pleuracentesis see THORACOCENTESIS.

pleural cavity the small space between the PLEURAe when they slide over each other as a person breathes in and out. Should gas or fluid enter the cavity because of infection or injury, the space increases and may hinder breathing.

pleurisy *or* **pleuritis** INFLAMMATION of the PLEURA, resulting in pain from deep breathing and shortness of breath. There is a typical frictional rub heard through a STETHOSCOPE. Pleurisy is often caused by PNEUMONIA in the adjacent lung and is always associated with disease in the lung, diaphragm, chest wall or abdomen, e.g. TUBERCULOSIS, ABSCESSES, bronchial CARCINOMA, etc.

plexus a network formed from intersecting NERVES and/or BLOOD VESSELS or lymphatic vessels.

PMS, PMT *see* PREMENSTRUAL TENSION.

pneumoconiosis a general term for a chronic form of LUNG disease caused by inhaling dust while working. Most of the cases are anthracosis (coal miner's pneumoconiosis), SILICOSIS and ASBESTOSIS.

pneumonia a bacterial infection of the LUNGS resulting in INFLAMMATION and filling of the ALVEOLI (*see* ALVEOLUS) with PUS and fluid. As a result, the lung becomes solid and air cannot enter. The symptoms vary, depending on how much of the lung is unavailable for RESPIRATION, but commonly there will be chest pain, coughing, BREATHLESSNESS, FEVER and possibly CYANOSIS. Pneumonia may be caused by several BACTERIA, VIRUSES or FUNGI, but bacterial infection is commonest. Bronchopneumonia affects the BRONCHI and BRONCHIOLES; lobar pneumonia the whole LOBES of the lung(s). ANTIBIOTIC treatment is usually effective, although it helps to know which is the infecting organism to provide the most specific treatment. (*See also* VIRAL PNEUMONIA).

pneumonitis INFLAMMATION of the LUNGS by chemical or physical agents.

pneumothorax air in the PLEURAL CAVITY, which enters via a wound in the chest wall or lung. When this happens, the lung collapses, but if the air is absorbed from the pleural cavity the lung reinflates.

polio the short term for POLIOMYELITIS.

poliomyelitis *or* **infantile paralysis** an infectious disease caused by a VIRUS that attacks the CENTRAL NERVOUS SYSTEM. The virus is taken in by mouth, passes through the ALIMENTARY CANAL and is excreted with the FAECES. The hands may be contaminated, leading to further spread. The INCUBATION period is seven to 12 days, and there are several types of condition, depending on the severity of the attack. In some cases the symptoms resemble a stomach upset or INFLUENZA; in others there is, in addition, some stiffness of muscles. Paralytic poliomyelitis is less common, resulting in muscle weakness and PARALYSIS, while the most serious cases involve breathing, when the DIAPHRAGM and related muscles are affected (bulbar poliomyelitis). IMMUNIZATION is highly effective, and the disease has almost been eradicated in most countries, but booster doses are advisable in countries with a high incidence of the disease.

polyneuritis *see* NEURITIS.

polyp a growth from a MUCOUS MEMBRANE and attached to it by a stalk. Most are BENIGN but may cause obstructions or infections. They commonly occur in the sinuses, nose or possibly the bladder or bowels. Their removal is usually straightforward, unless a more extensive operation proves necessary to reach the affected organ.

polyuria the passing of a larger than normal quantity of URINE, which is also usually pale in colour. It may be the result merely of a large fluid intake or of a condition such as DIABETES or a KIDNEY disorder.

pons (*pl* **pontes**) tissue that joins parts of an organ, e.g. the pons Varolii, a part of the BRAIN stem that links various parts of the brain stem, including the MEDULLA OBLONGATA, and THALAMUS.

pore a small opening, especially one of the minute openings in the SKIN through which fluids and minute substances are excreted or exhaled or by which they are absorbed.

porphyrin *see* HAEM.

portal vein a VEIN within the hepatic portal system that carries blood to the LIVER from other abdominal organs (stomach, spleen, intestine, etc). It is atypical in that it does not take blood directly to the heart but ends in a CAPILLARY network.

posterior a term meaning 'situated towards the back or at the back', the opposite of ANTERIOR.

post-viral fatigue syndrome *see* MYALGIC ENCEPHALOMYELITIS.

poultice *or* **fomentation** hot, moist material applied to the body to soften the skin, soothe irritations, ease pain or increase the circulation locally.

precancerous a term to describe any condition that is not MALIGNANT but may become so if left untreated.

pre-eclampsia the development of high BLOOD PRESSURE in PREGNANCY, sometimes with OEDEMA, which, unless treated, may result in ECLAMPSIA.

pregnancy the period of time, lasting approximately 280 days from the first day of the last menstrual period, during which a woman carries a developing FOETUS. Signs of a pregnancy include cessation of MENSTRUATION, increase in size of the BREASTS, MORNING SICKNESS and, later, the obvious sign of enlargement of the ABDOMEN. A foetal heartbeat and movements can also be detected.

Many of these changes are HORMONE-controlled, by PROGESTERONE (from the OVARY and PLACENTA).

premature birth a birth occurring before the end of the normal full term of PREG-NANCY. The definition refers to babies weighing less than 2.5 kg. In many cases the cause is unknown, but in some it may be because of PRE-ECLAMPSIA, kidney or heart disease or multiple pregnancy. Premature babies often require INCUBATOR care.

premenstrual tension (PMT) *or* **premenstrual syndrome (PMS)** the occurrence for up to ten days before MENSTRUATION of such symptoms as headache, nervousness and irritability, emotional disturbance, depression, fatigue with other physical manifestations such as swelling of legs and breasts, and constipation. The condition usually disappears soon after menstruation begins. The cause is not known, although the hormone PROGESTERONE is probably involved in some way.

premolar one of two teeth between the canines and molars on each side of the jaw.

prepuce *see* FORESKIN.

pressure sores *see* BED SORES.

preventive medicine the branch of medicine that seeks to prolong life by PROPHY-LAXISIS, by early diagnosis (e.g. CERVICAL SMEAR) or to prevent the occurence of a disease by encouraging a healthy lifestyle.

prickly heat *or* **heat rash** *or* **miliaria** an itchy RASH of small red spots that are minute blisters caused by the blocking of SWEAT GLANDS or SEBACEOUS GLANDS in the SKIN. Scratching may produce infection, but the condition itself is not serious.

process an anatomical term for a protuberance or projecting part of a bone or other part.

progesterone a steroid HORMONE that is vital in PREGNANCY. It is produced by the CORPUS LUTEUM of the OVARY when the lining of the UTERUS is prepared for the implanting of an egg cell. Progesterone is secreted under the control of other hormones (prolactin from the anterior PITUITARY GLAND and luteinizing hormone also from the pituitary, which stimulates ovulation and formation of the corpus luteum) until the PLACENTA adopts this role later in the pregnancy. The function of progesterone is to maintain the uterus and ensure that no further eggs are produced. Small amounts of this hormone are also produced by the testes (*see* TESTICLE).

prolactin *see* PITUITARY GLAND; PROGESTERONE.

prolapse a moving down of an organ or tissue from its normal position because of weakening of the supporting tissues. This may happen to the lower end of the bowel (in children) or the UTERUS and VAGINA in women who have sustained some sort of injury during childbirth. In the latter case, prolapse may result in the uterus itself showing on the outside. Surgery can shorten the supporting LIGAMENTS and narrow the vaginal opening.

prolapsed intervertebral disc *or* **slipped disc** the INTERVERTEBRAL DISCS provide cushioning for the BRAIN and SPINAL CORD and each is composed of an outer fibrous layer over a pulpy centre. A slipped disc is caused by the inner layer being pushed through the fibrous layer to impinge upon NERVES, causing pain (commonly LUMBAGO or SCIATICA). The PROLAPSE usually occurs during sudden twisting or bending of the SPINAL COLUMN and is more likely in middle age. Treatment involves bed rest on a flat, firm surface, probably with manipulation and physiotherapy at a later stage. If absolutely necessary, the disc can be removed, but this is now less common.

prone a term meaning 'lying face downwards'.

prophylaxis a treatment or action that is taken to avoid disease or a condition, e.g. taking a prophylactic medication to prevent ANGINA.

prostaglandin (PG) any of a group of compounds, derived from ESSENTIAL FATTY ACIDS, that act in a way that is similar to HORMONES. They are found in most body tissues (but especially SEMEN), where they are released as local regulators (in the UTERUS, BRAIN, LUNGS, etc). A number have been identified, two of which act antagonistically on BLOOD VESSELS, PGE causing dilation, PGF constriction. Certain prostaglandins cause contraction of the UTERUS in LABOUR, and others are involved in the body's defence mechanisms.

prostate gland a GLAND in the male reproductive system that is located below the BLADDER, opening into the URETHRA. Upon ejaculation, it secretes an alkaline fluid into the SEMEN, which aids sperm motility. In older men, the gland may become enlarged, causing problems with urination. In this case it is usually surgically removed in an operation called a prostatectomy.

prostatitis INFLAMMATION of the PROSTATE GLAND as a result of bacterial infection. The symptoms tend to be similar to a urinary infection although in the chronic form obstructions may form, necessitating surgical removal (prostatectomy).

prosthesis (*pl* **prostheses**) an artificial device fitted to the body, ranging from dentures to hearing aids, pacemakers and artificial limbs.

protein a large group of organic compounds containing carbon, hydrogen, oxygen, sulphur and nitrogen, with individual molecules built up of AMINO ACIDS in long polyPEPTIDE chains. Globular protein includes ENZYMES, ANTIBODIES, carrier proteins (e.g. HAEMOGLOBIN) some HORMONES, etc. Fibrous proteins have elasticity and strength and are found in MUSCLE, CONNECTIVE TISSUE and also CHROMOSOMES. Proteins are thus vital to the body and are synthesized from their constituent amino acids, which are obtained from DIGESTION of dietary protein.

proteinuria the condition in which PROTEIN (usually ALBUMIN) is found in the URINE. It is important because it may signify heart or kidney disease. Proteinuria may also occur with fever, severe anaemia and intake of certain drugs or poisons.

prothrombin *see* COAGULATION; THROMBIN; VITAMIN K.

pruritus another term for ITCHING, of whatever origin.

psilosis *see* SPRUE.

psittacosis a bacterial infection of parrots and budgerigars that can be transmitted to humans. It causes headache, shivering, nosebleeds, fever and lung problems. It is treatable with ANTIBIOTICS.

psoriasis a chronic SKIN disease, the cause of which is unknown and the treatment for which is PALLIATIVE. The affected skin appears as itchy, scaly red areas, starting usually around the elbows and knees. It often runs in families and may be associated with anxiety, commencing usually in childhood or adolescence. Treatment involves ointments and creams with some drugs and VITAMIN A.

ptyalin *see* MOUTH; SALIVA.

puberty the changes that occur in boys and girls around the age of 10 to 14, which signify the beginnings of sexual maturity and the subsequent functioning of reproductive organs. It is apparent through the appearance of SECONDARY SEXUAL CHARACTERISTICS, such as a deepening of the voice in boys and growth of BREASTS in girls. In addition, girls commence MENSTRUATION and in boys the size of TESTICLES increases. In both sexes body shape changes noticeably and body hair grows. The changes are initiated by PITUITARY GLAND hormones acting on the ovaries (*see* OVARY) and testes.

pubic pertaining to the pubes (*see* PUBIS), e.g. pubic hair.

pubis (*pl* **pubes**) one of the three BONEs, and the most anterior, that make up each half of the PELVIC GIRDLE.

pulmonary relating to the LUNGS.

pulmonary embolism a condition involving the blocking of the pulmonary ARTERY or a branch of it by an EMBOLUS. The clot usually originates from PHLEBOTHROMBOSIS of the leg. The seriousness of the attack relates to the size of clot. Large pulmonary emboli can be immediately fatal. Smaller ones may cause death of parts of the lung, PLEURISY and the coughing up of blood. ANTICOAGULANTS are used in minor cases; STREPTOKINASE may be used to dissolve the clot, or immediate surgery may be necessary. Several embolisms may produce PULMONARY HYPERTENSION.

pulmonary hypertension an increase in BLOOD PRESSURE in the pulmonary ARTERY because of increased resistance to the flow of blood. The cause is usually disease of the lung (such as BRONCHITIS, EMPHYSEMA, *see also* PULMONARY EMBOLISM), and the result is that the pressure increases in the right VENTRICLE, enlarging it, producing pain with the possibility of HEART failure.

pulmonary oedema gathering of fluid in the LUNGS, caused by, for example, MITRAL STENOSIS.

pulmonary stenosis a narrowing of the outlet from the HEART to the pulmonary ARTERY via the right VENTRICLE, which may be CONGENITAL or, more rarely, result from RHEUMATIC FEVER. Severe cases can produce ANGINA, fainting and enlargement of the HEART with eventual heart failure. Surgery is necessary to clear the obstruction.

pulp *see* TOOTH.

pulse the regular expansion and contraction of an ARTERY as a fluid wave of BLOOD passes along, originating with the contraction of the HEART muscle and blood leaving the left VENTRICLE. It is detected in arteries near the surface, e.g. the radial artery in the wrist, and decreases with a reduction in size so that the capillaries are under a steady pressure (hence why venous flow is also steady).

puncture a small hole in the skin made by a sharp object such as a needle, prickle or sting.

pupil the circular opening in the IRIS which permits light into the LENS in the EYE. *See also* LIGHT REFLEX.

purgative a drug or other treatment taken to evacuate the bowels. They may be grouped by their mode of action, LAXATIVES providing a gentle effect. Purgatives work by increasing the muscular contractions of the INTESTINE or by increasing the fluid content.

purine *see* NUCLEOTIDE.

pus the liquid found at an infected site (ABSCESS, ULCER, etc). It is white, yellow or greenish and consists of dead white blood cells (LEUCOCYTES), living and dead BACTERIA and dead tissue.

pustule an inflamed elevation of the SKIN, containing PUS.

putrid fever a former name for typhus fever (*see* RICKETTSIAE).

pyelitis INFLAMMATION of part of the KIDNEY, the renal PELVIS. The cause is usually a bacterial infection (commonly *E. coli*, *see* ESCHERIA) and sometimes it occurs as a complication of PREGNANCY. Symptoms include pain in the loins, high temperature, loss of weight, but it does respond to ANTIBIOTICS. Usually the infection is not limited to the pelvis but all the kidney is involved, hence a more accurate term is pyelonephritis.

pyloric stenosis a narrowing of the PYLORUS, which limits the movement of food from the STOMACH to the DUODENUM, resulting in VOMITING. It may be accompanied by distension and PERISTALSIS visible through the abdominal wall. A continuation of the condition causes weight loss and dehydration. It is often caused by an ULCER or CANCER near the pylorus, which requires surgery.

pylorus the lower end of the STOMACH where food passes into the DUODENUM and at which there is a ring of MUSCLE, the pyloric SPHINCTER.

pyrexia another term for FEVER.

pyridoxine *see* VITAMIN B6.

pyrimethamine *see* TOXOPLASMOSIS.

pyrimidine *see* NUCLEOTIDE.

pyrogen any substance that causes a rise in TEMPERATURE of the body. *See also* FEVER.

Q

Q fever an infectious disease that produces symptoms resembling PNEUMONIA, including a severe headache, high fever and breathing problems. It is caused by the organism *Coxiella burnetti* and is a disease of sheep, goats and cattle that can be passed to humans, mainly through unpasteurized milk. The disease is treated with drugs and lasts about two weeks.

quadriceps the large thigh muscle, which is divided into four distinct parts and is responsible for movements of the KNEE joint.

quadriplegia paralysis of all four limbs of the body.

quarantine a period of time in which a person (or animal) who has, or is suspected of having, an infectious disease is isolated from others to prevent the spread of the infection.

quartan fever the recurrent FEVER, which usually occurs every fourth day, associated with MALARIA.

quinine a colourless alkaloid, derived from the bark of certain (cinchona) trees, which is a strong ANTISEPTIC and especially effective against the malarial parasite. It was formerly widely used in the treatment of MALARIA but has now largely been replaced because it is toxic in larger doses. In small amounts it has a stimulating effect and is used in tonic water.

quinsy *or* **peritonsillar abscess** a complication of TONSILLITIS, when a pus-filled ABSCESS occurs near the tonsil, causing great difficulty in swallowing. It may require surgical lancing.

R

rabies *or* **hydrophobia** a very severe and fatal disease affecting the CENTRAL NERVOUS SYSTEM, which occurs in dogs, wolves, cats and other animals. Human beings are infected through the bite of a rabid animal, usually a dog. *See* page 112.

radial a term meaning 'pertaining to the RADIUS'.

radiation sickness any illness that is caused by harmful radiation from radioactive substances. This may be a complication of RADIOTHERAPY for cancer and produces symptoms of nausea, vomiting and sometimes itchiness of the skin. ANTIHISTAMINE drugs and TRANQUILLIZERS are used to alleviate the condition.

radical treatment treatment aimed at the complete cure of a condition (i.e. 'to the root'), rather than the alleviation of symptoms. In contrast, conservative treatment is directed towards the minimum interference necessary to keep a condition under control.

radiotherapy the therapeutic use of penetrating radiation, including X-RAYS, beta rays and gamma rays. These may be derived from X-ray machines or radioactive isotopes and are especially employed in the treatment of CANCER. The main disadvantages of radiotherapy is that there may be damage to normal, healthy surrounding tissues.

radium a radioactive metallic element that occurs naturally and emits alpha, beta and gamma rays as it decays. The gamma rays derived from radium are used in the treatment of CANCER.

radius (*pl* **radii**) the shorter outer bone of the forearm, the other being the ULNA.

rash an eruption of the skin, which is usually short-lived and consists of a reddened, perhaps itchy, area or raised red spots.

rat-bite fever two types of infectious disease that are contracted following the bite of a rat. The first type is caused by either of two kinds of BACTERIA and produces symptoms of fever, skin rash and joint and muscle pains. The second type is caused by a FUNGUS and produces similar symptoms and vomiting. Both diseases are treated with PENICILLIN.

receptor a SENSORY nerve ending that changes stimuli into NERVE IMPULSES to the brain. *See also* NERVOUS SYSTEM.

recessive gene a GENE the character of which will only be expressed if paired with a similar gene (ALLELE).

recombinant DNA DNA (deoxyribonucleic acid) containing GENES that have been artificially combined by the techniques of GENETIC ENGINEERING. Recombinant DNA technology has become synonymous with genetic engineering.

recrudescent a term used to describe a disease (e.g. HEPATITIS) that appears again after a period of abatement.

rectum the final portion of the large INTESTINE between the SIGMOID COLON and anal canal in which FAECES are stored prior to elimination.

red blood cell *see* ERYTHROCYTE.

referred pain *or* **synalgia** pain felt in another part of the body at a distance from the site at which it might be expected, e.g. certain HEART conditions cause pain in the left arm and fingers. The condition arises because some SENSORY nerves share common routes in the CENTRAL NERVOUS SYSTEM, hence stimulation of one causes an effect in another.

reflex action an unconscious movement that is brought about by relatively simple nervous circuits in the CENTRAL NERVOUS SYSTEM. In its simplest form it involves a single reflex arc of one RECEPTOR and SENSORY nerve, which forms a SYNAPSE in the BRAIN or SPINAL CORD with a MOTOR NERVE, which then transmits the impulse to a MUSCLE or GLAND to bring about a response. However some reflex actions are more complicated than this, involving several NEURONS. Examples are the plantar reflex of the toes when the sole of the foot is stroked, the knee-jerk reflex and the reflex PUPIL of the EYE, which contracts suddenly when a light is directed on its surface. The presence or absence of reflexes gives an indication of the condition of the nervous system and is a pointer to the presence or absence of disease or damage.

refractory a term used to describe a condition that does not respond to treatment.

regimen a course of treatment that usually involves several elements, including drugs, diet and lifestyle (such as the taking of exercise), aimed at curing a disease or promoting good health.

regression 1. in medicine, the term for the stage in the course of a disease when symptoms cease and the patient recovers. **2.** in psychiatry, a reversion to a more immature form of behaviour.

Reiter's syndrome a disease of unknown cause that affects men and produces symptoms of URETHRITIS, CONJUNCTIVITIS and ARTHRITIS. It may also produce other symptoms, including fever and diarrhoea, and it is suspected that the cause may be a VIRUS.

rejection in TRANSPLANTATION, when the IMMUNE system of the recipient individual rejects and destroys an organ or tissue grafted from a donor. Various drugs are given to the recipient to dampen down the immune system and reduce the risk of rejection.

relapse the return of the symptoms of a disease from which a person had apparently recovered or was in the process of recovering.

relapsing fever a disease caused by spirochaete bacteria of the genus *Borrelia*, which is transmitted to humans by lice and ticks. The disease is characterized by recurrent bouts of fever accompanied by headache, joint and muscle pains and nosebleeds. The first attack lasts for about two to eight days and further milder bouts occur after three to ten days.

remission a period during the course of a disease when symptoms have lessened or disappeared.

renal describing or relating to the KIDNEYS.

reproductive system the name given to all the organs involved in reproduction. In males these comprise the TESTICLES, VASA deferentia, PROSTATE GLAND, seminal vesicles, URETHRA and PENIS. In females, the reproductive system consists of the ovaries, FALLOPIAN TUBES, UTERUS, VAGINA and VULVA.

resection a surgical operation in which part of an organ, or any body part, is removed.

resistance 1. the degree of natural IMMUNITY that an individual possesses against a certain disease or diseases. **2.** the degree to which a disease or disease-causing organism can withstand treatment with drugs, such as a course of ANTIBIOTICS.

resonance the quality and increase of sound produced by striking the body over an air-filled structure. If resonance is decreased compared to normal, this is termed dullness and if increased hyper-resonance. Tapping the body, often the chest, to determine the degree of resonance, is called PERCUSSION.

respiration the whole process by which air is drawn into and out of the LUNGS, during which oxygen is absorbed into the bloodstream and carbon dioxide and water are given off. External respiration is the actual process of breathing and the exchange of gases that takes place in the lungs. Internal respiration is the process by which oxygen is given up from the blood CIRCULATION to the tissues, in all parts of the body, and carbon dioxide is taken up to be transported back to the lungs and eliminated. The process of drawing air into the lungs is known as inhalation or inspiration and expelling it out is exhalation or expiration. The rate at which this occurs is known as the respiratory rate, and it is about 18 times a minute in a static healthy adult.

respirator one of a number of different devices used to assist or take over RESPIRATION, especially when the MUSCLES that should normally be involved are paralysed, as in some forms of POLIOMYELITIS.

respiratory distress syndrome *or* **hyaline membrane disease** a condition usually arising in newborn babies, especially those who are PREMATURE, being particularly common in infants born between 32 and 37 weeks' GESTATION. It is characterized by rapid shallow laboured breathing. It arises because the lungs are not properly expanded and lack a substance (known as a surfactant) necessary to bring their expansion about. Adults may suffer from adult respiratory distress syndrome in which there is PULMONARY OEDEMA and a high mortality rate.

respiratory syncitial virus *or* **RS virus** the main cause of BRONCHIOLITIS and PNEUMONIA in babies under the age of six months.

respiratory system *or* **respiratory tract** all the organs and tissues involved in RESPIRATION, including the NOSE, PHARYNX, LARYNX, TRACHEA, BRONCHI, BRONCHIOLES, LUNGS and DIAPHRAGM, along with the MUSCLES that bring about respiratory movements.

resuscitation the reviving of a person in whom heartbeat and breathing have ceased. *See* ARTIFICIAL RESPIRATION; CARDIAC MASSAGE.

retina the layer that lines the interior of the EYE. The retina itself consists of two layers. The inner layer, next to the cavity of the eyeball, contains the light-sensitive cells, the RODS and CONES, and also NERVE fibres. This layer receives light directed on to its surface by the LENS. The outer layer of the retina, next to the choroid (MEMBRANE), contains pigmented cells that prevent the passage of light

retinol *see* VITAMIN A.

retroflexion the bending backwards of a part of an organ, particularly the upper portion of the UTERUS (*compare* RETROVERSION).

retroversion an abnormal position of the UTERUS in which the whole organ is tilted backwards instead of forwards, as is normally the case. A retroverted uterus occurs in about 20 per cent of women (*see* RETROFLEXION).

Retrovir the trade name of the antiviral drug ZIDOVUDINE.

retrovirus a type of VIRUS containing RNA (ribonucleic acid), which is able to introduce its genetic material into the DNA of body cells. These viruses are suspected as causal agents in the development of certain CANCERS.

Reye's syndrome a rare disorder, of unknown cause, that affects children and seems to follow on from a viral infection such as CHICKENPOX, often manifesting itself during the recovery phase. The symptoms include vomiting, high fever, delirium, convulsions, leading to coma and death, the mortality rate being about 25 per cent. Among those who survive, about half suffer some brain damage. It has been suggested that ASPIRIN may be implicated in the development of this condition, and this drug is not now recommended for children under the age of 12.

rhesus factor *or* **Rh factor** *see* BLOOD GROUP.

rheumatic fever a severe disease, affecting children and young adults, which is a complication of upper RESPIRATORY TRACT infection with BACTERIA known as *Haemolytic streptococci*. The symptoms include fever, JOINT pain and ARTHRITIS that progresses from joint to joint, a characteristic red rash, known as ERYTHEMA marginatum, and also painless nodules that develop beneath the skin over bony protuberances such as the elbow, knee and back of the wrist. In addition there is CHOREA and INFLAMMATION of the HEART, including the muscle, valves and membranes. The condition may lead to rheumatic heart disease in which there is scarring and inflammation of heart structures. The initial treatment consists of destroying the streptococci that cause the disease with ANTIBIOTIC drugs such as PENICILLIN. Other drugs are also used, such as non-steroidal anti-inflammatory drugs (*see* NSAID) and CORTICOSTEROIDS. Surgery may be required later in life to replaced damaged heart valves.

rheumatism a general term used to describe aches and pains in joints and muscles.

rheumatoid arthritis the second most common form of JOINT disease, after OSTEOARTHRITIS, which usually affects the feet, ankles, fingers and wrists. It is diagnosed by means of X-RAYS, which show a typical pattern of changes around the inflamed joints, known as rheumatoid erosions. At first there is swelling of the joint and INFLAMMATION of the SYNOVIAL MEMBRANE (the membraneous sac that surrounds the joint), followed by erosion and loss of CARTILAGE and BONE. In addition, a blood test reveals the presence of serum rheumatoid factor antibody, which is characteristic of this condition. The condition varies greatly in its degree of severity, but at its worst can be progressive and seriously disabling. In other people, after an initial active phase, there may be a long period of REMISSION. A number of different drugs are used to treat the disease, including ANALGESICS and ANTI-INFLAMMATORY agents.

Rh factor *or* **rhesus factor** *see* BLOOD GROUP.

rhinitis INFLAMMATION of the MUCOUS MEMBRANE of the NOSE, such as occurs with colds and allergic reactions.

rhodopsin *see* PIGMENT; ROD.

riboflavin *see* VITAMIN B2.

ribonucleic acid *see* RNA.

ribs 12 pairs of thin, slightly twisted and curved BONES that form the thoracic rib cage, which protects the LUNGS and HEART. The true ribs are the first seven pairs, which are each connected to the STERNUM at the front by a COSTAL CARTILAGE. The false ribs are the next three pairs and are indirectly connected to the sternum as each is attached by its cartilage to the rib above. The floating ribs are the last two pairs, which are unattached and end freely in the muscle of the thoracic wall. At the backbone, the head of each rib articulates with one of the 12 thoracic VERTEBRAE.

rickets a disease affecting children that involves a deficiency of VITAMIN D. This can be manufactured in the skin in the presence of sunlight, but dietary sources are important especially where sunlight is lacking. It is characterized by soft BONES that bend out of shape and cause deformities. Bones are hardened by the deposition of calcium salts and this cannot happen in the absence of vitamin D. Treatment consists of giving vitamin D, usually in the form of CALCIFEROL, and ensuring that there is an adequate amount in the child's diet. Vitamin D deficiency in adults causes OSTEOMALACIA.

rickettsiae (*sing* **rickettsia**) a group of microorganisms that share characteristics in common with both BACTERIA and VIRUSes and are parasites that occur in lice, fleas and ticks and other arthropods. They can be passed to humans by the bites of these animals and are the cause of several serious diseases including typhus, Rocky Mountain spotted fever and Q FEVER.

Rift Valley fever a disease, caused by a VIRUS, that formerly mainly affected domestic animals and rarely human beings in sub-Saharan Africa. A widespread outbreak in Egypt in 1977, however, caused many fatalities, and it now poses a threat to people throughout the Middle East. A new strain of virus of a more virulent type is thought to be responsible, and the infection is characterized by fever, muscle and joint pains, haemorrhages, headache, photophobia and loss of appetite. The virus is transmitted to humans by mosquitoes or by direct contact with the carcases of heavily infected animals. An effective VACCINE is available.

rigor a sudden bout of shivering and feeling of coldness that often accompanies the start of a FEVER.

rigor mortis the stiffening of the body that occurs usually within eight hours of death as a result of chemical changes in the MUSCLES. It generally passes off after about 24 hours.

ringworm an infection caused by various species of fungi (*see* FUNGUS) and known medically as tinea. It is classified according to the area affected, e.g. tinea capitis, which is ringworm of the scalp. Other areas affected are the beard, groin (tinea cruris or dhobie itch), nails and feet (ATHLETE'S FOOT). The infection is slightly raised, itchy and has a ring-like appearance. It is highly contagious, and the commonest form is athlete's foot. The ANTIBIOTIC drug griseofulvin, taken by mouth, is the normal treatment for ringworm and also antifungal creams applied to the affected areas.

RNA *or* **ribonucleic acid** a complex nucleic acid present mainly in the CYTO-PLASM of cells but also in the NUCLEUS. It is involved in the production of PROTEINS and exists in three forms, ribosomal (r), transfer (t) and messenger (m) RNA. In some viruses it forms the genetic material (*see also* DNA).

rod one of the two types of light-sensitive cell present in the RETINA of the EYE. The rods enable vision in dim light because of a PIGMENT called rhodopsin (visual purple). This pigment degenerates or bleaches when light is present and regenerates during darkness. In bright light all the pigment bleaches and the rods cannot function. Bleaching of the pigment gives rise to NERVE IMPULSES that are sent to the brain and interpreted.

rodent ulcer a slow-growing malignant ULCER that occurs on the face in elderly people, usually near the lips, nostrils or eyelids. Skin and underlying tissues and bone are destroyed if the ulcer is untreated. Normally, treatment is by means of surgery and possibly RADIOTHERAPY.

roseola any rose-coloured RASH such as accompanies various infectious diseases, e.g. MEASLES.

rotavirus one of a number of VIRUSES that commonly cause GASTROENTERITIS and DIARRHOEA in young children under the age of six. They infect the lining cells of the small INTESTINE.

RS virus *see* RESPIRATORY SYNCITIAL VIRUS.

rubella *see* GERMAN MEASLES.

rupture 1. the bursting open of an organ, tissue or structure, e.g. ruptured APPENDIX. **2.** a popular name for a HERNIA.

S

Sabin vaccine an oral VACCINE for POLIOMYELITIS. The appropriate VIRUS is cultured but rendered nonviolent while retaining its ability to stimulate production of ANTIBODIES.

sac a structure resembling a bag, e.g. the ALVEOLUS.

sacral nerves NERVES that serve the legs, anal and genital region and originate from the sacral area (SACRUM) of the SPINAL COLUMN. There are five pairs of sacral nerves.

sacral vertebrae the five VERTEBRAE that are fused together to form the SACRUM.

sacrum the lower part of the SPINAL COLUMN, comprising five fused vertebrae (SACRAL VERTEBRAE) in a triangular shape. The sacrum forms the back wall of the PELVIS and articulates with the COCCYX below, LUMBAR VERTEBRAE above and the HIPS to the sides.

Saint Vitus' dance the former name for Sydenham's CHOREA.

saliva an alkaline liquid present in the MOUTH to keep the mouth moist, aid swallowing of food and, through the presence of amylase ENZYMES (ptyalin), to digest starch. It is secreted by the SALIVARY GLANDS, and, in addition to ptyalin, contains water, MUCUS and buffers (to minimize changes in acidity).

salivary glands three pairs of glands – parotid, submandibular and sublingual – that produce SALIVA. The stimulus to produce saliva can be the taste, smell, sight or even thought of food.

Salk vaccine a VACCINE against POLIOMYELITIS administered by INJECTION. The VIRUS is treated to render it unable to cause the disease but it still prompts the production of ANTIBODIES.

salmonella infections FOOD POISONING caused by *Salmonella*, a genus of Gram-negative (*see* GRAM'S STAIN) rod-like BACTERIA. *See* page 92.

salpingitis INFLAMMATION of a tube, usually the FALLOPIAN TUBE, by bacterial INFECTION. It may originate in the VAGINA or UTERUS, or be carried in the BLOOD. PERITONITIS can ensue. Severe cases may cause a blockage of the Fallopian tubes, *de facto* STERILIZATION.

sandfly fever *or* **bartonellosis** a viral INFECTION passed to humans through the bite of a sandfly. It occurs in much of the tropics and subtropics during the warmer months. It is a short-lived infection that resembles INFLUENZA in its symptoms.

sanguineous containing blood, covered or stained with blood.

sarcoma *see* CANCER.

sarcomere *see* VOLUNTARY MUSCLE.

scab a crust that forms over an injury (scratch, sore, etc) during the body's healing processes. It consists of FIBRIN, dried blood, SERUM or PUS and epithelial cells (*see* EPITHELIUM). Healing occurs beneath the protective scab, which falls off when the process is complete. Scabs caused by INFECTIONS occur, e.g. on the face, with no previous sign.

scabies a skin INFECTION causing severe itching. It is caused by the mite *Sarcoptes scabiei*, which burrows into the skin and lays eggs, the resulting larvae causing the itching. The areas of the body affected are the skin between fingers, wrists, buttocks and genitals.

scalds *see* BURNS.

scaphoid bone a BONE of the WRIST, the outside one on the thumb side of the HAND.

scapula (*pl* **scapulae**) *or* **shoulder blade** a triangular BONE and one of a pair forming the PECTORAL GIRDLE.

scar the mark left after a wound heals. It is the result of damaged tissues not repairing completely and being replaced by a fibrous CONNECTIVE TISSUE.

scarlet fever an infectious disease, mainly of childhood, caused by the bacterium *Streptococcus*. Symptoms show after a few days and include sickness, sore throat, fever and a scarlet rash that may be widespread. ANTIBIOTICS are effective and also prevent any complications, e.g. inflammation of the kidneys.

schistosomiasis *or* **bilharziasis** a parasitic infection caused by blood flukes (*Schistosoma*). Humans are infected with the larvae of the fluke, which enter through the skin from infected water in tropical regions. The adults then settle in blood vessels of the intestine or bladder. Subsequent release of eggs causes ANAEMIA, DIARRHOEA, DYSENTERY, enlargement of the SPLEEN and LIVER and CIRRHOSIS of the liver. It can be treated with drugs but preventive measures are preferable. It affects millions of people worldwide, particularly in the Far and Middle East, South America and Africa.

Schwann cell *see* MYELIN.

sciatic pertaining to the HIP.

sciatica pain in the SCIATIC NERVE and therefore felt in the back of the thigh, leg and foot. The commonest cause is a PROLAPSED INTERVERTEBRAL DISC pressing on a nerve root, but it may also result from ankylosing SPONDYLITIS and other conditions.

sciatic nerve the major NERVE in the leg, passing down the back of the thigh from the base of the SPINAL COLUMN.

sclera the outer layer of the eyeballs, which is seen as white and fibrous except at the front of the EYE when it becomes the transparent CORNEA.

scleritis INFLAMMATION of the white of the eye (SCLERA).

scleroderma a condition in which CONNECTIVE TISSUE hardens and contracts. The tissue may be the SKIN, HEART, KIDNEY, LUNG, etc, and the condition may be localized or it may spread throughout the body, eventually being fatal. If the skin is affected, it becomes tough and patchily pigmented and may lead to stiff joints and wasting MUSCLES.

sclerosis hardening of tissue, usually after INFLAMMATION, leading to parts of organs being hard and of no use. It is applied commonly to such changes in the NERVOUS SYSTEM (MULTIPLE SCLEROSIS); in other organs it is termed FIBROSIS or CIRRHOSIS.

screening test a programme of tests carried out on a large number of apparently healthy people to find those who may have a particular disease, e.g. CERVICAL SMEARS.

scrofula TUBERCULOSIS of the LYMPH NODES in the neck, which form sores and scars after healing. It is now an uncommon condition, but drug treatment is effective.

scrotum the SAC that contains the TESTICLES and holds them outside the body to permit production and storage of sperm at a temperature lower than that of the abdomen.

scrub typhus *see* page 125.

scurvy a deficiency disease caused by a lack of VITAMIN C (ascorbic acid) as a result of a dietary lack of fruit and vegetables. Symptoms begin with swollen, bleeding gums and then SUBCUTANEOUS bleeding, bleeding into joints, ULCERS, ANAEMIA and fainting, diarrhoea and trouble with major organs. Untreated, it is fatal, but nowadays it is easily prevented, or cured should it arise, through correct diet or administration of the vitamin.

sebaceous cyst *or* **wen** a CYST formed in the duct of a SEBACEOUS GLAND of the skin.

sebaceous gland any of the minute GLANDS in the skin that secrete an oily substance called SEBUM. The glands open into hair FOLLICLES. Activity of the glands varies with age, PUBERTY being the most active period.

seborrhoea excessive production of SEBUM by the SEBACEOUS GLANDS, producing either a build-up of dry skin scales or oily deposits on the skin.

sebum the secretion, formed by the SEBACEOUS GLANDS, that forms as a thin oily film on the skin, preventing excessive dryness. It also has an antibacterial action.

secondary sexual characteristics the physical features that develop at PUBERTY. In girls, the BREASTS and genitals increase in size and PUBIC hair grows. Boys grow pubic hair and facial hair, the voice breaks and the genitals become adult size.

secretin a polyPEPTIDE hormone produced by the lining of the DUODENUM and JEJUNUM in response to acid from the stomach. It stimulates production of alkaline pancreatic juice, and BILE secretion by the liver.

secretion the material produced by a GLAND.

secretory otitis media *see* GLUE EAR.

section 1. in surgery, cutting, e.g. an abdominal section. **2.** in microscopy, a thin slice of a specimen as examined under a microscope.

sedative a drug that lessens tension and anxiety. Sedatives are hypnotic drugs, e.g. BARBITURATES, given in doses lower than would bring on sleep. They may be used to combat pain, sleeplessness, spasms, etc.

semen the fluid that contains the SPERM, which is ejaculated from the PENIS during copulation.

seminiferous tubule *see* TESTICLE.

senile dementia an organic mental disorder of the elderly involving generalized ATROPHY of the BRAIN. The result is a gradual deterioration with loss of memory, impaired judgement, confusion, emotional outbursts and irritability. The degree of the condition may vary considerably.

sense organ a bodily structure that reacts to stimuli and transmits them to the brain as NERVE IMPULSES.

sensitivity in a SCREENING TEST, the proportion of people with the disease who are identified by the test.

sensitization a change in the body's response to foreign substances. With the development of an ALLERGY, a person becomes sensitized to a certain ALLERGEN and then becomes hypersensitive. Similarly, it may be an acquired reaction when ANTIBODIES develop in response to an ANTIGEN.

sensory 1. of or relating to the senses, sensation or the SENSE ORGANS. **2.** of a NERVE, conveying NERVE IMPULSES to the BRAIN.

sepsis the destruction of tissues through putrefaction by BACTERIA-causing disease or TOXINS produced by bacteria.

septal defect a hole in the SEPTUM or partition between the left and right sides of the HEART, whether in the atria (*see* ATRIUM) or VENTRICLES. This condition is a CONGENITAL disorder caused by an abnormal development of the foetal heart. Whether the defect is atrial or ventricular, it allows incorrect CIRCULATION of the blood from left to right, from higher pressure to lower. This is called a shunt and results in too much blood flowing through the LUNGS. PULMONARY HYPERTENSION results, and a large shunt may cause heart failure. Surgery can correct the defect, although a small one may not require any treatment.

septic affected with SEPSIS.

septicaemia 1. a term used loosely for any type of blood poisoning. **2.** a systemic infection with PATHOGENS from an infected part of the body circulating in the bloodstream.

septic shock a form of shock that occurs because of SEPTICAEMIA. The toxins cause a drastic fall in BLOOD PRESSURE as a result of tissue damage and blood clotting. Kidneys, heart and lungs are affected, and related symptoms include fever, TACHYCARDIA or even COMA. The condition occurs most in those who already have a serious disease, such as CANCER, DIABETES or CIRRHOSIS. Urgent treatment is vital, with ANTIBIOTICS, oxygen and fluids given intravenously.

septum (*pl* **septa**) a planar dividing feature within a structure of the body; a partition, e.g. the nasal septum.

serositis INFLAMMATION of a SEROUS MEMBRANE.

serotonin an AMINE that acts as a vasoconstrictor (*see* VASOCONSTRICTION). It is present in the CENTRAL NERVOUS SYSTEM, blood PLATELETS and the INTESTINE. *See also* MAST CELL.

serous of or producing SERUM.

serous membrane a MEMBRANE lining a large CAVITY in the body. The membranes are smooth and transparent and the surfaces are moistened by fluid derived from BLOOD or LYMPH serum (hence the name). Examples are the PERITONEUM and the PERICARDIUM. Each consists of two layers: the visceral, which surrounds the organs, and the parietal, which lines the cavity. The two portions are continuous and the surfaces are close together, separated by fluid that permits free movement of the organs.

sertoli cells *see* TESTICLE.

serum 1. the clear, sticky fluid that separates from BLOOD and LYMPH when blood clotting occurs. In addition to water, serum contains ALBUMIN and GLOBULIN with salts, fat, sugar, UREA and other compounds important in disease prevention. **2.** a VACCINE prepared from the serum of a hyperIMMUNE donor for use in protection against a particular infection.

serum sickness a hypersensitive reaction that occasionally occurs several days after INJECTION of foreign SERUM, producing rashes, joint pains, fever and swelling of the LYMPH NODES. It is the result of circulating ANTIGEN material to which the body responds. It is not a serious condition.

sex chromosomes CHROMOSOMES that play a major role in determining the sex of the bearer. They contain GENES that control the characteristics of the individual, e.g. TESTICLES in males, ovaries (*see* OVARY) in females. Women have two X-CHROMOSOMES while men have one X-chromsome and one Y-CHROMO-SOME.

sex hormones steroid HORMONES responsible for the control of sexual development (primary and SECONDARY SEXUAL CHARACTERISTICS) and reproductive function. The ovaries (*see* OVARY) and TESTICLES are the organs primarily involved in hormone production, of which there are three main types: ANDRO-GENS, the male sex hormones; OESTROGENS and PROGESTERONE, the female sex hormones.

sex-linked disorders conditions produced because the GENES controlling certain characteristics are carried on the SEX CHROMOSOMES, usually the X-CHROMO-SOME. Some result from an abnormal number of chromosomes, e.g. KLINEFELTER'S SYNDROME affecting only men, and TURNER'S SYNDROME affecting only women. Other disorders, such as HAEMOPHILIA, are carried on the X-chromosome and these manifest themselves in men because, although the genes are RECESSIVE, there is no other X-chromosome to mask the recessive type, as is the case with women.

sexually transmitted diseases *see* VENEREAL DISEASES.

shin bone *see* TIBIA.

shingles *see* HERPES.

shock acute circulatory failure when the arterial BLOOD PRESSURE is too low to provide the normal blood supply to the body. The signs are a cold, clammy skin, PALLOR, CYANOSIS, weak rapid PULSE, irregular breathing and dilated pupils. There may also be a reduced flow of URINE and confusion or LETHARGY. There are numerous causes of shock, from a reduction in blood volume following a burn, external bleeding, dehydration, etc, to reduced heart activity, as in CORONARY THROMBOSIS, PULMONARY EMBOLISM, etc.

Certain other circumstances may produce shock, including severe allergic reactions (anaphylactic shock, *see* ANAPHYLAXIS), drugs overdose, emotional shock, etc.

short sight *see* MYOPIA.

shoulder blade *see* SCAPULA.

shoulder girdle *see* PECTORAL GIRDLE.

shunt *see* SEPTAL DEFECT.

Siamese twins *or* **conjoined twins** twins who are joined together physically at birth. The condition varies from superficial joining, e.g. by the umbilical vessels, to major fusion of head, torso and internal organs. The latter cases are inevitably very much more difficult to separate. The condition is caused by foetuses developing from the same OVUM.

sickle-cell anaemia a type of inherited, haemolytic ANAEMIA (*see* HAEMOLYSIS) that is genetically determined and is the most common hereditary disease in the world. It is caused by a RECESSIVE GENE and is manifested when this GENE is inherited from both parents. One AMINO ACID in the HAEMOGLOBIN molecule is substituted, causing the disease, which results in an abnormal type of haemoglobin being precipitated in the red blood cells (ERYTHROCYTES) during deprivation of oxygen. This produces the distortion of the cells, which are removed from the circulation, causing anaemia and JAUNDICE. Many people are carriers as a result of inheritance of just one defective gene and because this confers increased resistance to MALARIA, this gene remains at a high level.

side effect an additional and unwanted effect of a drug above the intended action. Sometimes it is harmful and may be the stronger than anticipated result of a drug or something quite different.

sigmoid colon the end part of the COLON, which is S-shaped.

silicosis a type of PNEUMOCONIOSIS caused by the inhalation of silica as particles of dust. The silica promotes FIBROSIS of the lung tissue, resulting in BREATHLESSNESS and a greater likelihood to contract TUBERCULOSIS. Workers in quarrying, mineral mining, sand-blasting, etc, are most susceptible.

sinew the TENDON of a MUSCLE.

sinoatrial node the natural HEART pacemaker, which consists of specialized MUSCLE cells in the right ATRIUM. These cells generate electrical impulses, contract and initiate contractions in the muscles of the heart. The AUTONOMIC NERVOUS SYSTEM supplies the node, and certain HORMONES also have an effect.

sinus 1. a cavity or channel. **2.** an air cavity in BONE, as in the bones of the FACE and SKULL. **3.** a channel, as in the dura mater, which drains venous blood from the BRAIN (*see also* MENINGES).

sinusitis INFLAMMATION of a SINUS, usually referring to the sinuses in the face that link with the nose and may therefore be caused by a spread of infection from the nose. Headaches and a tenderness over the affected sinus are typical symptoms, with a pus-containing discharge from the nose. Persistent infection may necessitate surgery to drain the sinus.

Sjögren's syndrome dryness of the mouth and eyes, associated with RHEUMATOID ARTHRITIS. The syndrome is the result of the destruction of the SALIVARY GLANDS (and LACRIMAL GLANDS).

skeleton the rigid, supporting framework of the body that protects organs and tissues, provides muscle attachments, facilitates movement, and produces red blood cells (ERYTHROCYTES). There are 206 BONEs, divided into the axial skeleton (head and trunk) and the appendicular skeleton (limbs). The types of bone are: long (e.g. HUMERUS), short (e.g. carpals, *see* CARPUS), flat (parts of the CRANIUM) and irregular (e.g. the VERTEBRAe).

skin the outer layer of the body, comprising an external EPIDERMIS, itself made up of a stratum corneum (horny layer) formed of flat cells that rub off, being replaced from below. Beneath this are two more layers (stratum lucidum and stratum granulosum), which act as intermediate stages between the stratum corneum and a still lower layer, the Malpighian layer. The Malpighian layer is where the epidermis is produced. The dermis lies beneath the epidermis, and there is subcutaneous tissue, composed mainly of fat. The SUBCUTANEOUS tissue contains glands (SWEAT, SEBACEOUS, etc), SENSORY receptors for pain, pressure and TEMPERATURE, NERVES, MUSCLES and blood capillaries. The skin is a protective layer against injury and parasites, and it moderates water loss. It is a medium of temperature control by means of the SWEAT GLANDS and blood capillaries and also the HAIRS (which provide insulation).

skull the part of the SKELETON that forms the head and encloses the BRAIN. It is made up of 22 BONES, forming the CRANIUM (eight bones) and 14 in the FACE, and all except the mandible (lower JAW) are fused along SUTURES, creating immovable JOINTS. The mandible articulates close to the ears. A large opening at the base of the skull (FORAMEN magnum) allows the SPINAL CORD to pass from the brain to the trunk of the body.

sleeping sickness *or* **African trypanosomiasis** a parasitic disease found in tropical Africa which is spread through the bite of tsetse flies. Initially the symptoms consist of a recurring fever, a slight rash, headache and chills. Then follows ANAEMIA, enlarged LYMPH NODES and pain in joints and limbs. Then after some time (possibly years), sleeping sickness itself develops. This is because of the parasites occupying minute blood vessels in the brain, resulting in damage and symptoms of drowsiness and lethargy. Death may follow from weakness or an associated disease.

slipped disc *see* PROLAPSED INTERVERTEBRAL DISC.

slough dead tissue, usually of limited extent, that, after INFECTION, separates from the healthy tissue of the rest of the body. In cases of GANGRENE it is possible for limbs to be lost.

slow virus one of several VIRUSES that show their effects some time after INFECTION, by which time considerable damage of NERVE tissue has occurred, resulting ultimately in death. Such a virus was found to cause scrapie in sheep and recently BOVINE SPONGIFORM ENCEPHALOPATHY in cows. In humans, a slow virus is thought to be the cause of CREUTZFELDT-JAKOB DISEASE and a type of MENINGITIS.

small intestine *see* INTESTINE.

smallpox a highly infectious viral disease that has nonetheless been eradicated. INFECTION results, after about two weeks, in a high fever, head and body aches and vomiting. Eventually red spots appear, which change to water and then pus-filled vesicles that, on drying out, leave scars. The person stays infectious until all scabs are shed. Fever often returns, with DELIRIUM, and although recovery is usual, complications often ensue, e.g. PNEUMONIA.

smooth muscle *see* INVOLUNTARY MUSCLE.

sneezing the involuntary REFLEX expulsion of air via the NOSE and MOUTH caused by irritating particles in the nose, e.g. pollen. It is also symptomatic of a COLD, MEASLES, HAY FEVER, etc. One sneeze can project many thousands of drops over several metres at great speed (>60 km/hour) and is therefore instrumental in the spread of INFECTIONS.

solar plexus a network of sympathetic nerves and ganglia (*see* GANGLION) behind the STOMACH. It is a major autonomic PLEXUS of the body where nerves of the SYMPATHETIC and PARASYMPATHETIC NERVOUS SYSTEM combine.

somatostatin *see* ISLETS OF LANGERHANS.

somatotrophin *see* GROWTH HORMONE.

somnambulism *or* **sleepwalking** walking and performing other functions during sleep with no recollection upon waking.

soporific sleep-inducing. *See also* HYPNOTICS.

sore a common term for an ULCER or open skin WOUND.

South American tryponosomiasis *see* Chagas' disease, page 122.

spasm a muscular contraction that is involuntary. Spasms may be part of a more major disorder (e.g. SPASTIC PARALYSIS, CONVULSIONS) or they may be specific, such as in CRAMP, COLIC, etc.

spasmolytic a drug that reduces SPASMS (in smooth MUSCLE) in a number of ways. It may generally depress the CENTRAL NERVOUS SYSTEM, act directly on the muscles in question, or modify the NERVE IMPULSES causing the spasm.

spastic colon *see* IRRITABLE BOWEL SYNDROME.

spasticity muscular hypertonicity (i.e. an increase in the state of readiness of MUSCLE fibres to contract; an increase in the normal partial contraction) with an increased resistance to stretch. Moderate cases show movement requiring great effort and a lack of normal coordination while slight cases show exaggerated movements that are coordinated.

spastic paralysis weakness of a limb characterized by involuntary muscular contraction and loss of muscular function. As with SPASTICITY, it is caused by disease of the NERVE fibres that usually control movement and REFLEXes.

sperm the mature male reproductive CELL or GAMETE. It has a head with the HAPLOID nucleus containing half the CHROMOSOME number and an acrosome (a structure that aids penetration of the egg). Behind the head comes a midpiece with energy-producing MITOCHONDRIA, and then a long tail that propels it forward. A few millilitres of SEMEN is ejaculated during intercourse, containing many millions of sperm.

spermatozoon (*pl* **spermatozoa**) the scientific name for SPERM.

sphenoid bone a BONE in the SKULL that lies behind the eyes.

sphincter a circular MUSCLE around an opening. The opening is closed totally or partially by contraction of the muscle, e.g. the anal SPHINCTER around the ANUS.

spina bifida a CONGENITAL malformation in newborn babies in which part of the SPINAL CORD is exposed by a gap in the backbone. Many cases are also affected with HYDROCEPHALUS. The symptoms usually include paralysis, incontinence, a high risk of MENINGITIS and mental retardation. There is usually an abnormally high level of ALPHA FETOPROTEIN in the AMNIOTIC FLUID and since this can be diagnosed and then confirmed by AMNIOCENTESIS, it is possible to terminate these pregnancies.

spinal anaesthesia 1. the generation of ANAESTHESIA by injecting the CEREBROSPINAL FLUID around the SPINAL CORD. Of the two types, the epidural (*see* EPIDURAL ANAESTHESIA) involves injecting into the outer lining of the spinal cord, while subarachnoid anaesthesia is produced by injecting between vertebrae in the LUMBAR region of the vertebral column. Spinal anaesthesia is useful for patients who have a condition that precludes a general ANAESTHETIC (e.g. a chest infection or heart disease). **2.** the loss of sensation in a part of the body as a result of spinal injury.

spinal column *or* **spine** *or* **backbone** *or* **vertebral column** the bony and slightly flexible column that forms a vital part of the SKELETON. It encloses the SPINAL CORD, articulates with other BONES, e.g. the SKULL and RIBS, and provides attachments for MUSCLES. It consists of bones, the VERTEBRAe, between which are discs of fibrocartilage (the INTERVERTEBRAL DISCS). From the top, the column comprises 7 cervical, 12 thoracic, 5 lumbar, 5 sacral and 4 coccygeal vertebrae. In adults the last two groups are fused to from the SACRUM and COCCYX respectively.

spinal cord the part of the CENTRAL NERVOUS SYSTEM that runs from the BRAIN, through the SPINAL COLUMN. Both GREY and WHITE MATTER are present, the former as an H-shaped core within the latter. A hollow core in the grey matter forms the central canal, which contains the CEREBROSPINAL FLUID. The cord is covered by MENINGES, and it contains both SENSORY and MOTOR NEURONS.

Thirty-one pairs of spinal nerves arise from the cord, passing out between the arches of the VERTEBRAE.

spine the SPINAL COLUMN.

spirochaete any of a group of spiral shaped BACTERIA that are the causal organisms of LYME DISEASE; RELAPSING FEVER and YAWS.

spleen a roughly ovoid (egg-shaped) organ, coloured a deep purple, that is situated on the left of the body, behind and below the stomach. It is surrounded by a peritoneal MEMBRANE and contains a mass of lymphoid tissue. MACROPHAGES in the spleen destroy microorganisms by PHAGOCYTOSIS. The spleen produces LYMPHOCYTES, LEUCOCYTES, PLASMA cells and blood PLATELETS. It also stores red blood cells (ERYTHROCYTES) for use in emergencies. Release of red blood cells is facilitated by smooth MUSCLE under the control of the SYMPATHETIC NERVOUS SYSTEM, and when this occurs, the familiar pain called STITCH may be experienced. The spleen removes worn-out red blood cells, conserving the iron for further production in the BONE MARROW. Although the spleen performs many functions, it can be removed without detriment and as a result there is an increase in size of the lymphatic GLANDS.

splenomegaly an abnormal enlargement of the SPLEEN, which occurs commonly with blood disorders and parasitic infections.

splint a support that holds a broken BONE in the correct and stable position until healing is complete.

spondylitis INFLAMMATION of the spinal VERTEBRAe – ARTHRITIS of the spine. Ankylosing spondylitis is a rheumatic disease of the SPINAL COLUMN and sacroiliac JOINTS (i.e. those of the SACRUM and ILIUM), causing pain and stiffness in the hip and shoulder. It may result in the spine becoming rigid (*see* KYPHOSIS).

spondylosis degeneration of JOINTS and the INTERVERTEBRAL DISCS of the spine, producing pain in the neck and LUMBAR region where the joints may actually restrict movement. OSTEOPHYTES are commonly formed and the space occupied by the discs reduced. PHYSIOTHERAPY may help sufferers, and collars or surgical belts can prevent movement and give support. Surgery may be required occasionally to relieve pressure on nerves or to fuse joints.

spongiform encephalopathy a neurological disease that is caused by a SLOW VIRUS and results in a spongy degeneration of the BRAIN with progressive DEMENTIA. Examples are CREUTZFELDT-JAKOB DISEASE and kuru (a progressive and fatal viral INFECTION seen in New Guinea Highland peoples, the incidence of which has decreased with the decline in cannibalism).

sprain an injury to LIGAMENTS (or MUSCLES or TENDONS) around a JOINT, caused by a sudden overstretching. Pain and swelling may occur, and treatment comprises, in the main, avoiding use of the affected joint.

sprue *or* **psilosis** essentially a composite DEFICIENCY DISEASE because of lack of food being absorbed as a result of a disease of the INTESTINE or a metabolic disorder that means fats cannot be absorbed. The symptoms include DIARRHOEA, inflamed TONGUE, ANAEMIA and weight loss. The condition was considered a disease of tropical climates but other versions have been seen. Treatment involves ANTIBIOTICS, folic acid (to combat the anaemia), vitamins and a high-protein diet. There may be an immediate improvement on returning to a temperate climate.

sputum SALIVA and MUCUS from the respiratory tract.

squint *or* **strabismus** an abnormal condition in which the EYES are crossed. There are two types: paralytic and nonparalytic. The paralytic type is the result of a muscular or neurological malfunction, while a nonparalytic squint is caused by a defect in the actual relative position of the eyes. Some squints can be corrected by surgery.

stagnant loop syndrome the condition when a segment of the small INTESTINE is discontinuous with the rest or when there is an obstruction, either of which causes slow movement through the intestines. The result is bacterial growth with malabsorption (*see* MALABSORPTION SYNDROME) and steatorrhoea (passage of fatty stools).

stapes *see* EAR.

staphylococcus (*pl* **staphylococci**) any of a group of minute spherical Gram-positive (*see* GRAM'S STAIN) BACTERIA of the genus *Staphylococcus* that are normally present on SKIN and MUCOUS MEMBRANES. *S. albus* may be found in superficial skin INFECTIONS. *S. aureus* is a more invasive, and therefore harmful, species and is a common cause of ABSCESSES.

starvation *see* MALNUTRITION.

steatorrhoea *see* STAGNANT LOOP SYNDROME.

stem cells *see* THYMUS GLAND.

stenosis (*pl* **stenoses**) the abnormal narrowing of a BLOOD VESSEL, heart VALVE or similar structure.

sterilization 1. the process of destroying all microorganisms on instruments and other objects by means of heat, radiation, etc. **2.** a surgical operation to render someone incapable of producing children. Men usually undergo a VASECTOMY while in women it can be achieved by cutting and tying the FALLOPIAN TUBES or removing them. The latter operation is performed via an INCISION in the abdominal wall or through the VAGINA.

sternum (*pl* **sterna**) *or* **breastbone** the long flat narrow vertical BONE situated in the centre of the anterior wall of the CHEST, extending from the neck to the ABDOMEN. The CLAVICLE and the first seven pairs of RIBS are attached to it.

steroid one of a group of compounds, resembling CHOLESTEROL, that are made up of four carbon rings fused together. The group includes the sterols (e.g. cholesterol), BILE acids, some HORMONES, and VITAMIN D. Synthetic versions act like steroid hormones and include derivatives of the glucocorticoids used as anti-inflammatory agents for RHEUMATOID ARTHRITIS; oral contraceptives, usually OESTROGEN and PROGESTERONE derivatives; and anabolic steroids, such as testosterone, used to treat OSTEOPOROSIS and wasting.

sterol *see* CHOLESTEROL; STEROID.

stertor noisy breathing, similar to SNORING, often heard in patients who are deeply unconscious.

stethoscope an instrument used to listen to sounds within the body, particularly the LUNGS and HEART.

stiffness a condition with numerous causes that results in a reduced movement in JOINTS and MUSCLES. The cause may be quite straightforward, e.g. physical injury, or it may be caused by disease, such as RHEUMATISM, MENINGITIS, or CENTRAL NERVOUS SYSTEM disorders.

stigma (*pl* **stigmata**) a mark or impression upon the SKIN, possibly one that is typical of a particular disease.

stillbirth the birth of any child that provides no evidence of life.

Still's disease a chronic ARTHRITIS affecting children and affecting several joints, with FEVER and a red RASH. Some cases develop into ankylosing SPONDYLITIS and there is often muscle wasting. The illness may affect the whole body, complicated by other conditions, e.g. enlargement of the SPLEEN and PERICARDITIS.

stimulus (*pl* **stimuli**) an agent that arouses or provokes a response in a SENSE ORGAN.

stimulant any drug or other agent that increases the rate of activity of an organ or system within the body. This assumes that the target organ is capable of increased activity and merely requires the necessary stimulus.

stitch a sharp pain in the side, often caused by CRAMP after hard exertion (*see also* SPLEEN).

stoma (*pl* **stomata**) an opening made in the abdominal surface to accommodate a tube from the COLON or ILEUM. This operation is undertaken because of malignancy or inflammatory bowel diseases, e.g. CROHN'S DISEASE.

stomach an expansion of the ALIMENTARY CANAL that lies between the OESOPHAGUS and the DUODENUM. It has thick walls of smooth MUSCLE that contract to manipulate food, and its exits are controlled by SPHINCTERS, the cardiac anteriorly and the pyloric at the junction with the duodenum (*see* PYLORUS). Mucosal cells in the lining secrete GASTRIC JUICE. The food is reduced to an acidic semi-liquid that is moved on to the duodenum.

stools *see* FAECES.

strabismus *see* SQUINT.

strangulation the constriction or closure of a passage or vessel. This may be because of INTESTINE twisting or herniation (*see* HERNA) of the intestine. Strangulation of a blood vessel and/or airway affects the organs being supplied and, if vital organs are affected, can prove fatal.

strangury the desire to pass water, which can be done only in a few drops and with accompanying pain. It is symptomatic of an irritation of the base of the BLADDER by a stone, cancer at this site or CYSTITIS or PROSTATITIS.

stratum (*pl* **strata**) a layer, especially of SKIN, e.g. the stratum corneum and stratum germiativum of the EPIDERMIS.

streptococcus (*pl* **streptococci**) a spherical bacterium (*see* BACTERIA) of the genus *Streptococcus*, which is Gram-positive (*see* GRAM'S STAIN) and forms chains. Many species are responsible for a variety of INFECTIONS, including SCARLET FEVER, ENDOCARDITIS and PNEUMONIA.

streptokinase an ENZYME that is produced by streptococci and causes FIBRIN to undergo LYSIS.

streptomycin an ANTIBIOTIC that is used in the treatment of TUBERCULOSIS and bacterial infections.

stress fracture a FRACTURE created by making excessive demands on the body, as commonly happens in sport. Treatment involves rest and ANALGESICS for the pain.

striated marked with small channels running parallel to each other, e.g. striated muscle (*see* VOLUNTARY MUSCLE).

stricture a narrowing of a passage in the body, e.g. the URETHRA, OESOPHAGUS, or URETER. It may result from INFLAMMATION, a SPASM, growth of a TUMOUR or pressure from surrounding organs. In many cases it is caused by ulceration and contraction of the subsequent scar tissue. With a urethral stricture, it becomes increasingly difficult to pass URINE.

stridor the noise created on breathing in when there is a narrowing of the upper RESPIRATORY TRACT, especially the LARYNX.

stroke *or* **cerebrovascular accident** *or* **apoplexy** the physical effects, involving some form of PARALYSIS, that result from an interruption to the BRAIN'S BLOOD supply. The effect in the brain is secondary, and the cause lies in the HEART or BLOOD VESSELS and may be a THROMBOSIS, EMBOLUS or HAEMORRHAGE. The severity of a stroke varies greatly, from a temporary weakness in a limb, or tingling, to paralysis, coma and death.

stye a bacterial INFECTION and INFLAMMATION of a GLAND at the base of an eyelash, resulting in a pus-filled CYST.

subarachnoid anaesthesia *see* SPINAL ANAESTHESIA.

subarachnoid haemorrhage bleeding into the SUBARACHNOID SPACE, often because of a ruptured cerebral ANEURYSM. Initial symptoms are a severe headache, stiff neck, followed by vomiting and drowsiness, and there may be a brief period of unconsciousness after the event. Brain damage is possible but severe haemorrhages may result in death.

subcutaneous a general term meaning 'beneath the SKIN'.

subdural a term meaning 'below the dura mater' and referring to the space between this and the arachnoid MENINGES around the BRAIN.

sublingual gland *see* SALIVARY GLAND.

submandibular gland *see* SALIVARY GLAND.

subnutrition *see* MALNUTRITION.

succus entericus *see* DIGESTION.

sudden infant death syndrome *or* **cot death** the sudden death of a baby, often occurring overnight, from unknown causes. A significant proportion (about 20 per cent in the UK) of infant deaths occur in this way. Although the cause is unknown, numerous suggestions have been put forward, from viral infection and allergic reaction to poor breathing control to overheating and mild infections. Research continues.

sulcus (*pl* **sulci**) *see* FRONTAL LOBE; TEMPORAL LOBE.

sulphonamide one of a group of drugs containing the chemical group -SO_2NH_2. These drugs do not kill BACTERIA but prevent bacterial growth and are thus very useful in controlling INFECTIONS. Some SIDE EFFECTS may occur but in general these are outweighed by the benefits.

sunstroke *see* HEATSTROKE.

supine the term used to describe the position in which someone is lying on his or her back, face upwards.

suppository medication prepared in a form that enables it to be inserted into the RECTUM (or VAGINA). It may be a lubricant, contain drugs for treatment in the area of the rectum or ANUS or for absorption. The suppository has to be inserted beyond the SPHINCTER muscle to ensure retention.

suppuration PUS formation, whether on the surface (ulceration) or more deep-seated (as with an ABSCESS).

suprarenal gland *see* ADRENAL GLAND.

surfactant *see* RESPIRATORY DISTRESS SYNDROME.

suture 1. in surgery, the means whereby a wound or incision is closed, using threads of silk or catgut. There are several types of suture to deal with different situations. 2. a type of JOINT across which there is no movement, e.g. in the SKULL, where there are several sutures.

sweat *see* PERSPIRATION.

sweat glands the GLANDS in the EPIDERMIS of SKIN that project into the dermis and are under the control of the SYMPATHETIC NERVOUS SYSTEM. The glands occur over most of the body but are especially abundant on the forehead, palms of the hands and soles of the feet and under the arms. *See also* PERSPIRATION.

Sydenham's chorea *see* CHOREA.

sympathetic the term used to describe a symptom or disease that occurs as a result of disease elsewhere in the body, e.g. injury of one eye and a related inflammation in the other, both being connected by the LYMPHATIC SYSTEM.

sympathetic nervous system with the PARASYMPATHETIC NERVOUS SYSTEM (and acting in opposition to it), this makes up the AUTONOMIC NERVOUS SYSTEM.

NORADRENALINE and ADRENALINE are the main NEUROTRANSMITTERS released by its nerve endings. Its functions include raising the heartbeat rate, constricting BLOOD VESSELS and inhibiting secretion of SALIVA.

symptom any evidence of a disease or disorder.

synalgia *see* REFERRED PAIN.

synapse the junction between two NERVE cells at which there is a minute gap. A NERVE IMPULSE bridges the gap via a NEUROTRANSMITTER (*see also* ACETYL-CHOLINE). The chemical diffuses across the gap that connects the AXON of one nerve cell to the DENDRITES of the next. Some BRAIN cells have many thousand synapses.

syncope *see* FAINTING.

syndrome a number of SYMPTOMS and signs that in combination together constitute a particular condition.

synovia *see* SYNOVIAL MEMBRANE.

synovial membrane *or* **synovium** the inner MEMBRANE of a capsule that encloses a JOINT that moves freely. It secretes into the joint a thick lubricating fluid (synovia), which may build up after injury to cause pain.

synovitis INFLAMMATION of the SYNOVIAL MEMBRANE that lines a JOINT capsule. The result is swelling with pain. It is associated with RHEUMATIC DISEASE, injury or INFECTION (e.g. chronic TUBERCULOSIS). The treatment depends on the cause of the condition, and often a sample of the synovia is taken for examination.

synovium *see* SYNOVIAL MEMBRANE.

syphilis an infectious, sexually transmitted disease (*see* VENEREAL DISEASE) caused by the bacterium *Treponema pallidum*, which shows symptoms in three stages. BACTERIA enter the body through MUCOUS MEMBRANES during sexual intercourse and an ULCER appears in the first instance. Within a short time the LYMPH NODES locally and then all over the body enlarge and harden and this lasts several weeks. Secondary symptoms appear about two months after infection and include fever, pains, enlarged lymph nodes and a faint rash, which is usually noticed on the chest. The bacterium is found in enormous numbers in the primary sores and any skin lesions of the secondary stage. The final stage may not appear until many months or years after infection and comprises the formation of numerous TUMOUR-like masses throughout the body (in skin, muscle, bone, brain, spinal cord and other organs such as the liver, stomach, etc). This stage can cause serious damage to the heart, brain or spinal cord, resulting in blindness, TABES DORSALIS and mental disability. CONGENITAL syphilis is much rarer than the former, ACQUIRED, type. It is contracted by a developing FOETUS from the mother and symptoms show a few weeks after birth. Treatment of syphilis is with PENICILLIN early in the development of the disease.

systemic a general term used to refer to the body as a whole.

systemic lupus erythematosus a chronic inflammatory disease of CONNECTIVE TISSUES, believed to be an AUTOIMMUNE DISEASE. Symptoms of the condition vary but generally include malaise, joint pain, red raised patches of skin and the involvement of internal organs as the disease progresses (including PULMONARY HYPERTENSION and haemolytic OEDEMA). Treatment is aimed at symptomatic relief as the disease itself cannot be cured. Anti-inflammatory drugs and immunosuppressives are used in conjunction with antibiotics to treat any infections that may arise. *See also* LUPUS.

systole the contraction of the HEART that alternates with the resting phase (DIAS-TOLE). It usually refers to ventricular systole (*see* VENTRICLE), which, at 0.3 seconds, is three times longer than atrial systole (*see* ATRIUM).

systolic pressure *see* BLOOD PRESSURE.

TAB 268

T

TAB (typhoid-paratyphoid A and B) a VACCINE obtained from SALMONELLA bacteria and used in the treatment of TYPHOID and the A and B strains of PARATYPHOID. If administered before a person is at risk, it can provide IMMUNITY for a year.

tachycardia increased rate of heartbeat, which may be caused naturally, as with exercise, or be symptomatic of disease.

talus (*pl* **tali**) the ankle bone, which articulates with the lower leg bones (TIBIA and FIBULA) above and also with the heel bone (calcaneus) below (*see* TARSUS).

target cell an abnormal form of ERYTHROCYTE (red blood cell), which is large and has a ringed appearance when stained and viewed microscopically, resembling a target. These cells are present in several kinds of ANAEMIA, including those caused by iron deficiency. They are also found when there is LIVER disease, a small SPLEEN, HAEMOGLOBIN abnormalities (haemoglobinopathies) and THALASSAEMIA.

tarsus (*pl* **tarsi**) a part of the foot in the region of the instep, consisting of seven BONES, chiefly the TALUS and the calcaneus (heel bone) and also the cuboid, navicular (boat-shaped) and three cuneiform (wedge-shaped) bones.

taste the perception of flavour brought about by CHEMORECEPTORS (the TASTE BUDS) situated on the TONGUE.

taste buds the SENSORY receptors responsible for the perception of TASTE, located in the grooves around the PAPILLAE of the TONGUE, in the EPIGLOTTIS, parts of the PHARYNX and the soft PALATE. The taste buds are stimulated by the presence of dissolved food in the SALIVA, and messages are sent via NERVES to the BRAIN where the information is interpreted and perceived.

taxis the returning to their normal position of displaced organs, parts of organs or bones by manipulation (*see* HERNIA).

T-cell *see* LYMPHOCYTE.

teeth *see* TOOTH.

temperature (of the body) the normal body temperature is around 37°C (98.4°F), but it varies considerably both between individuals and in one person throughout the day. In addition, temperature differences occur between various areas of the body, being lower in the skin than internally.

temple the side of the head above the level of the eye and the ear.

temporal the term used to describe the TEMPLE, e.g. temporal ARTERY.

temporal lobe one of the main areas of the CEREBRAL CORTEX in each of the CEREBRAL HEMISPHERES of the BRAIN, occurring in the TEMPORAL region of the SKULL. A cleft known as the lateral sulcus separates it from the FRONTAL LOBE.

temporal lobe epilepsy EPILEPSY that is centred within the TEMPORAL LOBE, caused by disease within the CEREBRAL CORTEX. It is characterized by hallucinations involving the senses of taste, smell, hearing and sight, and memory disturbances. During an attack, the person usually remains conscious, but not fully and normally aware, and afterwards may not have any memory of what has occurred.

tendinitis inflammation of a TENDON, which often results from excessive or unaccustomed exercise but may also result from INFECTION. Treatment involves rest, possibly splinting of an affected JOINT and CORTICOSTEROID injections and the taking of ANALGESIC drugs.

tendon a tough and inelastic white cord, composed of bundles of COLLAGEN fibres, that attaches a MUSCLE to a BONE. A tendon concentrates the pull of the muscle onto one point on the bone, and the length and thickness vary considerably. The fibres of a tendon pass into, and become continuous with, those of the bone it serves. Many tendons are enclosed in tendon sheaths lined with SYNOVIAL MEMBRANE containing synovia, which reduces friction and enables easy movement to occur.

tennis elbow a form of TENDINITIS affecting the TENDON at the outer part of the elbow, which becomes inflamed and painful. It is caused by hard and excessive use of the arm, and treatment involves rest and CORTICOSTEROID injections.

teratogen a substance or disease or any other factor that causes the production of abnormalities in a FOETUS. The drugs in this category include THALIDOMIDE and alcohol. GERMAN MEASLES is among the INFECTIONS.

teratogenesis the processes that result in the development of physical abnormalities in a FOETUS.

teratoma a TUMOUR that is composed of unusual tissues not normally found at that site and derived from partially developed embryological cells. Teratomas are most common in the OVARY and TESTICLE (particularly if the latter is undescended).

testicle *or* **testis** (*pl* **testes**) one of the pair of male sex organs that are situated within the SCROTUM and produce SPERM and secrete the hormone TESTOSTERONE. The testicles develop within the ABDOMEN of the FOETUS but descend around the time of birth into the SCROTUM.

testis (*pl* **testes**) *see* TESTICLE.

testosterone the male SEX HORMONE secreted by the testes (*see* TESTICLE). *See also* ANDROGEN.

tetanus *or* **lockjaw** a very serious and sometimes fatal infectious disease. *See* page 119.

tetany *see* PARATHYROID GLAND.

tetracyline an ANTIBIOTIC that is obtained both naturally and synethically and is used to treat rickettsial, viral and bacterial infections (e.g. RELAPSING FEVER).

thalamus (*pl* **thalami**) one of a pair of masses of GREY MATTER located within each side of the FOREBRAIN. Each is a centre for coordinating and relaying the SENSORY information concerned with all the senses, apart from that of smell.

thalassaemia *or* **Cooley's anaemia** an inherited form of ANAEMIA in which there is an abnormality in the HAEMOGLOBIN. There is a continuation in the production of foetal haemoglobin, and two forms of the disorder are recognized: thalassaemia major, in which the disorder is inherited from both parents (homozygous), and thalassaemia minor. The minor form is usually symptomless, but the major type causes, in addition to the severe anaemia, BONE MARROW abnormalities and enlargement of the SPLEEN. Treatment is by means of repeated BLOOD TRANSFUSIONS. The disease is widespread throughout the Mediterranean, Asia and Africa.

thalidomide a TERATOGENic drug that was formerly prescribed for treatment of MORNING SICKNESS in PREGNANCY. It was withdrawn when it was discovered that it caused developmental damage to the FOETUS, particularly malformation of limbs.

therapy the treatment of physical or mental illness.

thiabendazole *see* TOXOCARIASIS.

thiamine *see* VITAMIN B.

thigh the part of the leg above the knee.

thoracic pertaining to the CHEST, e.g. the thoracic duct (*see* LYMPH).

thoracocentesis *or* **pleuracentesis** the withdrawal, by means of a hollow needle inserted through the CHEST wall, of fluid from the PLEURAL CAVITY.

thorax the CHEST, the cavity of the body formed by the SPINAL COLUMN, RIBS and STERNUM and containing the LUNGS, HEART, etc.

threonine *see* ESSENTIAL AMINO ACID.

thrombin an ENZYME derived from prothrombin, its inactive precursor, which is formed and is active during the final stages of blood clotting (*see* COAGULATION).

thrombocyte *see* PLATELET.

thromboembolism the situation in which a blood CLOT (THROMBUS) forms in one part of the CIRCULATION, usually a deep VEIN in the leg (PHLEBOTHROMBOSIS), and a portion breaks off and becomes lodged elsewhere, causing a total blockage (EMBOLISM). The embolism often involves the pulmonary ARTERY or one of its branches, and this is known as PULMONARY EMBOLISM.

thrombolysis the dissolving of BLOOD CLOTs by ENZYME activity. Natural enzymes produced within the body have this effect but drug treatment, especially involving STREPTOKINASE, may be used to break up clots following PULMONARY EMBOLISM, CORONARY THROMBOSIS and PHLEBOTHROMBOSIS.

thrombophlebitis INFLAMMATION of the wall of a VEIN along with clot formation in the affected section of the vessel. This is a complication of PREGNANCY and may be dangerous, involving a deep vein THROMBOSIS that can result in PULMONARY EMBOLISM. The condition known as white leg (plegmasia alba dolens) is thrombophlebitis, especially of the FEMORAL vein, which can occur after childbirth.

thrombosis (*pl* **thromboses**) the process of clotting within a BLOOD VESSEL, producing a THROMBUS. It may occur within an ARTERY or VEIN, often one that is diseased or damaged, and can be very serious or even fatal, e.g. STROKE, CORONARY THROMBOSIS.

thrombus (*pl* **thrombi**) a BLOOD CLOT within a vessel that partially or totally obstructs the CIRCULATION.

thrush an INFECTION caused by the FUNGUS *Candida albicans*, which affects the MUCOUS MEMBRANES of the MOUTH and VAGINA, producing white patches. It is a popular name given to a group of infections known as candidiasis.

thumb the short, thick digit of the HAND. *See* PHALANGES.

thymine *see* NUCLEOTIDE.

thymus gland a GLAND, divided into two lobes, that is present in the neck and forms a vital part of the body's response to INFECTION. It is especially large in children and important in the development of the IMMUNE response and the production of lymphoid tissue. After PUBERTY, it gradually begins to shrink. BONE MARROW cells, known as stem cells, undergo maturation within the thymus, and one group, the T-LYMPHOCYTES, are dependent on the gland. These are very important cells in the body that produce ANTIBODIES.

thyroid gland a bilobed ENDOCRINE GLAND situated at the base and front of the neck. It is enclosed by fibrous tissue and well supplied with blood, and internally consists of numerous vesicles containing a jelly-like colloidal substance. These vesicles produce thyroid HORMONE, which is rich in iodine, under the control of thyroid-stimulating hormone (THYROTROPHIN STIMULATING HORMONE) released from the PITUITARY GLAND. Two hormones are produced by the gland, THYROXINE and triiodothyronine, which are essential for the regulation of METABOLISM and growth. *See also* CRETINISM, MYXOEDEMA and HYPERTHYROIDISM.

thyrotoxic adenoma a form of thyrotoxicosis or GRAVES' DISEASE.

thyrotoxicosis *see* GRAVES' DISEASE.

thyrotrophin-releasing hormone a HORMONE produced and released from the

HYPOTHALAMUS that acts on the anterior lobe of the PITUITARY GLAND, which then releases THYROTROPHIN-STIMULATING HORMONE (*see also* THYROID GLAND).

thyrotrophin-stimulating hormone a HORMONE produced and released by the anterior PITUITARY GLAND, which stimulates the THYROID GLAND to produce its hormones (*see also* THYROID GLAND).

thyroxine an important HORMONE produced by the THYROID GLAND and used medically to treat conditions resulting from underactivity of this gland, e.g. CRETINISM and MYXOEDEMA.

tibia (*pl* **tibiae**) *or* **shin bone** the larger of the two BONES in the lower leg, articulating above with the FEMUR and with the TALUS of the ankle below.

tic douloureux *see* TRIGEMINAL NEURALGIA.

tidal volume *see* LUNGS.

tinea *see* RINGWORM.

tinnitus any ringing or buzzing sound in the EAR that does not have a real external cause. Many disorders of the ear can cause this, e.g. hardened wax or MÉNIÈRE'S DISEASE, and also drugs, including ASPIRIN and QUININE, and there can be damage to the auditory NERVE. In many cases no underlying cause is found.

tissue one of the primary layers composing any of the parts of the body, consisting of a large number of CELLs with a similar structure and function, e.g. CONNECTIVE TISSUE.

T-lymphocyte *see* LYMPHOCYTE; THYMUS.

toe one of the five small digits at the extremity of the FOOT. *See* PHALANGES.

tocopherol *see* VITAMIN E.

tolerance the adaptation of the body to a particular drug or substance so that over a period of time there is a reduction in the response to a particular dose. Usually a larger dose must then be given to produce the same effect as before.

tongue the muscular and highly mobile organ attached to the floor of the MOUTH, the three main functions of which are manipulation of food during chewing prior to swallowing, taste and production of speech. The three areas of the tongue are the tip, body and root, and it is covered with a MUCOUS MEMBRANE that unites with that of the mouth and PHARYNX. It has a furred appearance because its surface is covered with minute projections called PAPILLAe, of which there are three different kinds: filiform, fungiform and circumvallate. There are grooves surrounding the papillae in which the TASTE BUDS occur. The tongue is well supplied with BLOOD and receives branches from five different NERVES on each side.

tonsillectomy surgical removal of the TONSILS.

tonsillitis INFLAMMATION of the TONSILS caused by bacterial or viral infection. The symptoms include a severe sore throat, causing painful swallowing, accompanied by fever and earache, especially in children. The tonsils are swollen and white in appearance because of infected material exuded from them, and GLANDS in the neck are enlarged. Treatment is by means of ANTI-BIOTICS, along with ANALGESICS for pain relief.

tonsils usually the two small masses of LYMPHOID TISSUE situated on either side at the back of the mouth (the palatine tonsils). However, another pair occur below the TONGUE, which are the lingual tonsils, while the ADENOIDS are the pharyngeal tonsils. All are part of the body's protective mechanism against INFECTION.

tooth (*pl* **teeth**) a hard structure used for biting and chewing. Each tooth consists of a root embedded in a socket within the jawbone to which it is attached by the fibrous periodontal membrane. The projecting part of the tooth, called the crown, is covered with a hard resistant layer of enamel (composed primarily of calcium phosphate and calcium carbonate). The root is covered with a thin hard layer of CEMENTUM. Most of the interior of the tooth consists of DENTINE, a hard ivory-like substance that surrounds the inner core or pulp. The pulp contains blood vessels and nerve fibres and is connected with the dentine by means of fine cellular processes. There are four different types of teeth: canine, INCISOR, premolar and MOLAR.

tophi (*sing* **tophus**) see GOUT.

torsion a twisting, particularly an abnormal state of the whole or part of an organ that impairs the NERVE and BLOOD supply. Examples are a torsion of a loop of bowel or of the spermatic cord of the TESTICLE. Surgery is usually required to correct a torsion.

torticollis *see* WRYNECK.

touch the sense that is conferred by specialized SENSORY receptors present in the SKIN (and also in MUSCLEs and other areas of the body), which enable sensations of pain, temperature, pressure and touch to be perceived. The SENSE ORGANS involved are specially adapted to respond to particular sensations conveying their messages to the brain along different NERVE pathways.

toxaemia blood poisoning resulting from the TOXINs produced by rapidly multiplying BACTERIA at a localized site of INFECTION, such as an ABSCESS. Symptoms are varied, including fever, vomiting and diarrhoea and a general feeling of being unwell. The source of the infection has to be treated with ANTIBIOTIC drugs. Toxaemia of PREGNANCY involves two relatively rare conditions known as ECLAMPSIA and PRE-ECLAMPSIA.

toxicology the scientific study of poisons and their effects.

toxic shock syndrome a state of acute SHOCK as a result of SEPTICAEMIA and caused by TOXINs produced by staphylococcal BACTERIA (*see* STAPHYLOCOCCUS). The symptoms include high fever, skin rash and diarrhoea and can prove rapidly fatal if not adequately treated with ANTIBIOTICS, especially PENICILLIN and CEPHALOSPORIN, along with fluid and salt replacement. The syndrome is associated with the use of tampons by women during MENSTRUATION, particularly if a tampon is left in place too long, but can also occur in other people and is in all cases rare.

toxin a poison produced by BACTERIA and by many species of plant and also present in snake venom. In the body, a toxin acts as an ANTIGEN and provokes the production of special ANTIBODIES, called antitoxins. The antitoxins produced may be used in IMMUNIZATION to protect against the disease, as with TETANUS and DIPHTHERIA. An endotoxin is contained within the bacterial cell and released only when the organism dies and decays. Endotoxins do not provoke antitoxin production (*see* TOXOID).

toxocariasis a disease caused by the larvae of roundworms, which normally infect the domestic dog (*Toxicara canis*) and cat (*Toxicara cati*) but can be passed to humans if they swallow material contaminated with eggs in infected faeces. Those most at risk are children, especially at a young age when hands may become infected while playing. Once swallowed, the larvae, which hatch from the eggs, travel around the body in the circulation and can cause considerable damage, e.g. to the LUNGS and LIVER. Also, the larvae may lodge in the RETINA of the EYE, causing INFLAMMATION and the production of abnormal granulated tissue called granuloma. Symptoms of the infection include muscular pain, fever, skin rash, respiratory problems, vomiting and convulsions. Treatment is with drugs, such as diethylcarbamazine and thiabendazole.

toxoid a preparation of TOXIN that has been treated with chemicals so that it cannot cause disease but is able to provoke the production of antitoxin. This is the basis of VACCINES against DIPHTHERIA and TETANUS.

toxoplasmosis an infectious disease caused by a protozoan organism known as *Toxoplasma*. The INFECTION is either transmitted by eating undercooked meat or through direct contact with contaminated soil or, especially, with infected cats. This form of the infection is mild and causes few ill effects. However, a much more serious form of the disease can be passed from a mother infected during PREGNANCY to her unborn baby. The newborn infant may suffer from HYDROCEPHALUS, mental retardation, blindness or may even be stillborn. Treatment is by means of SULPHONAMIDE drugs and pyrimethamine.

trachea the windpipe, the part of the air passage that is situated between the LARYNX and the BRONCHI.

tracheitis INFLAMMATION of the TRACHEA, often accompanying a viral infection of the upper respiratory tract. The symptoms include a persistent painful cough and sore chest, and it often accompanies BRONCHITIS and also DIPHTHERIA.

tracheostomy *or* **tracheotomy** a surgical procedure in which a hole is made in the TRACHEA to allow direct access of air to the lower respiratory passages. This may be performed in an emergency if there is an obstruction in breathing, but is usually carried out in hospital, especially on patients in intensive therapy who require long-term artificial VENTILATION. This is to avoid the damage to the trachea that is caused by the long-term use of an endotracheal breathing tube (inserted through the nose or mouth) which would normally be used first. Once the opening has been made, a double tube is inserted and held in place by tapes around the neck. The inner tube can be freely withdrawn and replaced and needs to be kept scrupulously clean and free from any obstruction.

tranquillizer a drug that has a soothing and calming effect, relieving stress and anxiety. Minor tranquillizers such as diazepam are widely used to relieve these symptoms, which may arise from a variety of causes. There is a danger of dependence with long-term use. Major tranquillizers are used to treat severe mental illnesses.

transdermal drug *see* DOSAGE.

transfusion *see* BLOOD TRANSFUSION.

transplantation the transfer of an organ or tissue from one person to another (allotransplant) or within the body of an individual (autotransplant), i.e. skin and bone grafting. The person from whom the organ is obtained is known as the donor and the one who receives it is known as the recipient. Organ transplants involving the KIDNEY, HEART, BONE MARROW, CORNEA, LUNGS and LIVER have all become more common. Success varies but is improving in all areas, especially with the advent of immunosuppressive drugs to prevent organ rejection by the recipient's immune system. *See also* IMMUNOSUPPRESSION and GRAFT.

trauma 1. an event that causes physical damage, such as a FRACTURE. **2.** an emotional shock brought about by a harmful and upsetting circumstance.

tremor an involuntary movement that may involve the whole of a MUSCLE or only part of it and produce fine trembling or more pronounced shaking. Tremors are classified according to the type of movement produced and are a symptom of many diseases, including CHOREA, MULTIPLE SCLEROSIS and PARKINSONISM.

trench fever an infectious disease caused by *Rickettsia quintana*, which was epidemic among troops in the First World War and still occurs in Mexico. It is transmitted to humans by the body louse and causes fever, rash, leg aches and general weakness.

triceps a three-headed MUSCLE, present in the upper arm, that extends the forearm.

trichomoniasis either of two types of INFECTION caused by a protozoan organism that either attacks the digestive system, causing DYSENTERY (*Trichomonas* *hominis*), or causes vaginal inflammation and discharge (*Trichomonas vaginalis*). In the latter case the infection can be transmitted to a male sexual partner. The ANTIBIOTIC drug metronidazole is highly effective.

trichorrhoea the medical name for the falling out of HAIR, which may be caused by disease, such as TYPHOID FEVER or SCARLET FEVER, or has no apparent cause.

tricuspid valve a VALVE that has three flaps or cusps and controls the passage of BLOOD from the right ATRIUM to the right VENTRICLE of the HEART and normally prevents back flow.

trigeminal nerve the fifth and largest of the CRANIAL NERVES, which has three divisions: the mandibular, maxillary and ophthalmic nerves. The ophthalmic and maxillary are SENSORY nerves and the mandibular has both sensory and MOTOR functions. Hence the trigeminal nerve is involved in the relaying and perception of sensations (temperature, touch, pain, etc) from the whole of the FACE and MOUTH and also in controlling the muscles involved in chewing.

trigeminal neuralgia *or* **tic douloureux** a severe form of NEURALGIA that can affect all the divisions of the TRIGEMINAL NERVE. It affects women more commonly than men, especially those over the age of 50. It causes severe pain of a burning or cutting nature, which can be constant or spasmodic and may be provoked by simple actions such as eating or by heat or cold. The skin of the face may be inflamed and the eye red and watery and the neuralgia is usually confined to one side. The condition is debilitating in that the pain is intense and interferes with sleeping and eating, but the ANTICONVULSANT drug carbamazepine is proving to be highly beneficial.

triglycerides fats consisting of three FATTY ACID molecules combined with GLYCEROL, which are the form in which the body stores fat. Triglycerides are derived from the DIGESTION of fats in food.

trihexyphenidyl hydrochloride *see* BENZHEXOL.

triiodothyronine *see* THYROID GLAND.

trophic a term used to describe nutrition. For example, trophic FRACTURE occurs when the BONE is weakened as a result of poor nourishment in the person concerned.

trypanosomiasis *see* SLEEPING SICKNESS.

trypsin an important ENZYME involved in the DIGESTION of PROTEINS. Its inactive precursor, trypsinogen, is secreted by the PANCREAS and converted to trypsin in the DUODENUM by the action of another enzyme, called enteropeptidase.

tryptophan *see* ESSENTIAL AMINO ACID; PELLAGRA.

tubercle 1. a small rounded knob on a BONE, e.g. on the RIBS. **2.** a minute nodular tissue mass (LESION) that is characteristic of TUBERCULOSIS.

tuberculin *see* MANTOUX TEST.

tuberculosis a group of INFECTIONS caused by the BACILLUS *Mycobacterium tuberculosis*, of which PULMONARY tuberculosis of the LUNGS (consumption or phthisis) is the best-known form. The pulmonary disease is acquired by inhalation of air containing the organism from an infected person or dust laden with BACTERIA. People infected in this way can show no symptoms but still be carriers. In the lungs, the infection causes formation of a primary TUBERCLE, which spreads to LYMPH NODES to form the primary complex. The disease may wax and wane for years as the body's natural IMMUNE system acts against the infection. If the infection is severe, symptoms include fever, wasting, night sweats and the coughing up of blood. The bacteria may enter the bloodstream and spread throughout the body, setting up numerous tubercles in other tissues (MILIARY tuberculosis). The organism may also be acquired by eating contaminated food, especially milk, in which case the production of a primary complex in abdominal lymph nodes can lead to PERITONITIS. Tuberculosis affects people throughout the world (about 6,000 new cases each year in England and Wales). Many people acquire the infection and recover without suspecting its presence, and the disease is curable with ANTIBIOTICS, e.g. STREPTOMYCIN. In addition, BCG VACCINATION as a preventative measure is given to children in the UK, in addition to X-RAY screening to detect carriers.

tubule a small tube-like structure in the body, as in the KIDNEY, testis (*see* TESTICLE), etc.

tumour an abnormal swelling in any part of the body, which consists of an unusual growth of tissue and may be MALIGNANT or BENIGN. Tumours tend to be classified according to the tissue of which they are composed, e.g. FIBROMA (mainly fibrous tissue) and MYOMA (largely muscle fibres).

Turner's syndrome a genetic disorder affecting females in which there is only one X-CHROMOSOME instead of the usual two. Those affected therefore have 45 instead of 46 CHROMOSOMES, are infertile (as the ovaries are absent), MENSTRUATION is absent and BREASTS and body hair do not develop. Those affected are short, may have webbing of the neck and other developmental defects. The heart may be affected and there can be deafness and intellectual impairment. In a less severe form of the disorder, the second X-chromosome is present but abnormal, lacking in normal genetic material.

tympanic membrane the eardrum, which separates the middle and outer EARS and vibrates in response to sound waves, transmitting the vibrations to one of the ear OSSICLES (the malleus).

typhoid fever a severe infectious disease of the digestive system that is caused by the bacterium *Salmonella typhi* and causes symptoms, including a rise in TEMPERATURE, a rash on the abdomen and chest, headache and nosebleeds. The temperature rise occurs in a characteristic fashion known as a step-ladder temperature. In severe cases there may be ulceration of the intestinal wall, leading to PERITONITIS if an ULCER bursts or HAEMORRHAGE from the bowels and INFLAMMATION of the LUNGS, SPLEEN and BONES. In these cases the disease can prove to be fatal. The infection is acquired through ingesting contaminated food or water, so preventative measures involving high standards of hygiene and sanitation are important. Drug treatment is by means of ANTIBIOTICS. Inoculation with TAB VACCINE confers temporary IMMUNITY.

typhus a disease that is characterized by FEVER, debility and RASH and is spread by body lice. *See* RICKETTSIAE and page 124.

tyrosine *see* DOPA; PHENYLKETONURIA.

U

ulcer a break on the SKIN surface or on the MUCOUS MEMBRANE lining within the body cavities that may be inflamed and fails to heal. Ulcers of the skin include BED SORES and varicose ulcers (which are caused by defective CIRCULATION). For ulcers of the alimentary tract, *see* DUODENAL ULCER, GASTRIC ULCER and PEPTIC ULCER.

ulna (*pl* **ulnae**) one of the two BONES making up the forearm. It is the inner and longer of the two bones (the other being the RADIUS). It articulates with the radius at both ends and also with the HUMERUS above and indirectly with the wrist below.

umbilical cord the cord connecting the FOETUS to the PLACENTA, containing two arteries (*see* ARTERY) and one VEIN. It is approximately 60 cm long, and after birth it is severed and the stump shrivels to leave a scar, the navel or umbilicus.

umbilicus the navel (*see* UMBILICAL CORD).

undulant fever *see* BRUCELLOSIS.

ungual a term meaning relating to the fingernails or toenails.

unguent the term in pharmacy for an ointment.

unguis a fingernail or toenail.

uracil *see* NUCLEOTIDE.

uraemia a condition in which there is excess UREA in the blood because of KIDNEY disease or failure. Waste products are usually excreted by the kidneys, but accumulation in the blood leads to headaches, drowsiness and lethargy, nausea and vomiting and diarrhoea. Eventually, without treatment, death follows. HAEMODIALYSIS may be necessary or even renal TRANSPLANTATION.

urataemia the presence in the blood of urate compounds (*see* URIC ACID), associated with GOUT, when urates are deposited in the body.

urate *see* GOUT; URIC ACID.

urea a metabolic byproduct of the chemical breakdown of PROTEIN and the form in which excess nitrogen is removed from the body in URINE. It is formed in the LIVER and taken in the blood to the KIDNEYS. The amount excreted daily is 30–35 g. Although urea is not poisonous in itself, an excess in the BLOOD (uraemia) implies a defective kidney, which will cause an excess of other waste products that may be poisonous.

ureaplasma microorganisms responsible for diseases such as PROSTATITIS, nonspecific URETHRITIS, infertility and NEONATAL death. The latter can be associated with infection of the PLACENTA by *Ureaplasma urealyticum*.

ureter the tubes joining the KIDNEYS to the BLADDER, through which URINE passes. The muscular ureter walls contract to force urine into the bladder.

ureteritis INFLAMMATION of the URETER, which usually occurs with BLADDER inflammations.

urethra the duct carrying URINE from the BLADDER out of the body. It is about 3.5 cm long in women and 20 cm in men. The male urethra runs through the PENIS and also forms the ejaculatory duct.

urethritis INFLAMMATION of the mucous lining of the URETHRA, which may be associated with CYSTITIS, often being the cause of the latter. The commonest cause of urethritis is GONORRHOEA (specific urethritis). Alternatively, it may be caused by INFECTION with microorganisms (nonspecific urethritis). The symptoms include pain on passing URINE and a discharge, and inflammations in other organs such as the BLADDER and TESTICLE are possible. SULPHONAMIDE and ANTIBIOTIC drugs are effective once the infecting organism is identified.

uric acid an organic acid that contains nitrogen and is the end-product of the METABOLISM of PROTEIN. It occurs in the URINE but in small amounts (less than 1 gram). It is formed in the liver and excreted by the kidneys, but in excess, salts (urates) form and occur as stone in the urinary tract. Deposits of urates in joints is a feature of GOUT.

urinary organs the system responsible for the extraction of components from the BLOOD to form URINE, its storage and periodic discharge from the body. The organs are the KIDNEYS, URETERS, BLADDER and URETHRA.

urinary tract the system of ducts that permits movement of URINE out of the body from the kidneys, i.e. the URETERS, BLADDER and URETHRA.

urination *or* **micturition** the discharge of URINE from the body via the URETHRA. It is begun by a voluntary relaxation of the SPHINCTER muscle below the BLADDER.

urine the body's fluid waste excreted by the KIDNEYS. The waste products include UREA, URIC ACID and creatinine (produced by muscles), with salt, phosphates and sulphates and ammonia also present. In a solution with about 95–96 per cent water, there may be 100 or more compounds but the vast majority occur only in trace amounts. Many diseases alter the quantity and composition of urine, and its analysis is standard procedure to assist DIAGNOSIS of diseases.

urine retention the condition when URINE is produced by the KIDNEYS but it is retained in the BLADDER. This may be because of an obstruction or a weakness in the bladder (less common). Enlargement of the PROSTATE GLAND is a common cause of blockage. It may also be caused by a STRICTURE caused by an injury scar or ulceration.

urinogenital a collective descriptive term relating to all organs and tissues involved in excretion and reproduction because they are closely linked anatomically and functionally.

urticaria *or* **nettle rash** an allergic reaction in an individual exposed to a substance to which he or she is hypersensitive, in which the response is manifested on the skin. Raised red patches develop, which may last for hours or days. There is intense itching. The sensitivity may be to certain foods, e.g. shellfish, and the effect may occur anywhere on the body but commonly erupts on the face and trunk. If it also affects the tongue or throat, there is danger of a blockage of the airway, which needs urgent attention.

uterine relating to the UTERUS.

uterus *or* **womb** a roughly pear-shaped organ within the cavity of the PELVIS that is specialized for the growth and nourishment of a FOETUS. FALLOPIAN TUBES connect to the upper part and the lower part joins the VAGINA at the CERVIX. It has a plentiful blood supply along with lymphatic vessels and nerves. During PREGNANCY it enlarges considerably and the smooth MUSCLE walls thicken. Contractions of the muscular wall push the foetus out via the vagina at childbirth. If there is no PREGNANCY, the lining undergoes periodic changes (MENSTRUATION).

uvea the middle pigmented layer of the EYE, consisting of the IRIS, choroid and ciliary body.

uveitis INFLAMMATION of any part of the UVEA of the EYE. The iris and ciliary body are often both inflamed (anterior uveitis), producing a painful condition, unlike posterior uveitis (when the choroid is affected). The cause of both types is usually different and may follow from affected areas elsewhere in the eye. All types lead to visual impairment, and symptoms may include blurred vision with discomfort or pain, and diseases or conditions with which it is known to be linked are ARTHRITIS, TUBERCULOSIS, SYPHILIS, and viral and parasitic INFECTIONS.

V

vaccination the production of IMMUNITY to a disease by INOCULATION with a VACCINE or a specially prepared material that stimulates the production of ANTIBODIES. It was used initially to refer only to cowpox virus (which also protected against SMALLPOX) but now is synonymous with INOCULATION in immunizing against disease.

vaccine a modified preparation of a bacterium (*see* BACTERIA) or VIRUS that is no longer dangerous but will stimulate development of ANTIBODIES and therefore confer IMMUNITY against actual INFECTION with the disease. Other vaccines consist of specific TOXINS (e.g. TETANUS) or dead bacteria (e.g. CHOLERA and TYPHOID). Live but weakened organisms are used against SMALLPOX and TUBERCULOSIS.

vagina the lower part of the female reproductive tract that leads from the UTERUS to the outside. It receives the erect PENIS during sexual intercourse, the SEMEN being ejaculated into the upper part from where the SPERMS pass through the CERVIX and UTERUS to the FALLOPIAN TUBES. The vagina is essentially a muscular tube lined with MUCOUS MEMBRANE.

vaginismus a sudden and painful contraction of muscles surrounding the VAGINA in response to contact of the vagina or VULVA, e.g. an attempted intercourse. It may be caused by a fear of intercourse or by an INFLAMMATION.

vaginitis INFLAMMATION of the VAGINA as a result of infection or deficiency in diet or poor hygiene. There may be itching, a discharge and pain on urination.

vagus nerve the tenth CRANIAL NERVE, which comprises MOTOR, SENSORY, vasodilator and secretory fibres. It supplies the MUSCLES for swallowing, and fibres go to the heart, throat, lungs and stomach and other organs in the abdomen. It also carries the taste sensation from the mouth.

valine *see* ESSENTIAL AMINO ACID.

valve a structure within an organ or vessel that restricts flow to one direction, whether the fluid be BLOOD or LYMPH. The valves comprise cusps on the vessel wall. The cusp is like a membranous pocket that fills with blood and prevents backward flow by distending and closing the valve.

valvular heart disease a disease that affects mainly the aortic VALVE and MITRAL VALVE, which may narrow (*see* AORTIC STENOSIS and STENOSIS) or weaken. Aortic valve disease is associated more with old age while mitral valve disease is rheumatic in origin. *See also* MITRAL INCOMPETENCE.

valvulitis INFLAMMATION of a VALVE, particularly in the HEART. It is commonly caused by RHEUMATIC FEVER.

vaporizer a device that produces a mist of liquid medication for INHALATION. It is commonly used in the treatment of ASTHMA.

varicose ulcer an ULCER on the lower leg that is difficult to heal because of poor CIRCULATION.

varicose veins VEINS that have become stretched, distended and twisted. The superficial veins in the legs are often affected, although it may occur elsewhere. Causes include congenitally defective VALVES, OBESITY, PREGNANCY and THROMBOPHLEBITIS. Elastic support is a common treatment.

variola a name for SMALLPOX.

vas (*pl* **vasa**) a vessel or duct, especially one carrying BLOOD, LYMPH or SPERM.

vascular relating to BLOOD VESSELS; supplied with blood vessels.

vasculitis INFLAMMATION of the BLOOD VESSELS, which may cause damage to the linings and narrowing. It may result from several conditions, including acute NEPHRITIS and SERUM SICKNESS.

vas deferens (*pl* **vasa deferentia**) one of the two tubes that join the testes (*see* TESTICLE) to the ejaculatory duct via the PROSTATE GLAND. It carries SPERM to the URETHRA on ejaculation, aided by contraction of its muscular wall.

vasectomy the cutting of the VAS DEFERENS, which is performed on both ducts, causing sterility, although the effect is not immediate.

vasoconstriction the narrowing of BLOOD VESSELS with a consequent reduction in blood supply to the tissues. A variety of circumstances can cause vasoconstriction, including cold and shock.

vasodilation *or* **vasodilatation** the increase in diameter of BLOOD VESSELS, producing a lowering of BLOOD PRESSURE and increased flow.

vasopressin *or* **antidiuretic hormone** a HORMONE of the PITUITARY GLAND that constricts BLOOD VESSELS and reduces URINE secretion by increasing the quantity of water reabsorbed by the KIDNEY.

vasovagal attack fainting, precipitated by a slowing of the HEART and a fall in BLOOD PRESSURE. This may be as a result of SHOCK, severe pain, fear, etc, and is caused by excessive stimulation of the VAGUS NERVE, which participates in the control of breathing and the circulation.

vasovasostomy the reversal of VASECTOMY.

vector commonly, an insect that carries parasitic microorganisms between people or from animals to people, e.g. mosquitoes carrying malaria.

vein one of the numerous BLOOD VESSELS carrying deoxygenated blood to the right ATRIUM of the HEART (the one exception is the PULMONARY vein). Each vein has three tissue layers, similar to the layers of the heart. Veins are less elastic than arteries and collapse when cut. They also contain VALVES to prevent back flow.

vena cava (*pl* **venae cavae**) either of two major VEINS carrying blood from other veins to the right ATRIUM of the HEART. The inferior vena cava takes blood from the body below the DIAPHRAGM, and the superior vena cava takes blood from the head, neck, arms and thorax.

venereal diseases *or* **sexually transmitted diseases** diseases transmitted by sexual intercourse. These include AIDS, SYPHILIS, GONORRHOEA, nonspecific URETHRITIS, etc.

venom the poisonous substance produced by snakes, scorpions, etc, that in humans may produce only localized pain and swelling, or in serious cases cause more general effects and even death.

venous pertaining to a VEIN or containing veins, e.g. venous blood, which is distinguishable from arterial blood by its darker colour.

ventilation the means whereby air passes into and out of the LUNGS, aided by movement of the DIAPHRAGM. Artificial ventilation is the use of a machine (VENTILATOR) to regulate and perform a person's breathing. This may be during an operation. Also, damage to the relevant part of the brain, chest injury, lung disease or nerve and muscle disorders may all require the use of artificial ventilation.

ventilator the machine used to provide an air supply to the LUNGS of patients who cannot breathe normally for themselves. Blood gases and other body functions can be monitored at the same time.

ventral the term used to describe anything relating to the front, abdominal part of the body or a hollow structure.

ventricle 1. one of the two major chambers within the HEART. They are thick-walled and muscular and form the main pumping chamber. The right ventricle receives BLOOD from the right ATRIUM and the VENAE CAVAE, and its outflow is the pulmonary ARTERY. The left ventricle takes blood from the pulmonary VEIN via the left atrium, and its outflow is the AORTA. **2.** cavities within the BRAIN, filled with CEREBROSPINAL FLUID.

ventricular fibrillation a rapid ARRHYTHMIA of the VENTRICLE, which is dangerous.

venule a tiny VEIN that collects blood from the capillaries (*see* CAPILLARY).

vermiform appendix *see* APPENDIX.

verruca a term for WART.

verrucose covered with WARTS.

vertebra (*pl* **vertebrae**) any of the bones making up the SPINAL COLUMN. Each has a cavity (the vertebral canal or FORAMEN) and various PROCESSes for attachment of MUSCLES or articulation of adjacent vertebrae. The SPINAL CORD passes through the vertebral canal. *See also* INTERVERTEBRAL DISC.

vertebral canal *see* VERTEBRA.

vertebral column *see* SPINAL COLUMN.

vertigo a condition in which a person has a false sensation of imbalance and of the surroundings moving. It is commonly a sensation of spinning but may be as if the ground is tilting. The semicircular canals of the ear are fundamental in the maintenance of balance, and vertigo is generally the result of some problem with this mechanism or with the appropriate centres in the brain.

vesicle 1. a small bladder-like structure, cavity or cell, etc, in the body, usually containing fluid. **2.** a little SAC or CYST. **3.** a small BLISTER or PUSTULE on the SKIN.

vesicular breathing soft, normal sounds of breathing heard in the lung by means of a stethoscope. The sounds change when the lungs are diseased, and the different sounds help a doctor diagnose the condition.

vessel any tube that carries fluid, particularly blood or lymph.

vestigial the term applied to an organ that has progressively, over a long time, lost its function and structure to become rudimentary.

viable able to live separately.

villi (*sing* **villus**) *see* JEJUNUM.

viral pneumonia an acute lung INFECTION caused by one of a number of VIRUSes. Symptoms include fever, headache, muscle pains and a thick SPUTUM associated with a cough. It often occurs after a viral infection, and treatment mainly deals with the symptoms only.

virology the study of VIRUSes.

virulence the ability of BACTERIA or VIRUSes to cause disease, measured by the number of people infected, the speed with which they spread through the body, etc.

virus the smallest microorganism that is completely parasitic because it is capable only of replication within the CELLS of its host. Viruses infect animals, plants and microorganisms. Viruses are classified according to their nucleic acids and can contain double or single-stranded DNA or RNA. In an INFECTION, the virus binds to the host cells and then penetrates to release the viral DNA or RNA, which controls the cell's METABOLISM. It then replicates itself and forms new viruses. Viruses cause many diseases, including INFLUENZA (single-stranded RNA), HERPES (double-stranded DNA), AIDS (a RETROVIRUS, single-stranded RNA) and also MUMPS, CHICKENPOX and POLIOMYELITIS.

viscera (*sing* **viscus**) the term for organs within the body cavity, usually the ABDOMEN.

visceral pertaining to the VISCERA.

vision the capacity for sight. Light enters the EYE through the CORNEA and the aqueous HUMOUR. Next, it passes through the PUPIL, LENS and VITREOUS HUMOUR to impinge upon the RETINA. There the ROD and CONE cells detect light and send impulses to the nerve fibres, which are relayed to the visual cortex in the BRAIN via the optic nerve. Visual acuity is the sharpness of vision, dependent on a healthy retina and accurate lens.

vital capacity the largest volume of air that can be exhaled after breathing in deeply.

vitamin any of a group of organic compounds required in very small amounts in the diet to maintain good health. Deficiencies lead to specific diseases.

Vitamins are divided into two groups: vitamins A, D, E and K are fat-soluble, while C and B are water-soluble.

vitamin A *or* **retinol** a fat-soluble VITAMIN that must be in the diet as it cannot be synthesized in the body. It is essential for vision in dim light, growth and the maintenance of mucous tissue.

vitamin B a group of VITAMINS that, although they are not related chemically, are often found in the same types of food. *See also* FOLIC ACID.

vitamin B1 *or* **thiamine** a VITAMIN active in the form thiamine pyrophosphate, a deficiency of which leads to BERI-BERI.

vitamin B2 *or* **riboflavin** a VITAMIN important in tissue respiration (ENZYME reactions in CELLS) although a deficiency is not serious.

vitamin B3 *or* **pantothenic acid** a VITAMIN that occurs widely in foods and is therefore unlikely to be lacking in the diet.

vitamin B6 *or* **pyridoxine** a VITAMIN that is important in the METABOLISM of several amino acids.

vitamin B12 *or* **cyanocobalamin** an important VITAMIN in the synthesis of NUCLEIC ACIDS, maintenance of MYELIN surrounding nerve fibres and in the production of red blood cells (ERYTHROCYTES). A deficiency produces ANAEMIA and degeneration of the nervous system.

vitamin C *or* **ascorbic acid** a VITAMIN that is essential in maintaining CELL walls and CONNECTIVE TISSUE and a deficiency of which leads to fragility of TENDONS, BLOOD VESSELS and SKIN, all characteristic of SCURVY. The presence of ascorbic acid is believed to assist the uptake of iron during DIGESTION.

vitamin D a VITAMIN that occurs as two STEROID derivations: D2 or CALCIFEROL in yeast, and D3 or cholecalciferol, which is produced by the action of sunlight on the SKIN. It is vital in control of blood calcium levels. It prompts an increase in calcium takeup in the gut, increasing the supply for the production of BONE. It also affects phosphorus uptake. A deficiency leads to RICKETS and OSTEO-MALACIA.

vitamin E a group of compounds (tocopherols) thought to prevent damage to cell membranes. A deficiency is unusual because of its widespread occurrence in foods.

vitamin H *see* BIOTIN.

vitamin K a VITAMIN that is essential for the clotting of blood as it is involved in the formation of prothrombin (the inactive precursor of THROMBIN) in the liver. A deficiency rarely occurs because the vitamin is synthesized by BACTERIA in the large INTESTINE.

vitreous humour the jelly-like substance occurring between the LENS and the RETINA in the EYE.

vocal cords two MEMBRANES in the LARYNX that vibrate to produce sound when air is expelled over them. Tension in the cords is controlled by MUSCLES and TENDONS, thus changing the sound generated.

voluntary muscle *or* **striated muscle** MUSCLE that is under conscious control, e.g. those operating the skeleton. It consists of bundles of elongated fibres surrounded by CONNECTIVE TISSUE. A TENDON at the end of the muscle attaches it to the BONE. Each muscle fibre comprises smaller fibres (myofibrils) with alternating dark and light bands (sarcomeres), which produce the striated appearance and provide the contractile function. A flexor (or agonist) muscle contracts, becoming shorter and thus moving bones closer to each other. An extensor or antagonist muscle works in the opposite way.

volvulus a twisting of part of the INTESTINE, which usually results in some obstruction that may reduce the BLOOD supply, ending in GANGRENE. It may right itself spontaneously or may be righted by manipulation. However, surgery is often necessary.

vomiting *or* **emesis** the REFLEX ACTION wherein the stomach contents are expelled through the mouth because of the contraction of the DIAPHRAGM and abdominal wall muscles. Vomiting is caused by stimulus of the appropriate centre in the BRAIN, but the primary agent is usually a sensation from the stomach itself, e.g. a gastric disease or some irritant. Other causes may be the action of drugs, some effect on the inner EAR (e.g. MOTION SICKNESS), MIGRAINES, etc.

von Recklinghausen's disease a CONGENITAL disorder, neurofibromatosis, in which soft tissue TUMOURS form along NERVES and beneath the SKIN. There are often other anomalies, such as decalcification of BONES, FIBROSIS of the lungs and formation of KIDNEY stones (renal calculi).

vulva (*pl* **vulvae**) the external female GENITALIA, comprising two pairs of fleshy folds (LABIA) surrounding the opening of the VAGINA. Below them is the CLITORIS.

vulvitis INFLAMMATION of the VULVA.

vulvovaginitis INFLAMMATION of both the VULVA and VAGINA.

W

warfarin an ANTICOAGULANT given to reduce the risk of EMBOLISM. It may be administered orally or by INJECTION, and the significant SIDE EFFECT is bleeding, usually from the gums and other MUCOUS MEMBRANES.

wart *or* **verruca** a solid, BENIGN growth in the skin caused by a VIRUS. They are infectious and spread rapidly in schools, etc. There are several types: plantar, on the foot; juvenile in children; and venereal, on the genitals. Warts often disappear spontaneously but can be dealt with in several ways, e.g. CRYOSURGERY (freezing), LASER treatment and ELECTROCAUTERY.

water on the brain *see* HYDROCEPHALUS.

weal *or* **wheal** an area of the skin that is temporarily raised and coloured red, or pale with red margins. It may be caused by an ALLERGY, nettle rash (*see* URTICARIA) or a sharp blow, and in the former cases may be accompanied by itching.

webbed fingers *see* SYNDACTYLY.

Weil's disease *see* LEPTOSPIROSIS and page 100.

wen *see* SEBACEOUS CYST.

wheal *see* WEAL.

wheeze the sound produced by the long-drawn-out breathing associated with ASTHMA. It also occurs when bronchial tubes are narrowed, e.g. as in BRONCHITIS.

whiplash injury damage caused by the sudden jerking backwards of the head and neck, as in a road accident. A severe whiplash can cause death, but injury is the usual outcome. The VERTEBRAe, spinal cord, LIGAMENTS and NERVES in the neck may all be damaged. Treatment usually involves wearing a special collar to immobilize the affected area.

Whipple's disease a rare disease of the INTESTINES, resulting in malabsorption of food (*see* MALABSORPTION SYNDROME). Symptoms include ANAEMIA, weight loss, ARTHRITIS, skin pigmentation, chest pain and a nonproductive cough. It seems to be caused by microorganisms in the MUCOSA. It responds to ANTIBIOTICS.

white leg *see* THROMBOPHLEBITIS.

white matter nerve tissue in the CENTRAL NERVOUS SYSTEM, composed primarily of NERVE fibres in light-coloured MYELIN sheaths. In the BRAIN it occupies the central part of the CEREBRAL CORTEX.

whitlow INFLAMMATION in the finger tip and usually an ABSCESS affecting the fat and fibrous tissues that comprise the pulp of the finger.

whooping cough *or* **pertussis** an infectious disease caused by the bacterium *Bordetella pertussis*. The MUCOUS MEMBRANES lining the air passages are affected, and after a one to two week INCUBATION period, fever, catarrh and a cough develop. The cough then becomes paroxysmal, with a number of short coughs punctuated with the 'whooping' drawing in of breath. Nosebleeds and vomiting may follow a paroxysm. After about two weeks the symptoms abate, but a cough may continue for some weeks. Whooping cough is not usually serious, and IMMUNIZATION reduces the severity of an attack. However, a child may be susceptible to PNEUMONIA and TUBERCU-LOSIS during the disease.

Wilm's tumour a TUMOUR of the KIDNEY (nephroblastoma) in infancy. Early removal of the kidney, with RADIOTHERAPY and CHEMOTHERAPY, confers a high survival rate.

windpipe *see* TRACHEA.

wisdom tooth the last (third) molar TOOTH on each side of either JAW. The wisdom teeth normally erupt last, around the age of 20 to 25, although some remain IMPACTED in the jaw bone.

womb *see* UTERUS.

woolsorter's disease *see* ANTHRAX.

wound a sudden break in the body tissues and/or organs caused by an external agent. There are four types based on the result of the injury: INCISIONS, punctures, LACERATIONS and CONTUSIONS.

wrist the JOINT between the HAND and forearm. The wrist region comprises eight carpal bones and five metacarpal bones joined by strong ligaments. The wrist joint then articulates with the RADIUS and ULNA. The joint can move in all directions with little risk of DISLOCATION.

writer's cramp an involuntary contraction of the HAND muscles when writing but not when using those muscles to undertake other functions. A similar condition may arise with musicians (guitarists and pianists), typists and computer operators.

wryneck *or* **torticollis** the condition when the head is twisted to one side because of a SCAR contracting or, more commonly, excessive MUSCLE contraction.

XYZ

xanthelasma yellow fatty deposits in the eyelids and skin around the eyes. It often occurs in elderly people, when it is insignificant, but a severe case may be caused by a fat METABOLISM disorder.

xanthochromia a yellow colouring, e.g. the SKIN in JAUNDICE or the CERE-BROSPINAL FLUID when it contains HAEMOGLOBIN breakdown products.

X-chromosome the SEX CHROMOSOME present in males and females, although women have a pair and men just one (with one Y-CHROMOSOME). Certain disorders, such as HAEMOPHILIA, are carried as GENES on the X-chromosome.

xeroderma a condition of the skin that manifests itself as a dryness and rough-ness with the formation of scales. It is a mild form of ICHTHYOSIS.

xiphoid process *or* **xiphoid cartilage** the lowest part of the STERNUM. It is a flat CARTILAGE that is progressively replaced by BONE, a process completed sometime after middle age.

X-rays the part of the electromagnetic spectrum with waves of wavelength 10^{-12} to 10^{-9}m and frequencies of 10^{17} to 10^{21}Hz. They are produced when high-velocity electrons strike a target. The rays penetrate solids to a depth that depends on the density of the solid. X-rays of certain wavelengths will pene-trate flesh but not BONE. They are therefore useful in therapy and diagnosis within medicine.

yawning a REFLEX ACTION when the mouth is opened wide and air is drawn into the lungs and slowly released. It is usually, although not exclusively, associ-ated with tiredness or boredom.

yaws an infectious disease of the tropics caused by a SPIROCHAETE, *Treponema pertenue*, usually in unhygienic conditions. The bacteria enter through ABRA-SIONS, and after about two weeks, during which time there is fever, pain and itching, small TUMOURS appear, each with a yellow crust of dried SERUM. These may eventually form deep ULCERS. The final stages may not appear until several years later and include LESIONS of skin and bone. Fortunately, PENICILLIN works dramatically and effectively in this disease.

Y-chromosome the small SEX CHROMOSOME that carries a dominant GENE confer-ring maleness. Normal males have 22 matched CHROMOSOME pairs and one unmatched pair, comprising one X-CHROMOSOME and one Y-chromosome. During sexual reproduction, the mother contributes an X-chromosome, but the father contributes an X or Y-chromosome. XX produces a female offspring and XY a male.

yellow fever an infectious viral disease in tropical Africa and South America *see* page 121.

zidovudine an antiviral drug (trade name Retrovir) that is used to treat AIDS. Although it slows the growth of the HIV virus, it does not effect a cure.

Zollinger-Ellison syndrome an uncommon disorder resulting in DIARRHOEA and multiple PEPTIC ULCERS. The cause is a pancreatic TUMOUR or enlarged PANCREAS, which in turn leads to high levels of the hormone gastrin, which stimulates excess production of acidic GASTRIC JUICE, causing the ulceration. Surgery is usually effective.

zoonosis (*pl* **zoonoses**) an infectious animal disease that can be transmitted to humans. Some of the 150 or so diseases are: ANTHRAX, BRUCELLOSIS, BOVINE TUBERCULOSIS, RIFT VALLEY FEVER, RABIES, LEPTOSPIROSIS and TYPHUS.

zygomatic arch the arch of BONE on either side of the FACE, below the eyes.

zygomatic bone a facial BONE and one of a pair of bones that form the promi-nence of the cheeks.

zygote the CELL produced by the fusion of male and female germ cells (GAMETES) during the early stage of FERTILIZATION, i.e. an OVUM fertilized by a SPERM. After passing down the FALLOPIAN TUBE, it implants in the UTERUS, forming the EMBRYO.